INTERMEDIATE
Health & Social Care

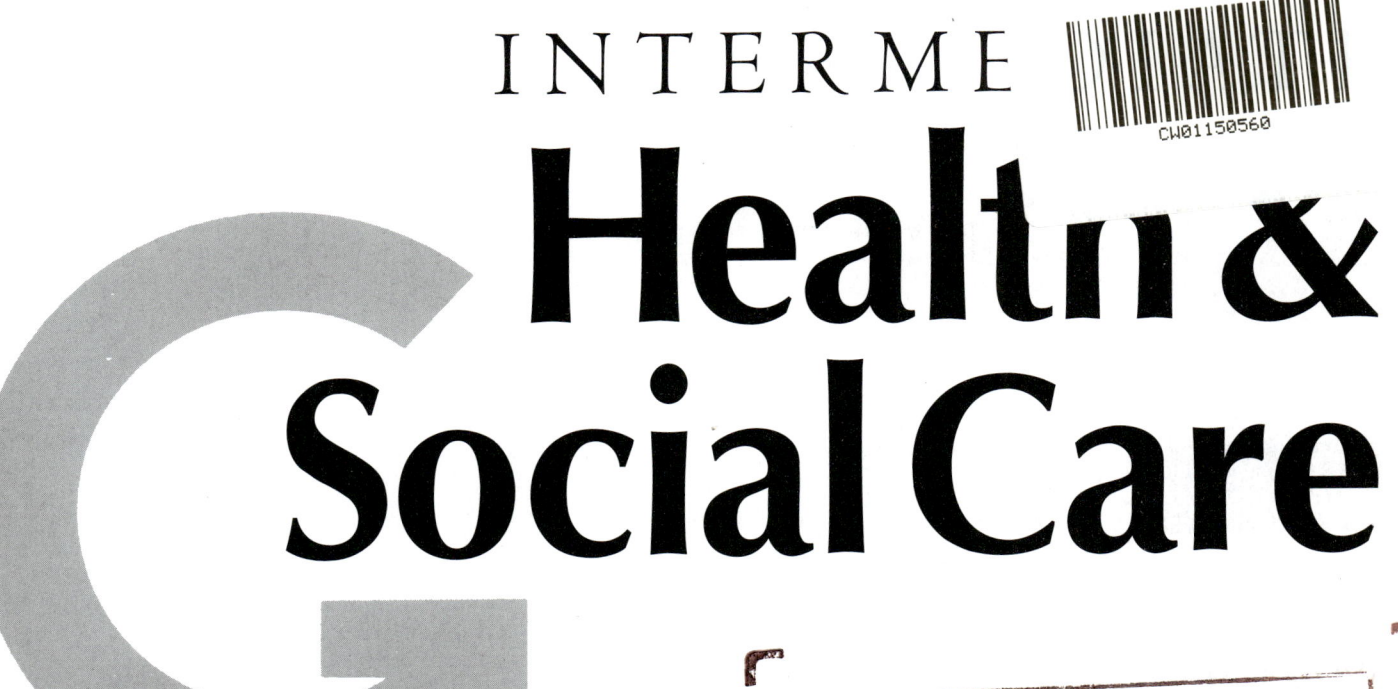

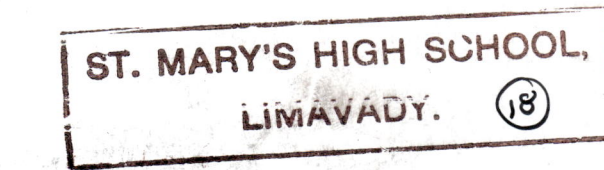

ST. MARY'S HIGH SCHOOL, LIMAVADY.

Anne Reddington & Peter Waltham

with contributions by

Alec Main, Anne-Marie Spry,
Sid Stace, Christine Wilkinson
and Christine Woodrow

Nelson

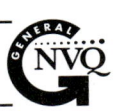

Thomas Nelson and Sons Ltd
Nelson House   Mayfield Road
Walton-on-Thames   Surrey
KT12 5PL   UK

Nelson Blackie
Wester Cleddens Road
Bishopbriggs
Glasgow
G64 2NZ   UK

Thomas Nelson Australia
102 Dodds Street
South Melbourne
Victoria 3205   Australia

Nelson Canada
1120 Birchmount Road
Scarborough   Ontario
M1K 5G4   Canada

© Anne Reddington, Peter Waltham 1995

First published by Thomas Nelson and Sons Ltd 1995

I(T)P   Thomas Nelson is an International Thomson Publishing Company

I(T)P   is used under licence

ISBN 0-17-4900007
NPN 9 8 7 6 5 4 3 2 1

All rights reserved. No paragraph of this publication may be reproduced, copied or transmitted save with written permission or in accordance with the provisions of the Copyright, Design and Patents Act 1988, or under the terms of any licence permitting limited copying issued by the Copyright Licensing Agency, 90 Tottenham Court Road, London W1P 9HE.

Any person who does any unauthorised act in relation to this publication may be liable to criminal prosecution and civil claims for damages.

Printed in Spain

The Intermediate GNVQ Health and Social Care Team

The authors

Anne Reddington was until recently the Assistant Director in Health and Social Care at Mid-Warwickshire College. She has written multiple choice questions for BTEC Unit Tests.

Peter Waltham has developed and taught vocational subjects and is now a freelance educational consultant in education and training. He is working for NCVQ and BTEC in developing vocational curricula for Health and Social Care including GNVQ. He is an external verifier for GNVQs and NVQs.

The main contributors
Alec Main is Co-ordinator of the Curriculum Materials Unit at Thomas Danby College in Leeds.
Ann-Marie Spry has broad experience in teaching and in curriculum development initiatives. She is a programme area manager for Health Science and Food Technology. She has written test questions for GNVQ Health and Social Care.
Sid Stace is a practising social worker currently working in the London Borough of Croydon. He has prepared reports on the Application of Prior Achievement in Health and Social Care NVQs and has written multiple choice questions for City and Guilds Unit Tests.
Christine Wilkinson teaches at St. Wilfreds Catholic High School. As a qualified first aid instructor she has taught first aid to groups of Health and Social Care students.
Christine Woodrow has been a maths and numeracy teacher for 20 years. During this time she has supported Health and Social Care students of various ages and levels. She is currently a GNVQ and Core Skills Co-ordinator in a growing Sixth Form College.

The advisers
Susan Cubitt is a student counsellor in several schools and tertiary colleges. She also trains college staff in the skills of counselling, towards maintaining and improving the physical and emotional well-being of students.
Ann Davey is Head of the GNVQ Faculty at John Ruskin College, Croydon and is actively involved in tutoring students in Health and Social Care.
Sue Dell is Head of Psychology at Alton College, Hampshire and is a member of the British Psychology Society.
Steve Harbourne is a Senior Lecturer at Alton College, and has extensive experience of GNVQ Health and Social Care at Intermediate and Advanced levels. He is an external verifier of Health and Social Care.
Trudi Hirons is a qualified nurse, midwife, health visitor and first aider as well as a lecturer in Health and Social Care. She is also an external verifier for GNVQs, CARE awards (NVQ) and a Chief Examiner for GNVQ Health and Social Care.
Peggy Munday is currently the Course Manager of Intermediate GNVQ Health and Social Care at Alton College, Hampshire, giving her an awareness of the needs of students following this programme.
Liz Shelley is the Nutrition and Dietetic Service Manager at the Royal Hampshire County Hospital. She has considerable experience in financial, personnel and quality management and is an adviser to the Health Commission on the effective use of resources in meeting nutritional needs.
Paul Smith is Head of Sociology at Alton College and has considerable teaching experience including GNVQ Health and Social Care.
Madge Storey is the co-ordinator for GNVQ at Tewkesbury School, which was a pilot school. She has taught students at both Intermediate and Advanced level GNVQ Health and Social Care.
Mary Wilkinson was until recently a lecturer in the Care Department of Evesham College. Currently she is a freelance lecturer and a practising McTimoney Chiropractor.

Thanks also to two first aid Instructors for their valuable advice on the first aid section.

Safety Adviser
Peter Borrows Chair, Safeguards in Science Committee, The Association for Science Education.

Acknowledgements

Illustrations and other printed matter
The authors and publishers are grateful to the following for permission to reproduce copyright material. If any acknowledgement has been omitted, this will be rectified at the earliest possible opportunity.

Figure 1.9, page 9: taken from the Department of Health booklet *The Health of the Nation*, HMSO, 1994. Crown copyright is reproduced with the permission of the Controller of HMSO.
Table 1.3, page 12: taken from the COMA report No. 41, *Dietary Reference Values for Food Energy and Nutrients for the United Kingdom*, HMSO, 1992.
Table 1.4, page 14: abstracted from table 3.1 in Appendix 1 of *Manual of Nutrition*, 10th edition, HMSO, 1995. Crown copyright is reproduced with the permission of the Controller of HMSO.
Figure 1.15, page 15: taken from *National Food Guide*, Health Education Authority, 1995. Reproduced with the permission of the Health Education Authority.
Figure 1.16, page 16: taken from *National Food Guide*, Health Education Authority, 1995. Reproduced with the permission of the Health Education Authority.
Figure 1.18, page 18: taken from the COMA report No. 46, *Nutritional Aspects of Cardiovascular Disease*, HMSO, 1992. Crown copyright is reproduced with the permission of the Controller of HMSO.
Figure 1.21, page 19: taken from *The Health Guide*, Health Education Authority, 1993. Reproduced with the permission of the Health Education Authority.
Figure 1.35, page 28: based on artwork from Foulger, R. and Routledge, E., *The Food Poisoning Handbook*, Chartwell-Bratt (Publishing and Training) Ltd, 1981. Original artwork by Fred Pipes.
Figure 1.37, page 29: based on illustration in *Basic Food Hygiene Certificate Coursebook*, Health Education Authority, 1993. Reproduced with the permission of the Health Education Authority.
Figure 1.39, page 29: poster reproduced by permission of the Health Education Authority.
Table 1.8, page 40: based on table in Clarke, L., Sachs, B. and Waltham, P., *GNVQ Advanced Health and Social Care*, Stanley Thornes (Publishers) Ltd, 1994.
Figures 1.51, 1.52, 1.53, 1.57, 1.58, 1.59, 1.60, 1.61, 1.62, 1.63, 1.67, 1.68, 1.69 and 1.72 based on artwork in St John's Ambulance Association *First Aid Handbook*, 6th edition, Dorling Kindersley, 1994.
Case Study, page 94: taken from Davenport, G. C., *An Introduction to Child Development*, Unwin Hyman 1988. Reproduced courtesy of HarperCollins publishers.

Figure 2.37, page 103: taken from Central Statistics Office, *Social Trends*, HMSO. Crown copyright is reproduced with the permission of the Controller of HMSO.
Figure 2.39, page 105: based on figure from Oppenheim, C., *Poverty: the facts*, Child Poverty Action Group.
Figures 3.2 and 3.12, pages 119 and 125: based on figures in Clarke, L., Sachs, B. and Waltham, P., *GNVQ Advanced Health and Social Care*, Stanley Thornes (Publishers) Ltd, 1994.
Figure 3.5, page 120: taken from *The Guardian*.
Figure 3.13, page 126: reproduced by permission of Bradford Health.
Figure 3.15, page 127: reproduced by permission of North Middlesex Health Trust.
Figure 3.19, page 130: reproduced by permission of Thomson Directories Ltd.
Figure 3.20, page 131: reproduced by permission of Age Concern.
Figure 3.38, page 144: reproduced by permission of North Middlesex Health Trust.
Figure 4.22, page 188: based on artwork in Morris, D., *Manwatching*, Triad Granada, 1978. Used by permission of Elsevier Publishing.
Appendix 1, pages 216–219: taken from Ministry of Agriculture, Fisheries and Food, *Manual of Nutrition*, 10th edition, HMSO, 1995. Crown copyright is reproduced with the permission of the Controller of HMSO.

Photographs
John Birdsall Photography: pp. 22, 23 (bottom left), 66 (right), 69 (top), 98 (left), 123, 134, 135, 136, 145, 148, 149, 150 (bottom right), 168 (right), 183 (bottom), 190
J Allan Cash: pp. 25, 84 (bottom)
Len Cross: pp. 2 (left), 6 (left and bottom two), 10, 17, 32, 66 (left and middle), 84 (top), 93 (bottom), 98 (middle), 106, 116, 122, 123 (top right), 129, 132, 133 (top), 141, 151, 168 (top), 170, 174, 183 (top), 186, 187 (top), 187 (bottom), 198 (top), 199 (bottom), 205
Format/Maggi Murray: pp. 2 (top right), 23 (left), 123 (left), 133 (bottom), 134, 137
Sally & Richard Greenhill: pp. 91, 138, 199 (top)
National Medical Slidebank: p.11 (bottom)
Photo Co-op: p. 142
Photofusion: pp. 88, 98 (top), 102
Rex Features Ltd: pp. 6 (top right), 76, 168 (left), 193
Science Photo Library: pp. 2 (bottom), 11 (top), 20, 26, 27, 28, 29 (top and bottom), 69 (bottom left and right), 75, 150 (left)
Tony Stone: pp. 21, 79, 93 (top right)

Contents

How to use this book — xi
    The structure of the book — xi
    Finding information in the book — xii

Introduction — xiii
    Intermediate GNVQ Health and Social Care:
    What do health and care workers 'do'? — xiii
        Structure of the qualification — xiii
        Assessment — xiv
    Building up your GNVQ portfolio — xvii
        Knowledge, skills and understanding — xvii
        Activities and assignments — xvii
        A note to teachers and students — xxi

Unit 1   Promoting health and social well-being — 2
    Health and social well-being — 2
        The Elements — 3
    Investigate personal health — 4
        Lifestyles — 4
    Activity: Lifestyle profile — 4
        Physical activity — 5
        Sleep — 5
    Activity: Sleep patterns — 5
        Mental stimulation — 6
        Social interaction — 7
        Balanced lifestyles — 7
        Health risks — 8
    Activity: Health benefits and risks — 8
        Health of the Nation targets — 9
        Diet — 10
        A healthy diet — 10
        How the body uses the dietary components — 10
        Dietary recommendations — 12
    Activity: Calorie counting — 13
        Balancing your diet — 14
        Eating patterns — 15
        Health risks from dietary habits — 18
        Exercise — 20
        The ingredients of fitness — 21
        Drug use and abuse — 22
    Activity: Drug audit — 22
        Tobacco and alcohol — 22
        Controlled and illegal drugs — 24
        Other dangerous drugs — 25
        Solvent abuse — 25
        Sexual behaviour — 26
        Hygiene and health — 26

Contents

Activity: Then and now	26
Personal hygiene	27
Levels of hygiene	28
Activity: The not-too-hot pot	29
Hygiene requirements	30
How is hygiene maintained?	30
The immune system	31
Activity: Hygiene investigation	31
Actions to promote personal health	31
Personal health assessment	32
Activity: Checking your own fitness	32
Activity: Monitoring your diet	32
Developing your plan to improve your health	33
Making a personal health promotion action plan	34
Activity: A personal health action plan	34
Health promotion advice	35
Producing health advice	35
Activity: What advice do people need?	36
Health and safety	39
Risks and hazards	39
Activity: Hazards to personal safety	40
Activity: Areas of hazard	41
Activity: Designed for safety	41
Dealing with health emergencies	42
Assessing an emergency	42
Make the area safe	42
Assessing a casualty	43
The approach	43
The five checks (Safety, Shake and shout, A, B, C)	44
Activity: The five checks	45
Activity: Order of actions	45
Mouth-to-mouth resuscitation	45
Activity: Mouth-to-mouth resuscitation	47
Activity: Cardiac compression	47
Activity: The recovery position	48
How to examine a casualty	48
Activity: What's happened?	48
Examining the casualty	50
Activity: Examining a casualty	51
Wounds and the treatment of bleeding	51
Activity: Severe bleeding	53
Activity: Practise stopping bleeding	54
Activity: Finding pressure points	54
Shock	54
Contacting the emergency services	55
A final note	57
Assignment: Promoting balanced lifestyles	58
Assignment: Hazards around the school/college	61
Questions	63

Unit 2	Health and social well-being	66
	The Elements	67
	Life stages	67
	Personal development	69
	Physical development	69
	Growth in infancy and childhood	70
	Activity: Using growth data	70
	Growth in puberty	74
	Early adulthood	75
	Mid-life adult	75
	Menopause	75
	Old age	76
	Activity: Growth patterns	76
	Social, emotional and intellectual development	77
	Language development	80
	Case study: Adam, Eve and Sarah	80
	Case study: Lee	81
	Activity: Child watching	81
	Activity: Children's toys	82
	Case study: Kate	83
	Development beyond the early years	83
	Childhood 5+	84
	Activity: Starting school	85
	Adolescence	85
	Activity: Surviving adolescence	86
	Early adulthood	86
	Mid-life	87
	Old age	87
	Activity: Old age is not only about loss	87
	Self-concept	88
	Activity: Who am I?	88
	Activity: Analysing your own self-concept	89
	Self-concept and health and well-being	90
	Activity: Strengthening self-concept	90
	Major life events	91
	How people manage change	91
	Activity: Marriage ceremonies	92
	Relationships and their influence on health and well-being	92
	Family	93
	Activity: Family structures	93
	Case study: Mark	93
	Case study: The Twins	94
	Activity: Who is close to you?	95
	Relationships outside the family	96
	Activity: Relationships	96
	Changes in relationships	96
	Activity: Effects of change	97
	Group roles	97
	Accepting a society's culture	97
	Rules, laws and conventions	98

Contents

	Activity: Group norms	99
	Socialisation	99
	Reference groups	100
	Influences on socialisation	100
	Social stratification	101
	What do we mean by social class?	101
	Activity: Class work	101
	Group membership and health and social well-being	102
	Activity: Class difference in health care	103
	Standards of living	104
	Case study: Project Headstart	104
	Activity: Social class: is the model a good one?	106
	Assignment: Development and change	107
	Assignment: Relationships	109
	Assignment: Role in society	110
	Questions	113
Unit 3	**Health and social care services**	116
	The Elements	117
	Health and social care services	118
	Activity: Who delivers care? – 1	118
	The statutory sector	119
	Control at government level	119
	Health and social services	119
	The formation of the health services	120
	Subdivisions of the health services	123
	The formation of the social services	124
	The National Health Service and Community Care Act 1990	125
	Care planning	125
	Predicting care needs	125
	Activity: Care needs in your community	126
	NHS purchasers and providers	127
	The emergence of Health Commissions	128
	Social services purchasers and providers	129
	Individual care planning	129
	Care in the community	129
	Activity: Provision in your local area	130
	The range of social services	130
	The voluntary sector	131
	Activity: Voluntary services	131
	Private sector	132
	Complementary medicine	133
	Not-for-profit services	134
	Informal carers	134
	Case study: Peter's story	134
	Who needs care?	136
	Physical care needs	136
	Emotional needs	136

Activity: Recognition of the emotional needs of children	136
Social needs	137
Children and families	137
Care provisions for babies, children, young people, families, adults and elderly people	137
If help is needed, how can it be arranged?	139
Services for people with physical and sensory disabilities	140
Services for people with learning difficulties	141
Services for older people and their carers	141
Services for people with mental health needs	142
Access to health and social care	143
Cultural issues	143
Support for people with different needs	145
Who pays?	145
Activity: Who pays what?	146
Who cares?	146
Activity: Who delivers care? – 2	147
What do the workers 'do'?	147
Hospital and specialist services	148
Community-based health services	151
Social services personnel	152
Activity: Who supports the carers?	154
Stereotypes	155
Training for the caring services	155
Becoming a care worker in health or social care	155
Case study: Jill's route to social work	156
But what do they really 'do'?	156
Activity: Who delivers care?	159
Assignment: Caring for Peter	160
Assignment: Meeting the needs of clients	161
Assignment: Where do I go from here?	163
Questions	165

Unit 4	**Communication and interpersonal relationships in health and social care**	168
	The elements	169
	Why communicate?	169
	Activity: Life without communication	169
	Supportive communication	170
	Activity: Relationships	170
	Conversation	171
	Activity: Identifying pitfalls	172
	Listening and talking	172
	Activity: Listening	172
	Listening skills	172
	Activity: Chinese whispers	173
	How to listen	173
	Activity: Effects of different listening styles	173
	Activity: Active listening	174
	Reflecting and summarising	174

Activity: Reflecting and summarising	174
Verbal clues that help a conversation	176
Activity: Just imagine	177
Asking questions	177
Activity: Using open and closed questions	177
Activity: What does this mean?	181
Activity: What generation gap?	182
Non-verbal communication	182
Activity: Charades	182
Activity: Building a non-verbal dictionary	184
Activity: Permission to speak	185
Activity: Matching pairs	186
Personal space	186
Crossing the barriers	187
Activity: Give me space	187
Working in care organisations	188
Individuality	189
Activity: Time to think	189
Prejudice	190
Discrimination	191
Case study: A problem with direct discrimination	192
Case study: James	192
Working with people in health and social care	194
Case study: Harold's hip	194
Dependence	195
Power relationships	198
How people respond to care	198
Types of support	198
The importance of effective interaction	199
Communicating respect	199
Activity: Golden Park Home	200
Self-esteem	201
Independence and self-esteem	202
Ethical issues in care	202
Putting it all together	203
A check list	204
Activity: Practice role play	205
Assignment: A communication record	206
Assignment: Discrimination	207
Assignment: Working with clients	209
Questions	210
Glossary	212
Bibliography/useful addresses	214
Appendix I Table of nutrients	216
Appendix II The Value Base and individual rights	220
Appendix III Key legislation	224
Answers	231
Index	232

How to use this book

To do any work successfully you need the right tools. This book provides the tools you need for Intermediate GNVQ Health and Social Care. To get your GNVQ you will need to:
- show through your *coursework* that you have met the requirements of the qualification
- pass *tests* for the mandatory units.

In this book you will find information about the knowledge, skills and understanding needed to tackle both coursework and tests. You may need more specialised books or information from other sources to help you to achieve merit or distinction grades for your assignments.

The structure of the book

Units 1–4 link directly to the mandatory intermediate health and social care units 1–4. Each begins with an introduction which:
- describes the area of care work upon which the unit is based
- gives the titles of elements in the unit
- outlines what you need to do to achieve each element.

This introduction is followed by information and activities for the unit. *Focus boxes* in the margin are summaries that enable you to move through a section quickly. Throughout the units, words in **bold** type direct you to the focus boxes. Other words which need emphasis are in *italics*. You can turn to the main text if you want more information. The text also contains figures and tables which, together with the focus boxes, may be useful for revision as well as for coursework.

The units contain activities, assignments and case studies. These give you the opportunity to collect evidence for your portfolio. The activities themselves can be used to collect evidence of core skills.

Activities look like this:

A	**Life without communication**
Activity	Title of activity

They may also be used as an alternative, or in addition to, assignments to collect evidence for the Health and Social Care units. In the assignments the parts of the Intermediate GNVQ specifications covered are indicated.

At the end of each unit there are *questions* which you can use for a pre-test check. Try to answer these questions before the unit test. Check your answers with those at the end of the book.

Finding information in the book

There are three ways in which you might find the information you need in this book:
- the contents list at the front
- the index at the back
- by 'pressing' the appropriate button to another section.

Buttons in the margin direct you to relevant sections. They are a cross-referencing system which allows you to find the information you need quickly. When you do look up something don't forget to mark your place in the book so that you can get back to it!

Buttons look like this:

▶ The Value Base and individual rights, page 220

heading to look for in the text   page to turn to for further information

Introduction

Intermediate GNVQ Health and Social Care: What do health and care workers 'do'?

Intermediate GNVQ Health and Social Care is about what care workers do. Their work falls into broad categories. Care workers:
- *support* people (helping them to carry out their activities of daily living)
- *communicate* with people to provide emotional support (helping to maintain relationships)
- *promote* an individual's rights (for example, by maintaining dignity and choice for people being cared for).

Within Health and Social Care work it is expected that people support and work within the *Care Value Base*.

The value base components are:
- freedom from any type of discrimination
- maintaining confidentiality of information
- promoting and supporting individual rights to dignity, independence, choice and health and safety
- acknowledging individuals' personal beliefs and identity
- supporting individuals through effective communication.

Essential to all of this work is the ability to form relationships that demonstrate a caring attitude.

> The Value Base and individual rights, Appendix II, page 220

Structure of the qualification

Health and Social Care units

The Intermediate GNVQ Health and Social Care is divided into units, each based on the knowledge and skills that underpin the range of caring processes. Information needed for the four *mandatory units* is provided in this book. However, many of the methods and ideas will also be useful when you tackle your two *optional units*.

Each unit consists of *elements*. The titles of the elements tell you what you must do to achieve the unit. In turn, each element consists of:
- *performance criteria*: a checklist of things you need to do to show that you can meet the requirements of the element
- *range*: the particular situations in which the performance criteria are to be met.

Core skills

There are three core skill units that you must gain: *Application of Number, Communication, Information Technology*. They should be achieved within the Health and Social Care activities and assignments that you undertake.

The requirements of these units are laid out in the same way as the Health and Social Care units, with elements, performance criteria and range. There are five levels of core skills. For Intermediate GNVQ, you must achieve at least level 2. However, you should strive to get higher levels. This extra achievement will be recognised on your certificate. It is worth working for.

FOCUS
Intermediate GNVQ Health and Social Care consists of:
- 4 mandatory units
- 2 optional units
- 3 core skill units.

FOCUS
You will find that words in the performance criteria are explained in the range. For example:
- Performance criterion: 'explain the importance of a *balanced* lifestyle'
- Range: *Balanced* in terms of: activity (work, recreation), rest (sleep, inactivity).

FOCUS
Core skill units:
- Application of Number
- Communication
- Information Technology.

Application of Number
This involves gathering and working on data, solving problems (for example, using graphs and equations), interpreting and presenting data (for example, using symbols and diagrams). The nature of Health and Social Care means that you will have to look for opportunities to show your ability in this core skill.

Communication
Communication involves writing about Health and Social Care (using suitable illustrations such as diagrams and flow charts) and talking about Health and Social Care (using suitable visual aids such as posters or overhead projector transparencies). Of course, some people know more about health and social care than others and so you need to be able to communicate with people with different experiences and knowledge.

Information Technology
This core skill involves word processing and using databases and spreadsheets. It is an invaluable aid to storing and communicating data and ideas. You will have the opportunity to show that you can: retrieve information from databases, word process reports and use spreadsheets to handle data.

Assessment
There are two parts to the assessment:
Your *portfolio of evidence* is a collection of your *coursework*. It should contain evidence that you have carried out work to:
- meet the requirements of elements through the related performance criteria and range (and so achieve the units)
- meet the requirements of the core skill units
- show that you are worthy of a merit or distinction grade.

Unit tests are designed to allow you to show that you have covered all aspects of the mandatory units. For each Unit Test you will need to know about all the range categories given in the Unit Test Specs. If you do not pass a test you may take it again. Optional units do not have tests.

The activities and assignments given to you by your school or college will have opportunities to meet these requirements built into them. However, an important aim of a GNVQ programme is that you begin to identify opportunities to gather evidence yourself. This may be, for example:
- extension work you have suggested to an activity
- experience gained on a work placement
- extra core skills you have used in an activity because of the way you chose to do it
- an activity that you designed and carried out.

It is important that you understand the GNVQ specifications and are able to recognise that you collect relevant evidence. This can be presented to your teacher or lecturer and you can 'claim' the appropriate part of the GNVQ. You are taking control of your own programme.

Meeting performance criteria
Quite simply, your portfolio must show that you have met all the performance criteria for each element. You must show that the *breadth of the range* has been covered. This means showing that you understand the key features of each *range category* within a *range dimension*. Finally you must show for each element that you have looked *in depth* at those aspects of

> **FOCUS**
> You should have access to the full specifications for health and social care and core skill units, as well as the grading criteria for merit and distinction.

range which form part of the particular assignments you are tackling. This can be done by providing the evidence described in the evidence indicator.

This probably sounds very complicated! An example will help. Consider the following performance criterion and related range:

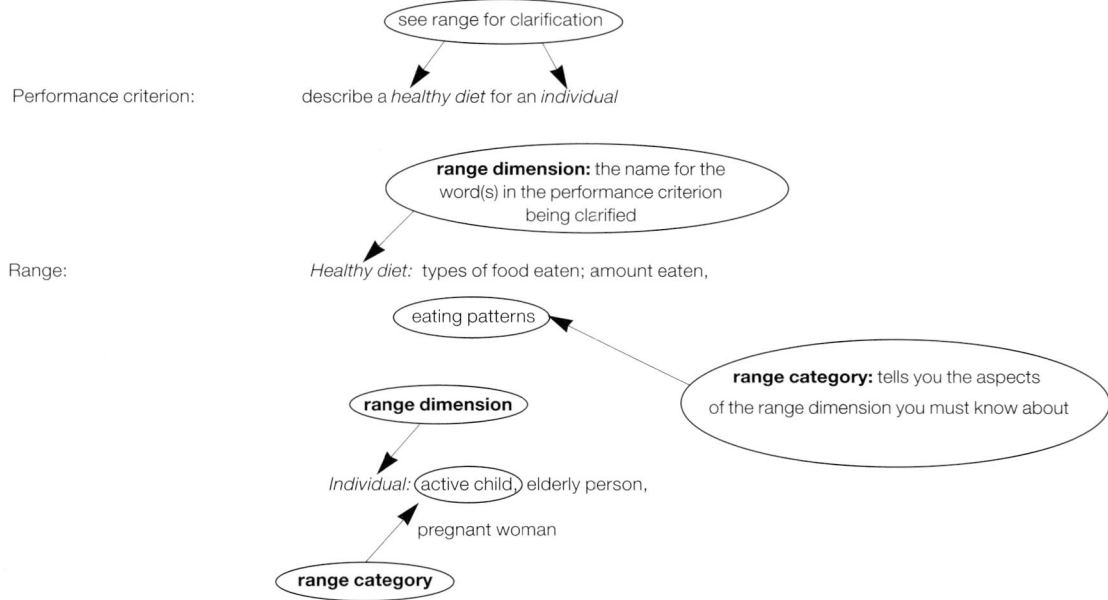

You would need to show that you can describe a healthy diet (in terms of the types of food eaten, the amount eaten and eating patterns) for an individual (who might be active, sedentary; a child, an elderly person, or a pregnant woman). You will need to understand the different needs of individuals in order to be able to do this. However, you would not be expected describe a healthy diet for each individual listed in the range category.

Evidence indicators

Each element has *evidence indicators*, showing the minimum amount of work you need to do. However, they are not prescriptive. Other types of evidence may be presented, provided they are comparable in *coverage* (performance criteria and range) and *sufficiency* (amount of evidence needed). You may find it useful, however, to start by using the evidence indicators in a prescriptive way until you are able to identify your own opportunities for generating evidence.

For example, consider these evidence indicators:

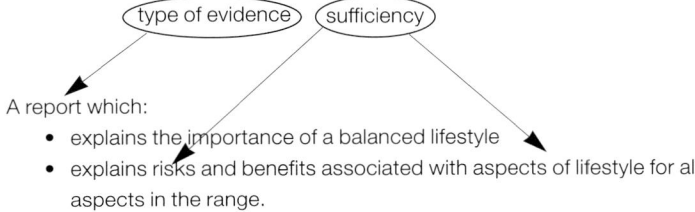

A report which:
- explains the importance of a balanced lifestyle
- explains risks and benefits associated with aspects of lifestyle for all aspects in the range.

The 'all' in the second sentence gives the sufficiency when related back to the range category. With some evidence indicators the number of range categories to be addressed may be stated. You may then select from the range. You may then however have to know all of the range category for the Unit Test.

Alternative types of evidence might be a poster or a talk accompanied by visual aids. It is always helpful to look at the core skill specifications because the form of the evidence can often be tailored to meet core skill requirements as well.

Whatever the form, there must be an explanation of a balanced lifestyle and of at least two risks and benefits as these words are plural, meaning more than one. Between them, the investigations must show that performance criteria and range have been covered to the same extent as the evidence indicators given in the specifications.

Grading

Individual units are not graded. Instead you will be awarded a grade for the whole qualification. At least a third of your evidence must meet the grading criteria for merit or the criteria for distinction. You will need to show that you can tackle activities using the knowledge, skills and understanding associated with Intermediate GNVQ Health and Social Care. The grading criteria also reflect the increasing responsibility that you are expected to take for the work you do. These are just the skills that employers are looking for.

There are four grading themes:

Planning
    1 drawing up plans of action
    2 monitoring courses of action

Information-seeking and information-handling
    3 identifying information needs
    4 identifying and using sources to obtain information

Evaluation
    5 evaluating outcomes and justifying approaches

Quality of outcomes
    6 synthesis of knowledge, skills and understanding
    7 command of language related to Health and Social Care.

Grading criteria reward independent work - your ability to make many of the decisions about what to do and how to do it.

FOCUS

Grading themes:
- **Planning**
- **Information-seeking and information-handling**
- **Evaluation**
- **Quality of outcomes.**

Building up your GNVQ portfolio

Knowledge, skills and understanding

Your GNVQ programme will consist of various activities, such as lectures, discussions, investigative work, problem solving exercises, debates, presentations, discussions, information searches (library and electronic) and so on. You will be given increasing responsibility for your work.

The activities and assignments you undertake will have been designed to help you to meet the requirements of elements and so achieve units. Your record of these activities and assignments will form the main part of your portfolio. You may be able to add relevant evidence from other sources such as work placements. To do this you will need to use the skills you develop, together with the underpinning knowledge and understanding, to apply to the task in hand.

Activities and assignments

In this section you will see how activities and assignments are designed so that you have opportunities to meet:

- requirements of the health and social care units
- requirements of the core skill units
- grading criteria.

It is helpful to think of opportunities to generate evidence as activities or assignments. For the purposes of your Intermediate GNVQ Health and Social Care and of this book, we will describe these as follows:

An *activity* is a structured piece of work which allows you to collect evidence for health and social care and core skill units. It is often a short piece of work which allows some or all of the performance criteria for one or more elements to be met. You are often given precise instructions and there may be less opportunity to meet the first five grading criteria relating to planning, information-seeking and information-handling and evaluation than there is in assignments. However, you can show 'quality of outcome'.

An *assignment* is more open-ended. It allows you to collect evidence for health and social care and core skill units. It also allows some or all of the grading criteria to be met. Assignments are not equally demanding. They may vary from *straightforward*, consisting of a number of separate tasks, to *complex*, where the tasks involved are interrelated. Complexity will also increase depending on the extent of planning and information use carried out. You will need to demonstrate a thorough grasp of the underlying knowledge, skills and understanding needed to meet the fourth grading theme.

This may be a little confusing, and some people may use the terms activity, task and assignment in different ways. Perhaps the important message is that some things you do will give you the chance to meet performance criteria and range requirements. However, you will not be able to show the skills associated with grading. On the other hand, some things will give you the opportunity to do both. For convenience, we are calling these activities and assignments respectively.

One example of an activity (*Using open and closed questions*) and one example of an assignment (*Working with clients*) will illustrate the idea.

> **FOCUS**
> Activities normally have precise instructions which you follow. Assignments require you to take more control. They can be broken down into tasks, but you will need to:
> - plan the approach and monitor how things are going
> - find and use information relevant to the problem
> - bring together the relevant knowledge, skills and understanding.

Introduction

Performance criteria addressed:
*demonstrate **listening and responding** skills to encourage communication with individuals in different **contexts***

Range
Listening and responding skills:
facial expression, body language, eye contact, sensory contact, posture, minimal prompts, paraphrasing, summarising, *questioning (open, closed)*, tone, pitch, pace of communication

▶ Activity: Using open and closed questions, page 177

A — Using open and closed questions

With a partner, take it in turns to find out about your partner's favourite foods, pastimes, rock group, etc.
You may ask only five closed questions that can be answered with a fixed range of responses. You may not ask directly, 'What is your favourite ...?'
After five questions write down what you think is your partner's favourite ...
Now ask five open questions about the same area.
How much more information about your partner's likes have you discovered?
(Think of the difference between the information gained from:
Do you like curries?
and
If you were going out for a meal what sort of restaurant would you choose?)

The instructions are precise. There is a clear link between the activity and the performance criteria and associated range. You would be able to gather evidence for your portfolio. Since no planning, information finding and use, or evaluation is involved, you would not be able to show that you are worthy of a merit or distinction in these grading themes.

The following assignment has these opportunities built into it.

Assignment

WORKING WITH CLIENTS

This assignment may take up to three weeks.

Setting the scene

You are working in a caring situation and have been asked to provide information for a new member of staff. This information is to be in the form of a list of important things for them to remember at work. You have also been asked to prepare an information sheet for new members of staff that builds on this list.

Note. You may be able to use work placement experience to help you to carry out this assignment. Make use of any skills that you have learned in the workplace to help you to prepare the list. If you can, talk to staff in a caring workplace to get a better understanding of the caring work role.

Task 1
Draft the list. Use the headings in Task 3 to guide you.

Task 2
Talk to people who are working in caring situations about the different headings on your own list. Ask them what they consider to be important information for a new worker. They may give you further ideas for your list.

Task 3
Use word processing or desk-top publishing to prepare an information sheet for new members of staff. You should include examples of things to do and things not to do. The information should address these five areas:
- the caring relationship
- different ways that people respond to care
- different types of support
- the basics for good communication
- the need for confidentiality and when it might be breached.

Opportunities to collect evidence
On completing these tasks you will have the opportunity to meet the following requirements for Intermediate GNVQ Health and Social Care
Unit 4
Element 4.3 PCs 1, 2, 3, 4, 5, 6

Core skills
This assignment develops communication core skills. Tasks 1 and 3 address written core skills communication, whereas task 2 addresses oral core skills communication and note-taking.

Grading
The themes of planning (in organising the sequence of your work and arranging to speak with people in the workplace), information seeking and information handling (in gathering and presenting appropriate material on the information sheet) may be demonstrated in this assignment. Quality of outcomes (in the use of appropriate language in a form that meets the needs of the junior staff member on the information sheet) may also be shown.

Assignments of this kind are a major source of evidence for the award of a merit or distinction grade. Let's see how you would be able to show that you are worthy of a distinction.

Criterion 1: Drawing up plans of action
You have a great deal to plan. You will need to work out what needs doing and how to do it. Your action plan will prioritise tasks and put them in a logical order. How you tackle one task may affect when and how you can do work on other parts of the assignment. If you are going to investigate a real work environment you will need to plan the visit. You need time to write up the assignment. There is much to think about!

Criterion 2: Monitoring course of action
Three weeks is not a long time. There is a lot to do and you may decide to change your plans depending on how things unfold. If you want to visit a work place, it may take time to set up. The resources you need for word processing or desk-top publishing may need to be booked. Therefore, you need to review your action plan regularly and be prepared to modify it if necessary.

Criterion 3: Identifying information needs
You will need various information in order to tackle the assignment, for example, a knowledge of the law and confidentiality and the care value base. When planning your work, all your information needs must be identified.

Criterion 4: Identifying and using sources to obtain information
Where can the required information be found? Sources (for example, text books) need to be identified. You must justify your selection in terms of its suitability for providing the relevant information.

Criterion 5: Evaluating outcomes and justifying approaches
Your overall information sheet contents should justify the approach you took. The alternative examples of what to do and what not to do should be discussed. You should also comment on how you might do things differently if you tackled the assignment again.

Criterion 6: Synthesis
Throughout the investigation you must show a grasp of the relevant caring skills and understanding. You can show this by explaining decisions taken. For example, 'This example of good practice was chosen because...'. Your planning, and the information sheet you produce will reflect your grasp of the subject matter.

Criterion 7: Command of 'language'
Finally, you will need to show that you can use language related to caring in an appropriate way.

Introduction

A note to teachers and students

Role play – Debriefing

The nature of activities and assignments in health and social care mean that you may look at emotional issues. This can be particularly true of role play work, where you put yourself in the shoes of somebody giving or receiving care. You may use role plays where you end up feeling very emotional. After any role play activity it is important to take time debriefing. This involves sharing your feelings and making sure that you recognise that the activity or assignment has ended. For example, you may need to take time to release your anger rather than take it out of the classroom and let it affect your normal daily relationships and activities.

Confidentiality

It is likely that you will be involved in gathering information from other people, for example by interview. It is essential that the person being interviewed has consented to the use of the information within the GNVQ. If no consent is given, then the information must remain confidential. Even where consent is given to use the information about an individual, it is normal for the person's name not to be mentioned.

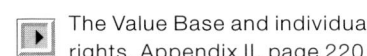
The Value Base and individual rights, Appendix II, page 220

Good luck with your studies and enjoy your Intermediate GNVQ Health and Social Care course.

1 | Promoting health and social well-being

Health and social well-being

In this unit we look at how people can keep healthy or become more healthy. The health of each individual contributes to an assessment of how healthy we are as a nation.

Although we are focusing on the health and social well-being of an individual, it is important to recognise that the needs of millions of individuals in the country as a whole amount to a pattern of demands that the country has to respond to as a whole. Every time somebody needs health and care support, it has a financial cost, an emotional cost and a social cost. Therefore we should all work to ensure that where health breakdown can be prevented, we do prevent it. The main way to do this is through health promotion.

Even so, health emergencies do occur. It is important for everyone to have some knowledge of life-saving skills and to be able to use them. The major skills are described in this chapter.

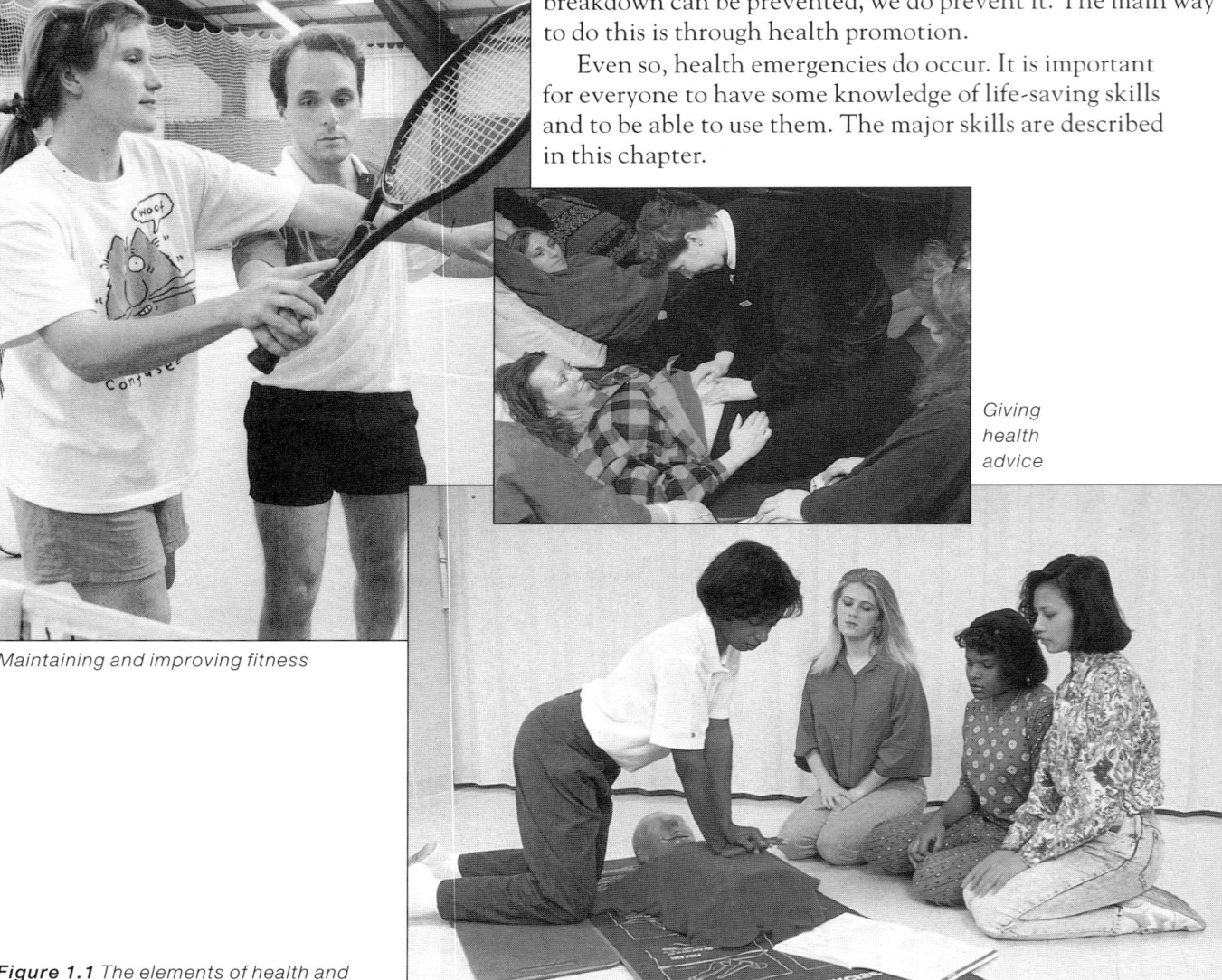

Maintaining and improving fitness

Giving health advice

Figure 1.1 *The elements of health and social well-being*

Learning how to cope in health emergencies

Promoting health and well-being

The Elements

Investigate personal health
- explain the importance of a balanced lifestyle
- explain the risks and benefits associated with aspects of lifestyle
- identify how the body uses each dietary component
- describe a healthy diet for an individual
- describe the effects of the use of substances on health and well-being
- explain good practice in maintaining hygiene.

In this unit you will examine the different ways in which health can be improved. This includes both means of promoting health and strategies to reduce harm. You will investigate the effect of lifestyles on the health of individuals and the practices likely to promote good health.

▶ Investigate personal health, page 4

Present advice on health and well-being to others
- assess an individual's health against standard measures
- produce a plan to improve an individual's health
- produce advice on maintaining health and well-being related to the needs of a target group
- present the advice to the target group on maintaining health and well-being
- assess the impact of the advice on the target group.

Using the knowledge gained in the first part of this unit, you will be guided to produce a plan to improve the health of another person and to work out and present advice to a particular group of people on how to maintain their health and well-being.

▶ Producing health advice, page 35

Reduce risk of injury and deal with emergencies
- explain hazards which could affect the health of individuals
- describe the methods of reducing risks of injury from hazards
- describe personal roles and responsibilities in dealing with health emergencies
- explain the physiological basis of life-saving techniques for dealing with health emergencies
- demonstrate the basic life-saving techniques in simulated health emergencies.

The third part of the unit will make you aware of common hazards to health and help you to learn about ways of reducing risk of injury. You will also identify hazards to personal health and the ways of reducing risk from these hazards. Finally, you will look at how to deal with emergencies including opening and maintaining an airway, placing someone in the recovery position, mouth to mouth resuscitation, heart-massaging techniques and controlling bleeding.

▶ Health and safety, page 39

Promoting health and well-being

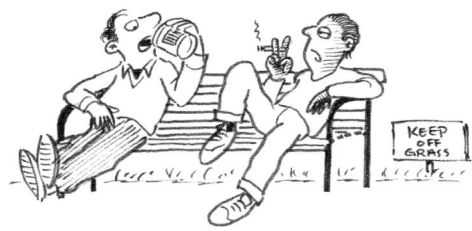

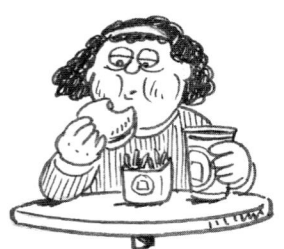

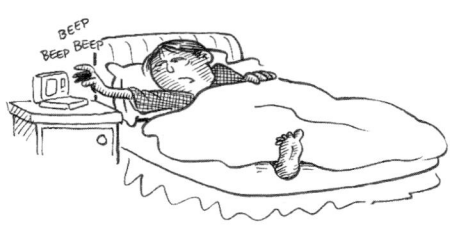

Figure 1.2 Are you happy with your lifestyle?

Investigate personal health

Lifestyles

Have you ever tried to lose weight or get fitter? Do you smoke or drink alcohol? Do you ever get up in the morning wishing that you could sleep for longer? Do you want to change your daily routines and become healthier?

Lifestyles clearly differ, and that is perfectly okay, but it is important to establish some features that relate lifestyle to health. The next activity gives you an opportunity to look at your lifestyle in terms of activity exercise, rest, work and leisure.

A   Lifestyle profile

For a week keep a record of what you do each day, and for how long. You may like to keep the record in the form of a diary.

At the end of each day try to classify each thing that you did as one of:
- exercise (makes your heart beat faster)
- rest, including sleep, reading, etc.
- work (college, school, paid, housework, etc.)
- recreation (leisure activities).

Work out how long you spent on each of these four categories. Round each one to the nearest hour. You may find it useful to draw up a table.

Category	Time spent	Time spent, to nearest hour

Note. This is an example of a 'data collection sheet' or 'observation sheet'. You may find it useful to devise one in other situations to make collecting data easier.

Look at your information for Saturday. For each category:
- work out what fraction of the total time it represented (this would normally be 24 h, but by rounding to the nearest hour you may get 23 or 25 h)
- convert each fraction to a percentage
- use this information to draw a pie chart.

You may find it helps to extend your table like this:

Category	Time spent	Time spent, to nearest hour	Fraction of the day	% of the day
Exercise				

Repeat this process for Sunday.

For your five weekdays work out the mean amount of time spent in each area (use the 'to the nearest hour' information). Remember the mean is found by adding together the total number of hours for a given category (eg exercise) and dividing by the number of days (5). Draw a pie chart for this information. Look at the three pie charts – do you see any similarities/differences? Write down your findings. Compare your results with others in your group. Look at the similarities and differences. Record your observations about similarities and differences in your pie charts and which activities make a contribution to health as a simple report.

The results of your discussion will probably be that everything that you have listed has an influence on your personal health. Some of the activities will be good for your health and others may have potentially bad effects. The important thing to recognise is that you should consider the balance of your activities in looking at your health. Twenty-four hours of college study, part-time employment stacking supermarket shelves, and nightclubbing would be a pattern as bad for your health as getting out of bed only to make another sandwich or open another packet of biscuits.

Physical activity

The importance of physical activity is in helping to maintain your fitness. This is not about becoming an athlete but about being physically active enough to stimulate your lungs, heart, circulation and muscles. In doing this you also stimulate your brain to produce chemicals which give you a feeling of well-being and reduce the risk of developing health problems.

> **FOCUS**
> Lifestyle patterns should be balanced in terms of:
> • activity – work, recreation
> • rest – sleep, inactivity.

Sleep

To balance the physical **activity**, it is important to get sufficient **rest** and sleep. Sleep is a period during which the body slows its activities. It is a time when the brain appears to process and store materials, although we know little of how this is done. There is no set amount of sleep that is required: we all have different needs, and they vary with age, temperature, excitement and season, as well as the physical activity of that day. However, it is essential and insufficient sleep leads to tiredness and increased reaction times, with consequent increased risks of injury.

A good indicator of having enough sleep is waking naturally (not needing an alarm) and not feeling tired.

A   Sleep patterns

1 Conduct a simple survey of how many hours of sleep fellow students and college staff have on average, whether they regard it as enough, whether they wake naturally and whether they wake without the need for an alarm. Decide how to present your findings.

2 In health and social care, major client groups are children and older people. How different are their sleep needs? Collect information for members of your group about relevant members of their families, friends or neighbours. Present a summary of the findings, using suitable graphs.

It is particularly important to have periods of dreaming sleep. Dreaming indicates that the brain is reprocessing information and this is best achieved naturally. Drug-controlled sleep (e.g. by sleeping pills or alcohol) does not promote good dreaming sleep.

Total loss of sleep (sleep deprivation) for several days causes significant damage to mental health. It leads to short-term memory loss, hallucinations and it can be a contribution to death.

It is unlikely that the occasional all-night party will have these dramatic effects but care needs to be taken to catch up on the shortage of sleep as soon as possible.

Mental stimulation

Work and recreation both contribute to mental, social and physical activity. We have already considered physical activity and its importance. Mental stimulation is also vital as it provides challenges and problems to solve, giving material for the brain to process. This helps you stay alert and to approach new situations in a confident way. In health and social care, where every client at any time can present you with a new need to meet, it is essential to be mentally alert, ready to respond in a suitable way.

Boredom is an indicator that you need more mental stimulation. Anyone beginning to feel bored should first of all take responsibility for it: I'm bored, what can I do about it? – not: I'm bored, who can I blame for that? Secondly, the bored person should look for stimulation, challenge, a demand, a problem: How could I persuade my parents to let me re-decorate my room, or choose my own time to come home at night? What's the solution to this crossword, Rubic-cube? Can I learn to have a conversation with an older person in Urdu?

Why not challenge yourself now? What could you tackle to keep yourself mentally stimulated?

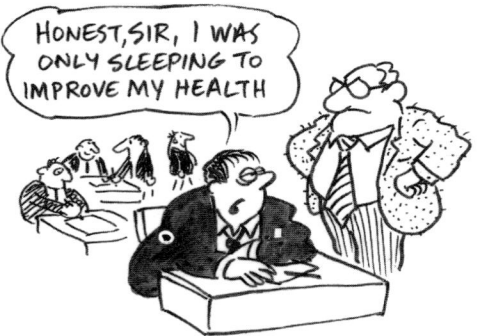

Figure 1.3 Lack of sleep can damage your education

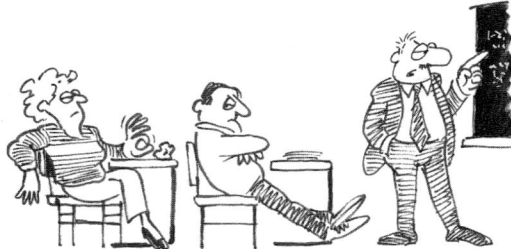

Figure 1.4 Boredom can be disruptive!

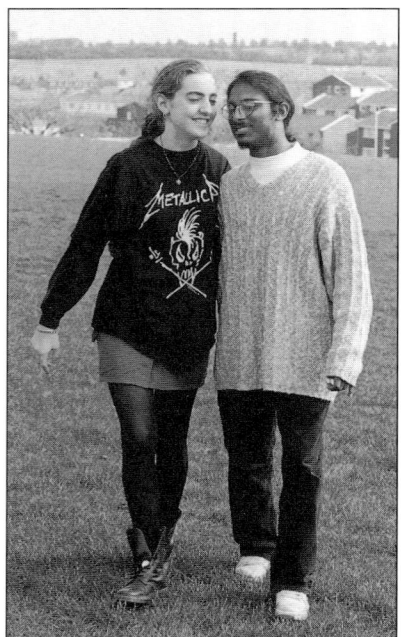

Figure 1.5 Examples of social interaction

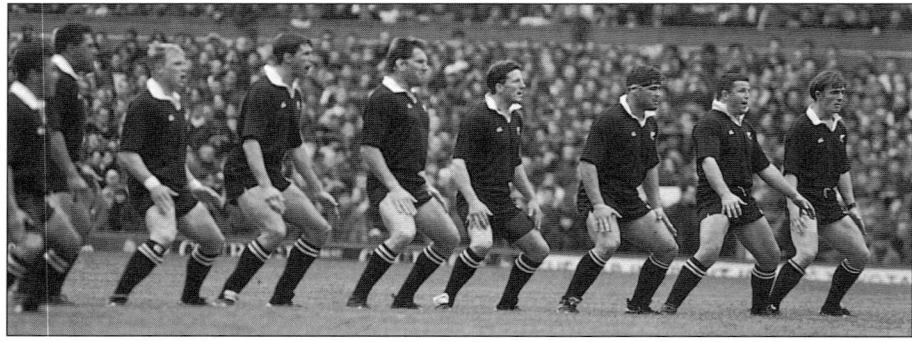

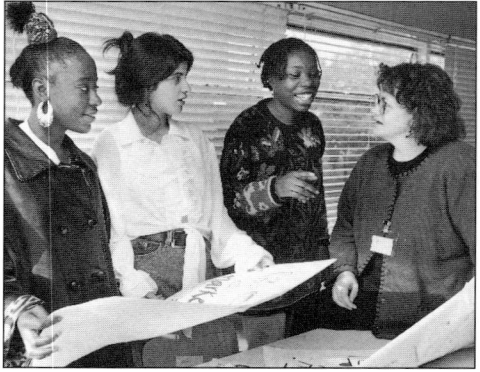

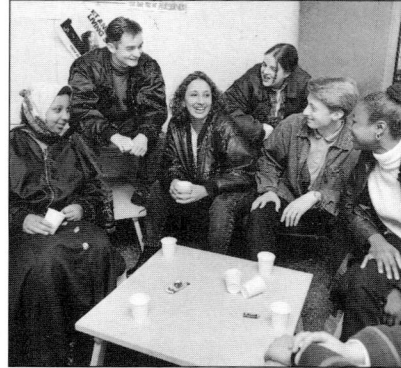

Social interaction

Social interaction serves a variety of functions, including:
- finding a partner
- working with others on problem solving
- providing opportunities to relax
- maintaining group structures.

Social interaction: *Any activity involving several people. The interaction may be very formal (e.g. a business meeting) or very informal (e.g. a party).*

We are social beings. It is very important for our health that we have regular contact and relationships with other people. This can be through leisure activities, friendships or situations in which activities are organised to bring people together, for example in day centres for elders.

As social animals, people who become isolated from social contact tend to become depressed. They withdraw, concentrating on their own thoughts and fears. These can become magnified and lead to severe mental ill-health. For this reason many people who live alone are encouraged to take part in some form of social interaction. This can be (for instance) in the form of planned visits by a person who befriends someone living alone, without family, friends or neighbours; someone with whom to have frequent contact and build a relationship.

Social activities contribute to your own feelings of self worth and belonging. Being in a group or with an individual can provide much support. It gives an opportunity to share ideas and worries. In doing so it helps reduce the risk of depression.

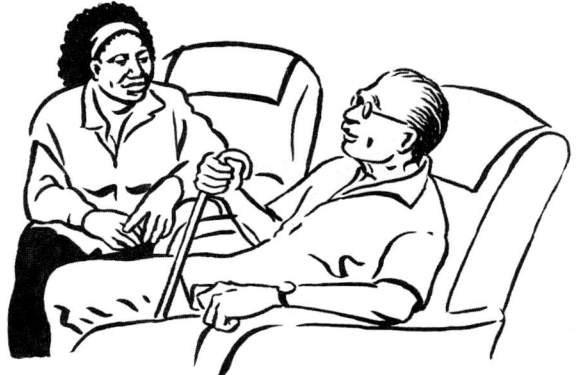

Figure 1.6 Regular, planned visits reduce the isolation of people living alone

▶ Group roles, page 97

Balanced lifestyles

The various factors which make up your lifestyle contribute to your mental, physical, emotional and social health and well-being. You will not recognise the value of many of the features of your lifestyle until the balance is upset. It is important to review the things that you do and try to keep the features in balance over a period of time. There will always be times when you choose to put things out of balance – but you should always recognise the need to compensate later on.

Going without sleep for an overnight party may help the social side of your lifestyle, but sleep requirements will need to be balanced quickly. Although you can tolerate working hard under stress for a short period, you will need to find time later to relax.

Some lifestyle features, however, are clearly a risk to your health. In the next section you will identify some of them.

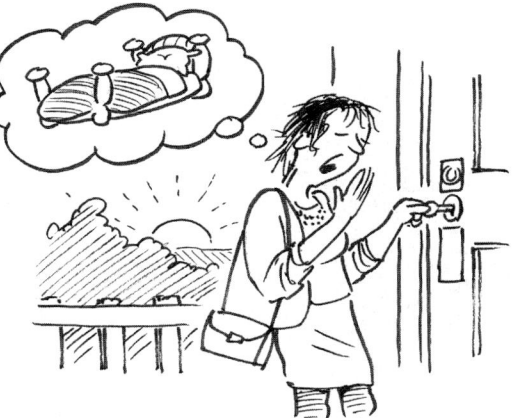

Figure 1.7 Great party but I need to catch up on my sleep!

Health risks

A — Health benefits and risks

Individually or in small groups, select a number of advertisements in newspapers and magazines for products or natural items that have some impact on health. Make a table of the different health benefits or risks that are associated with things being advertised.

What was being advertised	Benefit	Risk	Under my control?
apples	balanced diet	—	—
cigarettes	—	cancer and heart disease	Yes
blood donors needed	people needing blood	None	—

Figure 1.8 Your table should look something like this

In column 4 list the things that you have identified as risks to health that are under your control.
Identify the health risks that are likely to affect you personally.

In doing the activity you will have become more aware of **health risks** that are of concern. High on most people's lists of dangers to health will be drug abuse (including smoking and alcohol), illnesses such as cancer and those associated with HIV/AIDS, diseases associated with poor diet and lack of exercise and stress related diseases.

In Britain, the problem of health risks associated with lifestyle is so great that the Government, as part of the Health of the Nation Project, has set targets towards a better state of health. The targets are to encourage all individuals, and the health services, to improve the health of British people by the year 2000.

They have targeted six key areas:
- coronary heart disease and strokes
- cancers
- mental health
- accidents
- smoking
- HIV/AIDS and sexual health.

Health of the Nation targets

The Health of the Nation documents set targets for a range of health matters. Some of the targets are listed below:

Look after your heart campaign
Target: reduce premature deaths by 25% by the year 2000 (30% reduction for people under 65)

Strokes
Target: reduce premature deaths by 30% (25% in 65 – 74 age group)

Mental health
Target: move most psychiatric treatment to district-based services

Accidents
Target: reduce by 25% from 1980 levels accidents, that lead to death. This target is a World Health Organisation target and is also a global target.

HIV/AIDS and other sexually transmitted diseases
Target: reduce all levels (no target percentage). Increased information from research and for health promotion to be used.

Smoking: reduce all levels
Target percentages are age-specific:

Table 1.1 Target percentages for the reduction in smoking by the year 2000

	Male		Female	
Age	1988	2000	1988	2000
16-19	28	20	28	20
20-24	37	25	37	25
25-49	37	25	35	25
50-59	33	20	34	20
60 and over	26	15	21	15

FOCUS
Aspects of lifestyle:
- exercise
- diet – adequate and balanced
- sufficient rest
- avoidance of drug abuse including alcohol and tobacco
- safe sexual practice (including celibacy).

Health promotion
One of the ways that the targets for the health of the nation will be met is by increased health promotion. An example of part of a health promotion booklet is shown in Figure 1.9.

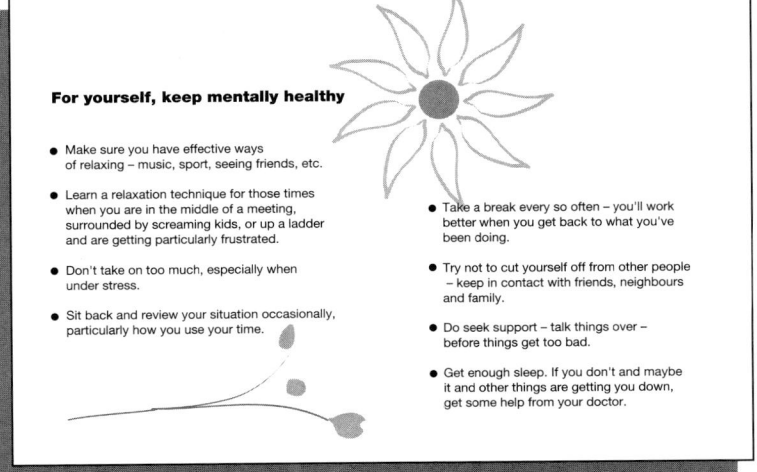

Figure 1.9 Extract from a booklet on mental health prepared by The Department of Health

Promoting health and well-being

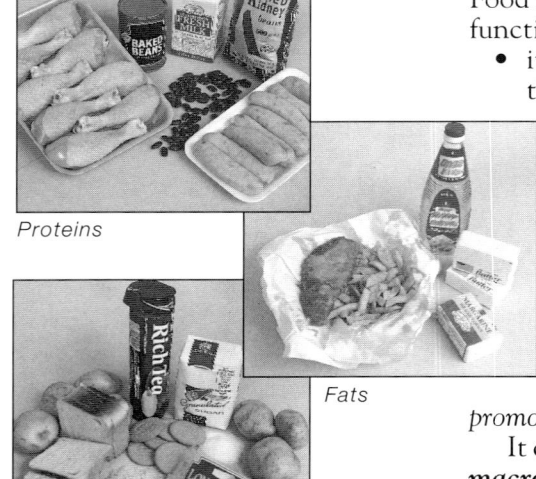

Proteins

Fats

Carbohydrates

Figure 1.10 *Proteins, fats and carbohydrates are macronutrients*
Proteins

FOCUS
Diet components:
- carbohydrates
- fats
- proteins
- vitamins and minerals
- water
- fibre.

FOCUS
Healthy diet:
- types of food eaten
- amounts eaten
- eating patterns.

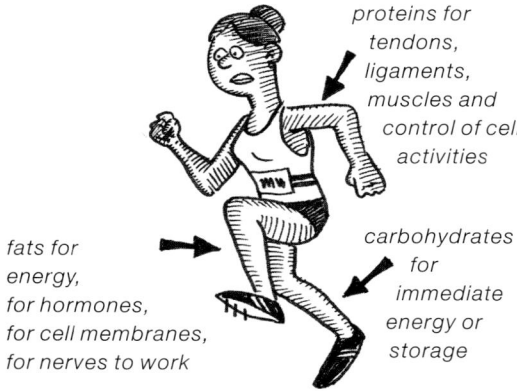

fats for energy, for hormones, for cell membranes, for nerves to work

proteins for tendons, ligaments, muscles and control of cell activities

carbohydrates for immediate energy or storage

Figure 1.11 *How the body uses nutrients*

Diet
Food is an essential part of a healthy lifestyle. It has several important functions:
- it provides us with the essential substances and nutrients needed to keep the body cells and tissues functioning normally
  - it is socially important – meal times can be a time when family relationships form
  - it is an essential part of celebrations and festive occasions
  - eating is a pleasurable experience
  - eating a healthy diet will reduce the risk of diseases such as coronary heart disease, cancers and strokes.

A healthy diet
In order to maintain health it is important to eat a **balanced diet**.

Balanced diet: *a diet consisting of sufficient nutrients to maintain and promote good health.*

It contains appropriate amounts of nutrients to meet the daily needs. The **macronutrients** are:
- proteins (for building body tissues)
- fats (for building cell structures and for energy)
- carbohydrates (for energy).

Macronutrients: *the nutrients we take in, in the largest quantities.*

The **micronutrients** are:
- vitamins – to help protect and regulate body functions
- minerals – to take part in body functions and as part of structures such as bone.

Micronutrients: *substances we need in smaller amounts.*

Also required as major components are:
- water – to provide a medium for chemical reactions in the body. To support, transport and to assist excretion
- fibre – to aid digestion, bind some toxic materials in foods and to ease passage of materials through the gut.

How the body uses the dietary components
See Figure 1.11, it gives an outline of the uses of the macronutrients: proteins, fats and carbohydrates. In more detail the uses are:

Proteins
Proteins are used to form:
- structural materials like cartilage, ligament and tendon
- muscles fibres
- enzymes that control the chemistry of the cells.

The proteins we eat are made up of individual building blocks, called amino acids, that are joined together in long chains. These chains are broken down (digested) to amino acid molecules. We absorb these building blocks and use them to produce our own proteins. Ideally, the food we eat contains just enough of the different amino acids necessary to build our own proteins. This never actually happens and so we normally eat too much. The amino acids that we cannot use are broken down to form a waste product (urea) and an energy-rich portion. This portion can either be used to provide energy, or is converted to the energy storage material, fat. Unwanted amino acids can also be converted into other, useful amino acids.

Carbohydrates
Carbohydrates come in three broad forms:
- small sugar molecules, for example sucrose (the sugar that comes from the supermarket!) and glucose
- large molecules of digestible starches

Table 1.2 Major vitamins and minerals required by humans

Vitamin	Functions	Major sources	Deficiency disease
A	Essential for black and white night vision	Carotene in plants is needed to make Vitamin A, liver	Night blindness
B_1	Required for energy production in cells	Yeast, rice, most plant and animal tissues	Beri-beri – muscle wastage and paralysis
B_6	Enables excess amino acids to be changed to other amino acids	All animal and plant tissues	Anaemia and vomiting
B_{12}	Required for correct red blood cell formation	Beef, kidney, liver	Pernicious anaemia (not treatable with Iron)
C	Helps cells to stick together	Citrus fruits, e.g. oranges, green vegetables	Scurvy – breakdown of membranes
D	Aids calcium absorption for skeletal growth and repair	Fish liver, egg yolk. Formed by action of UV light on skin	Rickets in children
E	Poorly understood	Lettuce, peanuts, egg yolk	Sterility only demonstrated in animals
K	Required for blood clotting	Leafy vegetables	Increased bleeding times
Mineral	**Functions**	**Major sources**	**Deficiency disease**
Calcium	Part of skeletal and tooth structure	Milk, cheese, fish	Poor skeletal growth
Chlorine	Required for activity of nerves and muscle	Cooking salt, cheese	Localised shortage linked to muscle cramps
Fluorine (trace)	Helps to prevent dental cavities	Drinking water, tooth paste	Weak tooth enamel
Iodine (trace)	Needed to make thyroid hormone	Sea fish, shell fish, iodised table salt	Goitre (enlarged thyroid gland)
Iron	Oxygen-carrying part of blood (haemoglobin)	Liver, eggs, cocoa powder. Not easily absorbed from plants, e.g. spinach	Anaemia
Nitrogen	Part of protein	Meat, fish, beans	Kwashiorkor
Potassium	Required for activity of nerves and muscle	Leafy vegetables, liver	Rare / not known
Sodium	Important for water balance in cells	Cooking salt, bacon, most foods	Localised deficiency causes muscle cramp

- indigestible large molecules (these form part of fibre).

The digestible starches and sugars are digested to produce simple sugars, for example glucose. These are then absorbed into the body. There are three main fates for the carbohydrates in the body, although all are part of producing energy for living:

- they travel in the blood to cells where they are used to produce energy for the cells to work
- they travel in the blood to muscles and the liver where they form an energy store of glycogen (a large starch-like molecule). This will eventually be used to provide energy for the cells
- they travel in the blood to the liver where they are converted to fat. This is then deposited in storage places, for example just under the skin. This fat is a long-term energy reserve and is formed as a consequence of taking in too much energy.

Fats

Fats are an interesting nutrient because it has so many roles. Fats are digested to form fatty acids and glycerol, but are then rebuilt into fats once they have been absorbed. They are then used:

- as a source of energy or an energy store
- as a component of cell membranes. Cells contain a large amount of membrane, which in turn contains a large amount of fat
- as a starting point for making many hormones such as oestradiol (an oestrogen) and testosterone. These biochemical pathways also produce cholesterol
- as a structural material forming myelin around nerve fibres. This acts as an insulator and also helps the nerves to transmit messages.

Fats are not just an energy-rich nutrient – they also have many other roles.

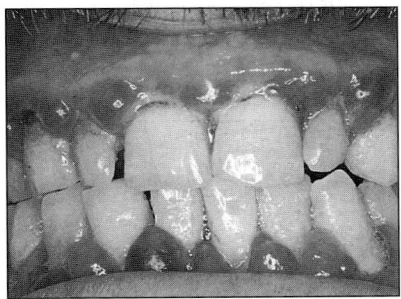

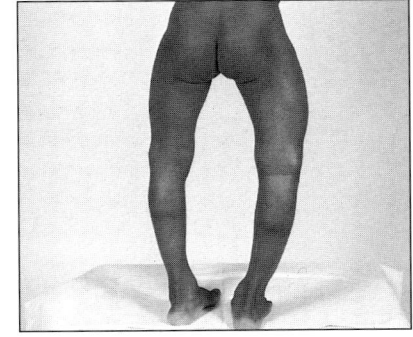

Figure 1.12 Lack of vitamins can cause such health problems as scurvy (top) or rickets (bottom) though these are less common in Great Britain now than earlier this century

Dietary recommendations

If you were to look back at nutritional guidance from the Second World War onwards you would see changes in dietary recommendations. Recommended nutritional intakes have changed over the years as our knowledge of the science of nutrition has increased. For example, during the Second World War the recommended consumption was one egg a day; now it is not more than two a week. In the 1930s and 1940s high amounts of fat on meat were recommended; now they are not. Nutritional information soon goes out of date, so it is always best to check that you are working with the most up-to-date information.

Table 1.3 Reference nutrient intakes (RNI)

Reference Nutrient Intakes (RNI): typical amounts (per day) of the various nutrients to form a balanced diet. The figures are related to the age and gender (sex) of an individual and represent figures that would supply 97% of the group with sufficient of a given nutrient.

	*Av. Wt (kg)	Energy (MJ)	Energy (kcal)	Protein (g)	Calcium (mg)	Iron (mg)	A (µg)	B_1 (mg)	B_6 (mg)	B_{12} (µg)	C (mg)	**D (µg)
Boys												
0–3 months	6.12	2.28	545	12.5	525	1.7	350	0.2	0.2	0.3	25	8.5
4–6 months	8.0	2.89	690	12.7	525	4.3	350	0.2	0.2	0.3	25	8.5
7–9 months	9.2	3.44	825	13.7	525	7.8	350	0.2	0.3	0.4	25	7.0
10–12 months	10.04	3.85	920	14.9	525	7.8	350	0.3	0.4	0.4	25	7.0
1–3 years	14.4	5.15	1230	14.5	350	6.9	400	0.5	0.7	0.5	30	7.0
4–6 years	19.3	7.16	1715	19.7	450	6.1	500	0.7	0.9	0.8	30	-
7–10 years	29.7	8.24	1970	28.3	550	8.7	500	0.7	1.0	1.0	30	-
11–14 years	45.5	9.27	2220	42.1	1000	11.3	600	0.9	1.2	1.2	35	-
15–18 years	64.0	11.51	2755	55.2	1000	11.3	700	1.1	1.5	1.5	40	-
Men												
19–50 years	75.0	10.60	2550	55.5	700	8.7	700	1.0	1.4	1.5	40	-
51–59 years	73.0	10.60	2550	53.3	700	8.7	700	0.9	1.4	1.5	40	-
60–64 years	74.0	9.93	2380	53.3	700	8.7	700	0.9	1.4	1.5	40	10.0
65–74 years	71.0	9.71	2330	53.3	700	8.7	700	0.9	1.4	1.5	40	10.0
over 75 years	69.0	8.77	2100	53.3	700	8.7	700	0.9	1.4	1.5	40	10.0
Girls												
0–3 months	5.7	2.16	515	12.5	525	1.7	350	0.2	0.2	0.3	25	8.5
4–6 months	7.44	2.69	645	12.7	525	4.3	350	0.2	0.2	0.3	25	8.5
7–9 months	8.55	3.20	765	13.7	525	7.8	350	0.2	0.3	0.4	25	7.0
10–12 months	9.5	3.61	865	14.9	525	7.8	350	0.3	0.4	0.4	25	7.0
1–3 years	13.85	4.86	1165	14.5	350	6.9	400	0.5	0.7	0.5	30	7.0
4–6 years	18.9	6.46	1545	19.7	450	6.1	500	0.7	0.9	0.8	30	-
7–10 years	29.7	7.28	1740	28.3	550	8.7	500	0.7	1.0	1.0	30	-
11–14 years	47.0	7.92	1845	41.2	800	14.8	600	0.7	1.0	1.2	35	-
15–18 years	55.0	8.83	2110	45.0	800	14.8	600	0.8	1.2	1.5	40	-
Women												
19–50 years	60.0	8.10	1940	45.0	700	14.8	600	0.8	1.2	1.5	40	-
pregnant	-	8.90	2140	51.0	700	14.8	700	0.9	1.2	1.5	50	-
lactating 1–3 months (average)	-	10.30	2460	56.0	1250	14.8	950	1.0	1.2	2.0	70	-
lactating 4+ months	-	10.50	2470	53.0	1250	14.8	950	1.0	1.2	2.0	70	-
51–59 years	63.0	8.0	1900	46.5	700	8.7	600	0.8	1.2	1.5	40	-
60–64 years	63.5	7.99	1900	46.5	700	8.7	600	0.8	1.2	1.5	40	10.0
65–74 years	63.0	7.96	1900	46.5	700	8.7	600	0.8	1.2	1.5	40	10.0
over 75 years	60.0	7.61	1810	46.5	700	8.7	600	0.8	1.2	1.5	40	10.0

* where weights are for a range of ages the weight at the top of the range is given for children and in the middle for adults

** Vitamin D figures assume that vitamin D is being produced by the action of sunlight on the body. Some people may need to supplement this in the diet (e.g. pregnant women and elderly people)

Figures for average weight and vitamin D adapted from the COMA report N0. 41. Dietary Reference Values for Food Energy and Nutrients for The United Kingdom. HMSO, 1992 (revised 1994)

The reference nutrient intakes are only part of the information required to determine a balanced diet. They provide guidelines for broad categories of people. They identify the fact that **dietary requirements / nutritional requirements** vary with age and gender (sex). For example, if a woman is pregnant or breast-feeding a child (lactating), then her needs are for calcium increase.

In elderly people deficiency in Vitamin C (ascorbic acid) is quite common due to lack of fresh fruit and vegetables in their diet. Elderly people may also develop osteoporosis, in which calcium is lost from the bones, which leaves the bones weak. An elderly person's diet should be high in calcium and Vitamin D which can help to prevent osteoporosis. This condition is not only diet-related, hormonal levels and exercise also affect the calcium content of the bones.

Nutrient needs also vary with the amount of exercise a person takes. This exercise can be related to the work done (e.g. manual labour) or to sporting activities. A person who undertakes little physical activity (has a sedentary occupation) will need less energy than an active person. Careful study shows that energy requirements per kilogram of body weight are greatest in babies where growth is most rapid. Elderly people, where activity is low, growth has ceased and repair of tissues is limited, require least energy per kilogram of body weight.

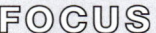

Individual's dietary requirements are affected by:
- activity
- age
- pregnancy.

▶ Menopause, page 75

A   Calorie counting

1 Look at the information provided in Table 1.3. In particular look at:
- energy
- protein
- calcium.

You have a bowl of cornflakes weighing 50 gm, with 125 ml whole milk. What percentage of the RNI would be provided for these three areas if you were:

(a) a boy aged 17

(b) a woman aged 70?

2 Throughout the day we use up the calories we take in from food. The likely calorie usage (in kcal per hour) for males and females is:

▶ Table of nutrients, Appendix I, page 218

Activity	Male	Female
Sleep	65	50
Lightly active (sitting/reading/writing, etc.)	85	70
Moderately active	200	160
Very active (hard walking/strenuous physical exercise, etc.)	340	270

If a person had 8 hours sleep, 9 hours of light activity and 7 hours of moderate activity, what would be the calorie requirement for:

(a) a male

(b) a female?

Look back at the diary you produced in the Lifestyle activity (page 4). Estimate your calorie use for your Saturday, Sunday and an average weekday.

Without using the tables provided, estimate (make a reasonable guess about) the number of calories you consume in a day.
Now write down your food intake for a typical day. Think about the food you normally eat each day. Are some days very different? Be honest! Don't forget drinks and snacks. Use the energy section of the extended table of nutrients in Appendix I to check your estimate of the number of kcals you consume on a typical day. Comment on your findings.

Promoting health and well-being

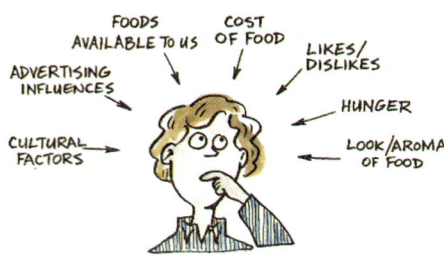

Figure 1.13 Many different factors influence your food intake

Balancing your diet

Eating a balanced diet is not, for some people, easy. Our food intake is affected by many factors.

In addition we do not choose nutrients, we choose food, and, as we have seen, all foods vary in their composition.

No single food contains all the nutrients we need. Different foods contain different mixtures of proteins, fats, carbohydrates, minerals and vitamins.

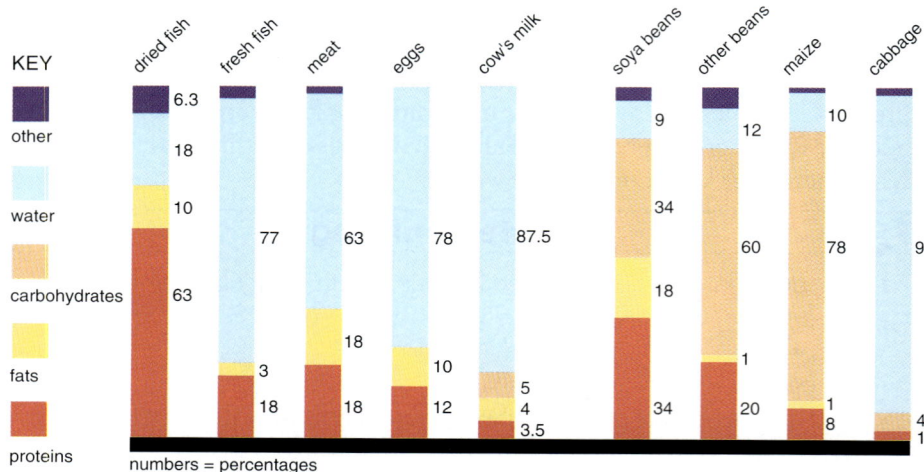

Figure 1.14 Different nutrients in some well-known foods

▶ Appendix I has a fuller list, page 216.

In order to determine if your diet is balanced you will need to know the nutritional content of the food and the reference nutrient intakes. There are several books that include this information in detail. Computer programmes are also available. Figure 1.14 gives some examples of the nutrient content of some common foods.

Table 1.4 Table of nutrients (Composition per 100 g raw edible weight, except where stated)

Food	Inedible waste%	Water (g)	Energy (kJ)	Energy (kcal)	Protein (g)	Fat (g)	Saturated fatty acids(g)	Carbo-hydrate(g)	Total sugars (g)	Fibre NSP(g)	Calcium (mg)	Iron (mg)	Sodium (mg)	Vitamin A (µg)	Thiamin (mg)	Vitamin C(mg)
Wholemeal bread, average	0	38.3	914	215	9.2	2.5	0.5	41.6	1.8	5.8	54	2.7	550	0	0.34	0
Weetabix	0	5.6	1498	352	11.0	2.7	0.4	75.7	5.2	9.7	35	7.4	270	0	0.9	0
Cheesecake, frozen	0	44.0	1017	242	5.7	10.6	5.6	33.0	22.2	0.9	68	0.5	160	0	0.04	0
Whole milk, average	0	87.8	275	66	3.2	3.9	2.4	4.8	4.8	0.0	115	0.06	55	55	0.03	1
Yogurt, low fat, fruit	0	77.0	382	90	4.1	0.7	0.4	17.9	17.9	0	150	0.1	64	11	0.05	1
Cottage cheese, plain	0	79.1	413	98	13.8	3.9	2.4	2.1	2.1	0.0	73	0.1	380	46	0.03	0
Eggs, chicken, fried in vegetable oil	0	70.1	745	179	13.6	13.9	4.0	0.0	0.0	0.0	65	2.2	160	215	0.07	0
Bacon, rasher, lean and fat, grilled, back	0	36.0	1681	405	25.3	33.38	13.2	0.0	0.0	0.0	12	1.5	2020	0	0.43	0
Chicken, roast, meat only	0	68.4	621	148	24.8	5.4	1.6	0.0	0.0	0.0	9	0.8	81	0	0.08	0
Sausages, pork, grilled	0	45.1	1320	318	13.3	24.6	9.5	11.5	1.8	0.7	53	1.5	1000	0	0.02	0
Haddock, steamed, flesh only	24	75.1	417	98	22.8	0.8	0.2	0.0	0.0	0.0	55	0.7	120	0	0.08	0
Potato crisps	0	1.9	2275	546	5.6	37.6	9.2	49.3	0.7	4.9	37	1.8	1070	0	0.11	27
Cauliflower, boiled in unsalted water	0	90.6	117	28	2.9	0.9	0.2	2.1	1.8	1.6	17	0.4	4	10	0.07	27
Yam, boiled in unsalted water	0	64.4	568	133	1.7	0.3	0.1	33.0	0.7	1.4	12	0.4	17	0	0.14	4
Apples, eating, average, raw, flesh and skin	11	84.5	199	47	0.4	0.1	0.0	11.8	11.8	1.8	4	0.1	3	3	0.03	6
Mangoes, ripe, raw, flesh only	32	82.4	245	57	0.7	0.2	0.1	14.1	13.8	2.6	12	0.7	2	300	0.04	37
Peppermints	0	0.2	1670	392	0.5	0.7	N	102.2	102.2	0.0	7	0.2	9	0	0.0	0
Coffee, instant powder	0	3.4	424	100	14.6	0.0	0.0	11.0	6.5	0.0	160	4.4	41	0	0.00	0
Tomato ketchup	0	64.8	420	98	2.1	0.0	0.0	24.0	22.9	0.9	2.5	1.2	1120	38	1.00	2
Beer, bitter, keg	0	93.5	129	31	0.3	0.0	0.0	2.3	2.3	0.0	8	0.01	8	0	0	0

One simple way of checking the overall balance of the diet is to compare your average daily diet with the food groups shown in The Balance of Good Health (the National Food Guide).

By choosing a variety of foods from the first four food groups every day, you can easily ensure that you get the range of nutrients your body needs to remain healthy. Foods in the fifth food group – fatty and sugary foods – are not essential to a healthy diet, but add extra choice and palatability. The main nutrients provided by each food group are shown.

The Balance of Good Health encourages people to eat more fruit and vegetables than most people currently do (five portions or more is recommended) and it also suggests that we eat more carbohydrate foods such as bread, other cereals and potatoes.

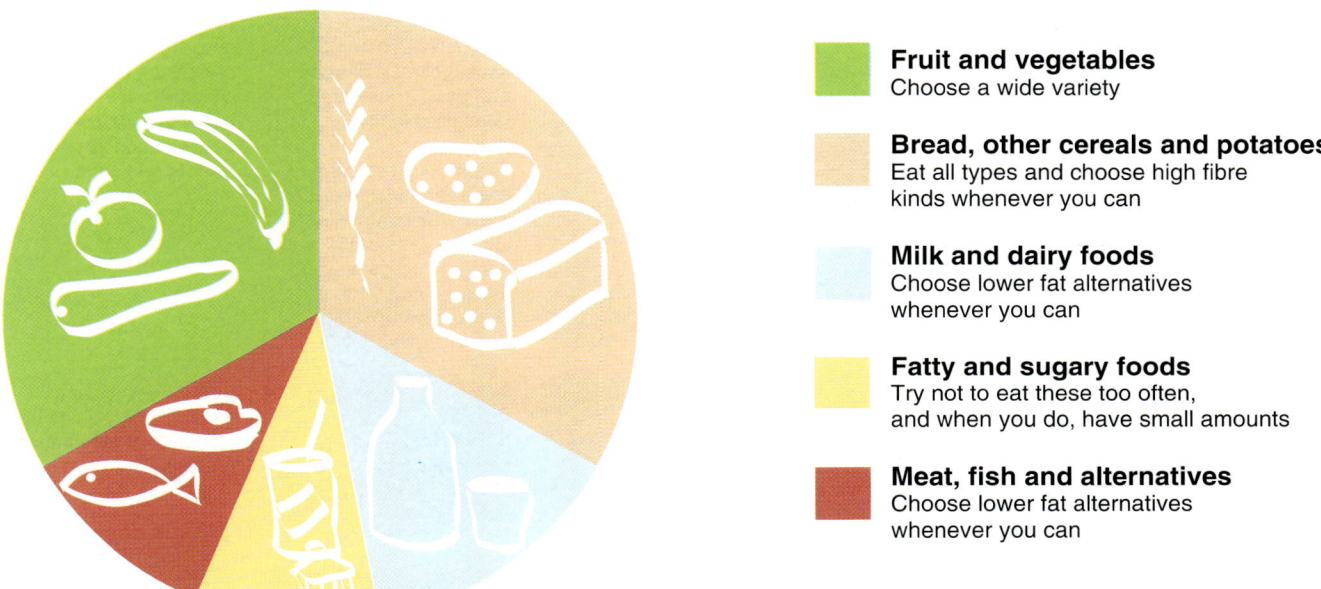

Figure 1.15 The balance of good health

Eating patterns

One thing that is not identified by looking at overall nutrient intakes is the pattern of eating. The traditional pattern in the UK is for three meals a day to be consumed, with between-meal snacks being consumed to a greater or lesser extent. This pattern has been criticised, in particular the between-meal snacks, as the energy content of snack foods is often too high. However, this view has been challenged and a pattern of grazing (small regular intakes of food) is becoming more acceptable so long as the balance of nutrients is correct. What this pattern does is to spread the load on the digestive system. Possibly it reflects our evolutionary origins as a hunter/gatherer species: it is thought that our ancestors moved around gathering seeds, fruits and vegetables and hunting animals for meat.

A balanced diet has social and psychological aspects. Most of us eat many of our meals with family, friends or colleagues. This can influence what we eat, and our enthusiasm about eating at all. How far are your eating habits influenced by your social relationships? Do you eat fish and

Promoting health and well-being

BREAD, OTHER CEREALS & POTATOES	FRUIT AND VEGETABLES	MILK AND DAIRY FOODS	MEAT, FISH AND ALTERNATIVES	FATTY AND SUGARY FOODS
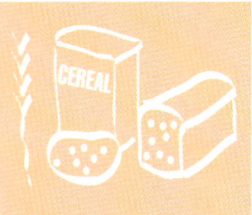	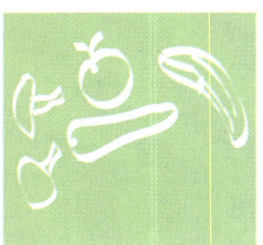	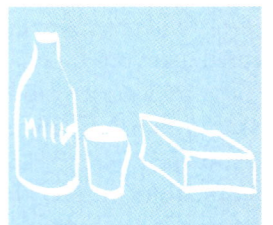		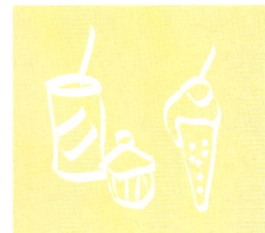
WHAT'S INCLUDED				
Other cereals means things like breakfast cereals, pasta, rice, oats, noodles, maize, millet and cornmeal. Beans and pulses can be eaten as part of this group.	Fresh, frozen and canned fruit and vegetables and dried fruit. A glass of fruit juice can also contribute. Beans and pulses can be eaten as part of this group.	Milk, cheese, yoghurt and fromage frais. This group does not include butter, eggs and cream.	Meat, poultry, fish, eggs, nuts, beans and pulses. Meat includes bacon and salami and meat products such as sausages, beefburgers and paté. These are all relatively high fat choices. Beans, such as canned baked beans and pulses are in this group. Fish includes frozen and canned fish such as sardines and tuna, fish fingers and fish cakes.	Margarine, low fat spread, butter, other spreading fats, cooking oils, oily salad dressings or mayonnaise, cream, chocolate, crisps, biscuits, pastries, cake, puddings, ice-cream, rich sauces and fatty gravies, sweets and sugar.
MAIN NUTRIENTS				
Carbohydrate (starch) 'Fibre' (NSP*) Some calcium and iron B Vitamins	Vitamin C Carotenes Folates 'Fibre' (NSP*) and some carbohydrate	Calcium Protein Vitamin B12 Vitamins A and D	Iron Protein B Vitamins, especially B12 Zinc Magnesium	Some vitamins and essential fatty acids but also a lot of fat, sugar and salt.
HOW MUCH TO CHOOSE				
Eat lots.	Eat lots.	Eat or drink moderate amounts and choose lower fat versions whenever you can.	Eat moderate amounts and choose lower fat versions whenever you can.	Eat fatty and sugary foods sparingly – that is, infrequently and/or in small amounts.
WHAT TYPES TO CHOOSE				
Try to eat wholemeal, wholegrain, brown or high fibre versions where possible. Try to avoid: • having them fried too often (eg. chips) • adding too much fat (eg. thickly spread butter, margarine or low fat spread on bread) • adding rich sauces and dressings (eg. cream or cheese sauce on pasta).	Eat a wide variety of fruit and vegetables. Try to avoid: • adding fat or rich sauces to vegetables (eg. carrots glazed with butter, roast parsnips) • adding sugar or syrupy dressings to fruit (eg. stewed apple with sugar, chocolate sauce on banana).	Lower fat versions means semi-skimmed or skimmed milk, low fat (0.1% fat) yoghurts or fromage frais, and lower fat cheeses (eg. Edam, Half-fat Cheddar, Camembert). Check the amount of fat by looking at the nutrient information on the labels. Compare similar products and choose the lowest – for example 8% fat fromage frais may be labelled low fat but is not actually the lowest available.	Lower fat versions means things like meat with the fat cut off, poultry without the skin and fish without batter. Cook these foods without added fat. Beans and pulses are good alternatives to meat as they are naturally very low in fat.	Some foods from this group will be eaten every day, but should be kept to small amounts, for example; margarine, low fat spread, butter, other spreading fats, cooking oils, oily salad dressings or mayonnaise. Other foods from this group really are occasional foods, for example; cream, chocolate, crisps, biscuits, pastries, cake, puddings, ice-cream, rich sauces and fatty gravies, sweets and sugar.

Figure 1.16 The five food groups

* 'Fibre' is more properly known as non-starch polysaccharides (NSP)

chips to keep a friend company, when you'd planned a salad sandwich? Do you manage on crisps and a cola when your friends want to 'save themselves for a meal later'? How far are the foods eaten, and the mealtimes themselves, a compromise in your family? Do you sometimes eat more than you had appetite for because you felt lonely?

We shall be looking later at this link between food and relationships, between diet and social stimulation, when we consider (for instance) the importance of lunch clubs and day centres for older people.

Eating as a social activity
A second feature of a balanced diet that needs to be considered is the psychological aspect of eating. As we have already identified, eating has a major importance as a social activity. A balanced diet ideally recognises this and involves dining with friends. The benefits to social and mental health should be considered when identifying what constitutes a balanced diet.

The role of dietary fibre in health maintenance
It seems odd that something that is not digested has an important role in health. Fibre provides bulk to the material passing through the digestive system. In doing so it speeds up movement through the system, reducing the time that any toxic materials remain in contact with the lining of the gut. The waste also passes through in a softer form, because it contains more water because less water has been reabsorbed. This is particularly important in the large intestine where waste material can spend a long time before being passed out as faeces. Softer materials reduce the physical damage to the lining of the large intestine.

The two major effects of speed of passage and softness of material mean that cancer-producing chemicals do not come into contact with damaged intestine lining. This is thought to be one of the reasons why a high fibre diet reduces the risk of cancers of the large intestine.

It is important to ensure that the fibre comes from a variety of sources and is not just added to the diet as bran. In particular there is some evidence that fibre from oats and beans may provide protection from heart disease. The way this protection works is not yet understood and the evidence is not fully accepted.

The identification of the role of fibre in cancer prevention was based on studies of populations in Africa and North America. It was noticed that cancer of the large intestine was almost non-existent in the population studied in Africa while it was a major cause of death in North America. The link was made between the time that food spent in the digestive system and the incidence of the cancer. The high fibre African diet meant that food took less than a day to pass through the digestive system. In the low fibre American diet the figure was close to two days. The link between low fibre diets and cancer was identified.

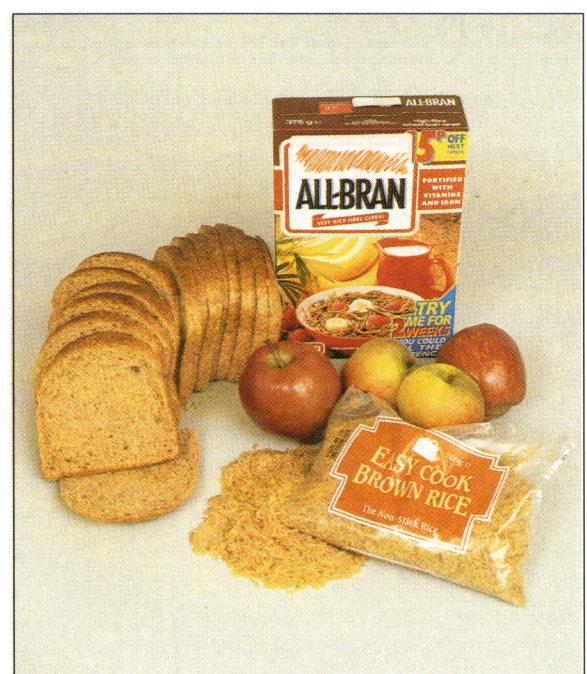

Figure 1.17 High fibre foods

Health risks from dietary habits

The broad pattern of the British diet is shown below. Since the Second World War there has been a decline in the amount of food energy (calories) obtained from carbohydrates, and an increase in calories from fats and this has not changed significantly for the last twenty years, even though there have been changes in the types and quantities of foods eaten.

There have been many Government reports linking unhealthy diet with diseases such as coronary heart disease, stroke and some cancers. In 1983 a discussion paper was prepared for the National Advisory Committee on Nutrition Education (NACNE). It was called 'Proposals for nutritional guide-lines for health education in Britain'.

The most recent report, published in 1994, (COMA Report No 46, Nutritional Aspects of Cardiovascular disease) gives key recommendations for a healthy diet.

The recommendations focus particularly on fats and the importance of their role in increasing the risk of heart disease. The amount of fat eaten, of any kind, should be reduced. In particular, we should cut down on our consumption of saturated fats. Saturated fats come from animal sources, such as butter or lard, but they are also found in processed foods such as biscuits, cake, pies and pastry. There are two other types of fats, one is polyunsaturated fat (found mainly from plant sources such as sunflower and soy, but also from fish), the other is monounsaturated fat (found mainly from plant sources such as olives). We should eat about the same amount of these fats.

Foods which seem to have a beneficial effect on heart disease are fibre, found in oats and pulses (peas and beans) and Vitamins A, C and E.

This reduction in total fat intake should also help to decrease the percentage of people who are obese. The Government report also suggests that we should go back to obtaining more of our energy from carbohydrate foods such as bread, pasta, rice, cereals, fruit and vegetables.

The other recommendations are concerned with dietary fibre, salt and alcohol. We have already looked at the benefits of dietary fibre (page 17).

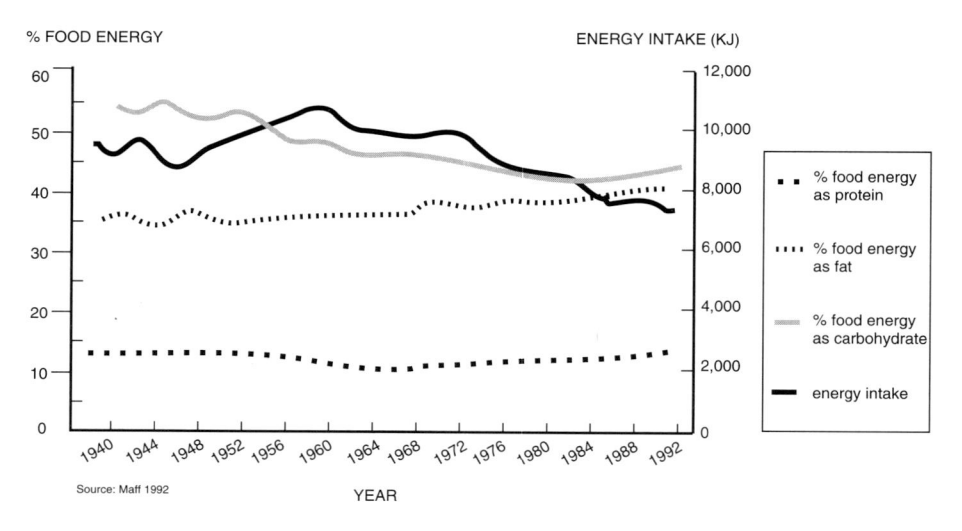

Figure 1.18 *Changes in the amount of daily food energy obtained from carbohydrate, fat and protein*

Salt has a role in increasing blood pressure, but not everybody is equally at risk. The recommendation to reduce salt intake applies to all, through adding less salt to meals, less in cooking and less in processed foods.

Excess alcohol consumption is also linked with high blood pressure and the risk of stroke as well as increasing energy intake. The added benefit relating to reduced alcoholism in this country is hard to calculate. There have been some studies that identify alcohol in moderation (one glass of wine per day) as having a positive beneficial effect on health.

Malnutrition from under-eating

The benefits system means that starvation in the UK is rare. However, eating disorders such as anorexia nervosa and bulimia (an illness that involves eating and then inducing vomiting), mean that individuals literally starve themselves. In extreme cases this causes death. However, the reasons for this are mainly psychological – they are not due to lack of food.

More common are deficiencies in the micronutrients (vitamins and minerals), the most common being iron deficiency – anaemia. This often occurs with people who change their dietary habits without thinking about the need to check on the balance of their diet, or as a result of disease. In particular, people who turn from eating meat to being vegetarian and people trying to lose weight can unintentionally reduce their iron intake and this may cause anaemia.

Malnutrition from over-eating

Our weight is known to influence our health. Much research evidence has been produced which links being overweight with life-threatening diseases such as coronary heart disease, stroke and certain cancers, all of which are major causes of death in the modern world.

The basic principle associated with over-eating is that more energy is consumed than used, so the excess energy consumed is stored as fat. This means that the individual moves outside the ideal height to weight ratio.

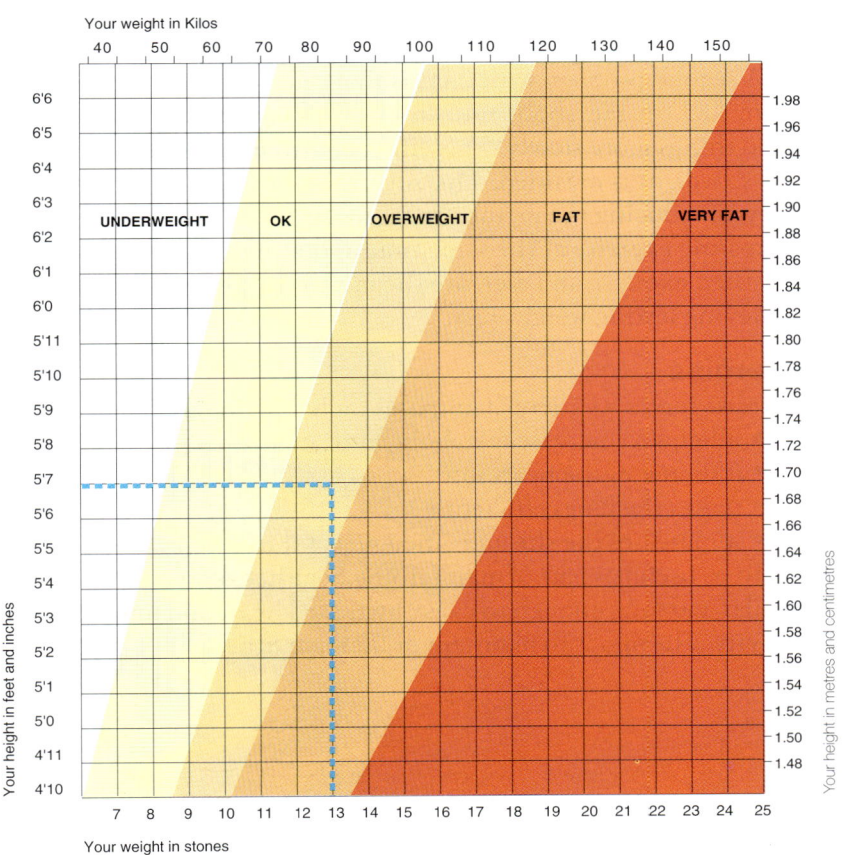

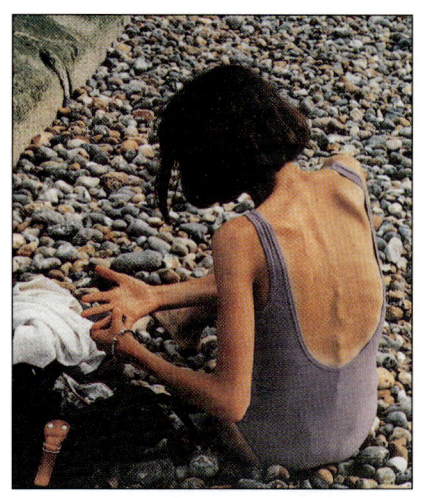

Figure 1.19 Anorexia nervosa is an illness that leads to dangerous malnutrition

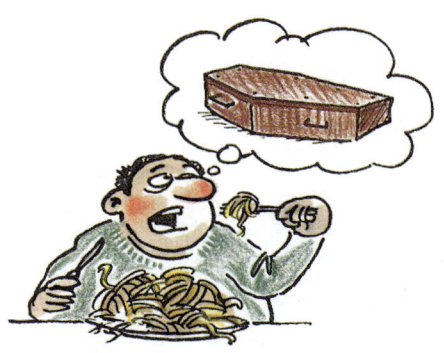

Figure 1.20 Malnutrition from over-eating can be dangerous

Are you the right weight for your height?

The information on this chart is designed for adult men and women only.
Make a straight line up from your weight (without clothes), and a line across from your height (without shoes). Put a mark where the two lines meet. This tells you whether you need to lose or gain weight.

☐ UNDERWEIGHT
Maybe you need to eat a bit more. But go for well-balanced nutritious foods and don't just fill up on fatty and sugary foods. If you are very underweight see you doctor about it.

☐ OK
Your weight is in the desirable range for health. You're eating the right quantity of food but you need to be sure that you're getting a healthy balance in your diet.

☐ OVERWEIGHT
Your health could suffer. You should try to lose weight.

☐ FAT
It is really important to lose weight

☐ VERY FAT
Being this overweight is very serious. You urgently need to lose weight. Talk to your doctor or practice nurse. You may be referred to a dietitian.

For example, a person who is 5'7 tall and weighs 13 stones is overweight.

Figure 1.21 Height-weight chart

Promoting health and well-being

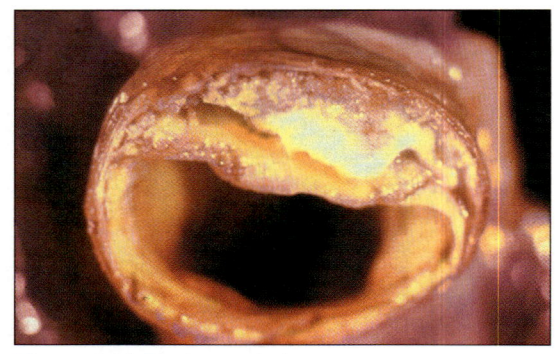

Figure 1.22 Cholesterol plaques on the wall of an artery (cross section)

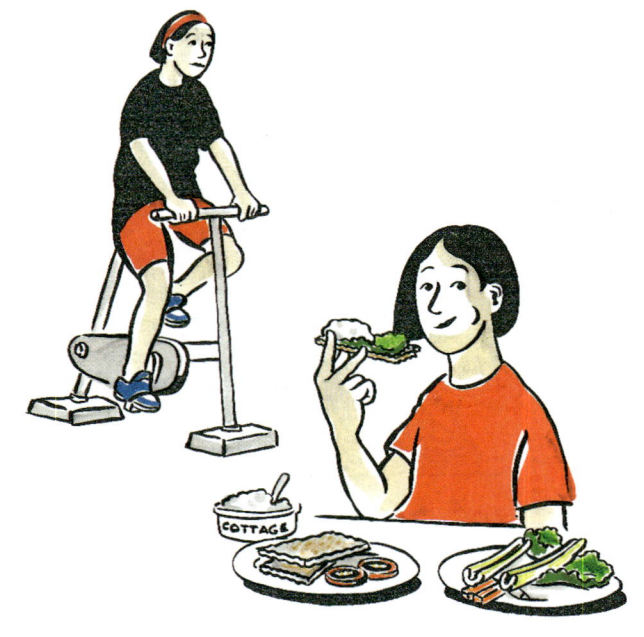

Figure 1.23 Exercise and diet together improve the effects of the diet alone

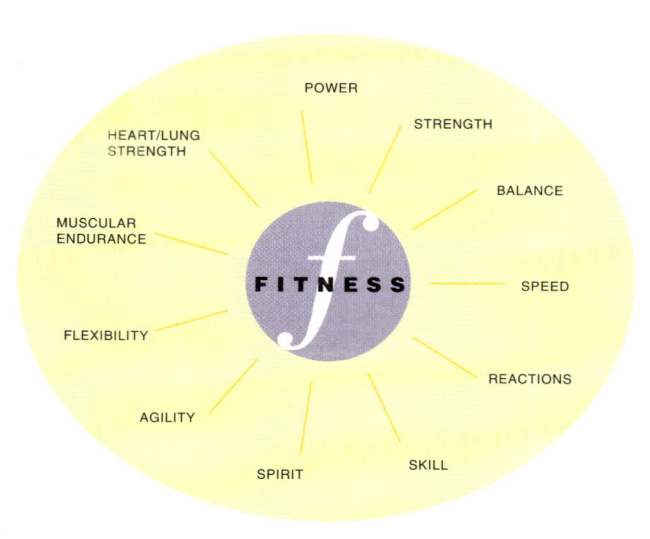

Figure 1.24 Physical fitness is a blend of a number of things

The risks of being overweight

The effects of being overweight include:
- increased pressure and wear on joints
- an increased strain on the heart in pumping blood
- increased risk of build up of fatty plaques on the artery walls, leading to increased risk of heart attacks.

The more overweight (obese) you are, the greater the risks. There is some evidence, however, that to be slightly overweight is less damaging than constantly dieting, as dieting can increase levels of stress.

How to deal with being overweight

The answer to being overweight is not as simple as saying 'eat less', or 'go on a diet'. Clearly the cause of overweight is normally taking in too much food and not using all the energy supplied. However, people eat for many reasons and the reasons they do so need to be understood before a weight-reducing diet is likely to work. Eating for comfort, eating out of habit, eating in emotional distress and for social reasons, can all have links with overeating.

Achieving lasting weight loss

Quick weight reduction diets often work in the short term, but the person's eating habits are not re-educated and so as soon as the diet is stopped, resuming old eating habits means the weight is put on again. This causes a cycle of diet and weight gain that can be more damaging to health than being slightly overweight. A better approach, long term, would be to look at reducing the fat and sugar content of the diet, i.e. healthy eating.

A second problem with diets is that reduced food intakes mean that the metabolic rate drops. This means the body starts to do things more slowly. This effect continues after the diet and so weight is regained. This survival mechanism by the body, of reducing the metabolic rate, can be overcome by increasing exercise at the same time as dieting. The two together, exercise and diet, are the most effective way of achieving lasting weight loss.

Exercise

Exercise serves a variety of purposes including the following:
- it helps to increase metabolic rate and the use of energy
- it increases the heart rate
- it uses the lungs efficiently
- it increases the size and efficiency of the muscles.

To be useful as part of maintaining health, exercise should be regular and long enough to cause increased heart and lung activity. The aim is to maintain or increase fitness.

Promoting health and well-being

The ingredients of fitness

The minimum level of fitness we should all aim for is:
- to keep the heart and lungs working efficiently
- to have muscles strong enough to support us and enable us to move ourselves and carry out everyday activities
- to have joints flexible enough to let us carry out a full range of movements
- to carry out physical work efficiently with the minimum of effort
- to be able to react by moving to protect ourselves from danger
- to have the reserve strength to cope with new situations.

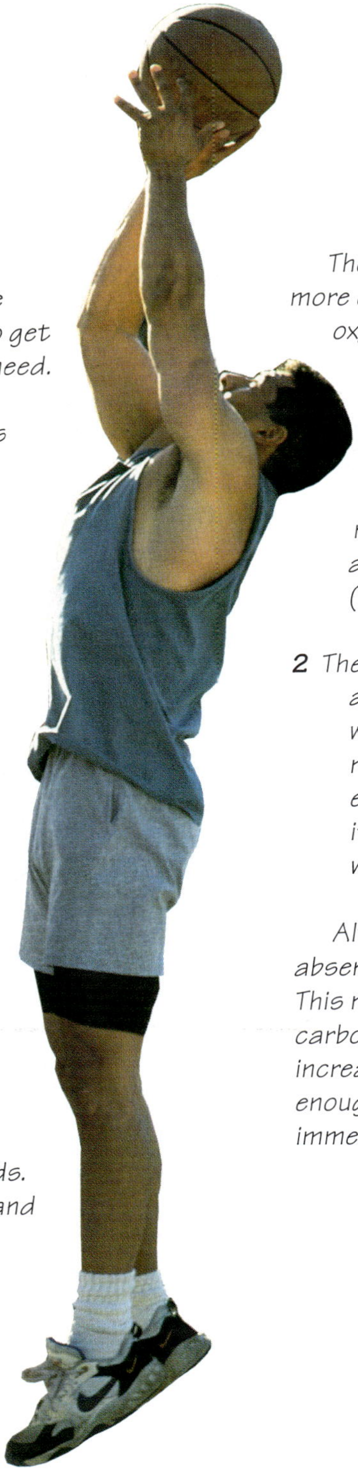

The circulatory system must circulate the blood (and therefore oxygen) more quickly. It must also get more blood to the areas most in need.

The blood supply to the brain is constant.

Respiratory system causes faster and deeper breathing. The more carbon dioxide in the blood, the more rapidly and deeply we breathe.

Exchange of gases is more efficient in the lungs during exercise.

Blood flow is reduced to the areas of the body not in urgent need. It is increased to those areas in greatest need.

Anticipation of exercise causes hormonal releases which prepare the body for action.

Adrenalin is released into the bloodstream by the adrenal glands. This stimulates the respiratory and cardiovascular systems.

The aerobic production of ATP (energy) is much more efficient than if ATP has to be produced without oxygen. There are two reasons for this:

1. *The system is able to use stored fat as a source of energy rather than having to rely only on carbohydrate in the form of muscle glycogen. Not only does fat carry twice as much energy per gram as carbohydrate, but we also have much greater stores of it available. (Stores of muscle glycogen are limited.)*

2. *The presence of oxygen also enables much greater amounts of fuel to be released from carbohydrate without a build-up of lactic acid. A carbohydrate molecule can produce over 12 times the amount of energy if oxygen is present than if the muscle is working anaerobically.*

Although carbohydrate can be burned up in the absence of oxygen, this is not the case for fat. This means that the muscles will revert to using carbohydrate as fuel whenever the intensity of exercise increases to such an extent that enough oxygen is not available for immediate muscular needs.

Figure 1.25 What happens to our body when we exercise?

Promoting health and well-being

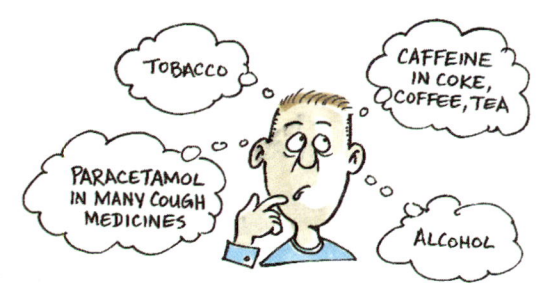

Figure 1.26 Some of the drugs you may be using yourself

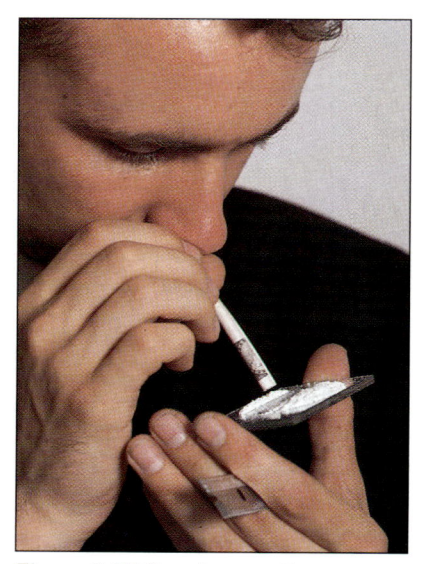

Figure 1.27 Cocaine snorting

Figure 1.28 Passive smoking is almost as harmful as smoking the tobacco yourself

Drug use and abuse

Drugs are available in three ways:
- those that are prescribed by a doctor and obtained from a pharmacist (prescribed drugs)
- those that can be purchased without a prescription (over-the-counter-drugs)
- those it is illegal to possess other than in special circumstances (controlled drugs).

A   Drug audit

Many over-the-counter medicines contain drugs that are much cheaper in their B.P. equivalent form. Look at cold remedies to see what their contents are and produce a table to show them.

Various drugs are known to be harmful to health. These include legal drugs such as tobacco and alcohol, the medically prescribed tranquilisers, misused chemicals such as solvents, and illegal drugs such as heroin, ecstasy, cocaine, cannabis, and other psychotropic drugs.

Psychotropic drugs: *drugs that change mood or alter the way our senses work, e.g. they may cause hallucinations.*

The list of dangerous substances is immense and they present varying risks and effects.

Tobacco and alcohol

These two legal drugs lead to many deaths in the UK. Both are socially acceptable. However, many people now feel that tobacco is less socially acceptable than it used to be.

Table 1.5 The effects of tobacco on health

Use	Drug	Effects	Dangers
smoked or chewed	nicotine	addictive constricts arterioles, blood vessels brings about a feeling of relaxed well-being	chemicals in tobacco are known to cause cancer (particularly lung cancer) lung tissues damaged irreparably by smoke (smoking is the cause of 90% of the structural damage to lungs called emphysema) increased risk of heart disease increased risk of chest and throat infections bronchitis, the inflammation of the lungs and tubes to the lungs, is caused by smoking carbon monoxide in the smoke reduces the ability of the blood to carry oxygen pregnant women may miscarry there is a greater risk of premature birth, stillbirth and low birth weight

The risk from smoking is not just to the user but also to unborn children and the victims of passive smoking.

Passive smoking: *being exposed to the tobacco smoke of a smoker. This has a similar range of effects to actually smoking the tobacco. The effect is controlled by the amount of exposure.*

Table 1.6 The effects of alcohol on health

Use	Drug	Effects	Dangers
in drinks containing various percentages of the drug	ethyl alcohol, (an excretory product of yeast)	addictive a clinical depressant taken, often in social settings to release inhibitions	The dangers of alcohol vary according to the amount consumed **Low consumption** may be beneficial in terms of preventing heart disease increased reaction times (we take longer to react to a situation like an emergency) which increases the risk of accidents **Moderate consumption** increased weight caused by extra energy intake some mental impairment reduced sexual potency **Excessive consumption** damage to the liver (cirrhosis) stomach disorders increased depression and stress reduced ability to cope with infections increased risk of heart disease damage to the brain structure increased risk of cancers danger of injury linked to loss of ability to balance sexual impotence

It is important to monitor your intake of alcohol very carefully and stay in the safe range. People who become addicted to alcohol should not drink alcohol at all.

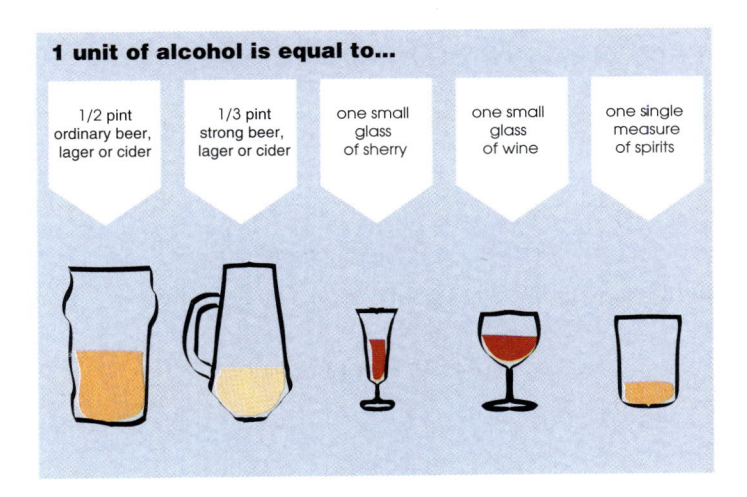

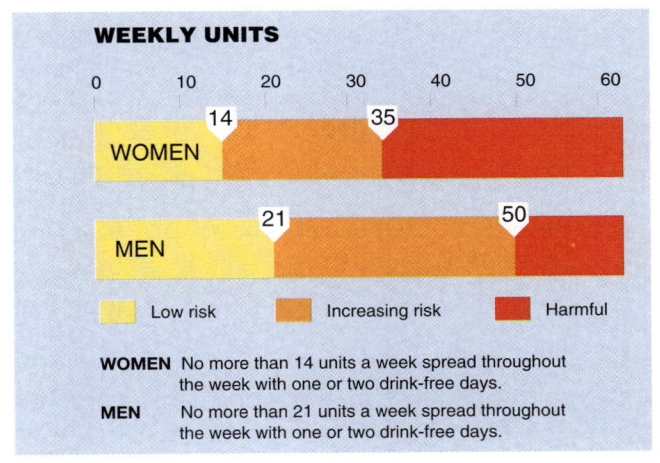

1 unit of alcohol is equal to...
- 1/2 pint ordinary beer, lager or cider
- 1/3 pint strong beer, lager or cider
- one small glass of sherry
- one small glass of wine
- one single measure of spirits

WEEKLY UNITS

WOMEN: 14 (low risk threshold), 35 (harmful threshold)
MEN: 21 (low risk threshold), 50 (harmful threshold)

Low risk | Increasing risk | Harmful

WOMEN No more than 14 units a week spread throughout the week with one or two drink-free days.
MEN No more than 21 units a week spread throughout the week with one or two drink-free days.

Figure 1.29 Sensible alcohol limits

Controlled and illegal drugs

These are drugs that have been identified by parliament as being such a danger that their use, possession and sale are illegal. In some cases the drugs may be prescribed for medical use.

Although many people use illegal drugs and some claim that they do no more damage then legal drugs like alcohol and tobacco, it is essential to realise that no matter what your views are on this matter, being associated with the sale and/or use of illegal drugs would mean that you might get a criminal record. You might also suffer the damage that most of them cause.

Table 1.7 Some illegal drugs and their effects

Drug	Use	Effects	Dangers
cannabis	smoked with tobacco or baked in biscuits	mildly hallucinogenic; increased talkativeness; relaxing	may cause psychological dependency; risks associated with tobacco smoking
amphetamines	sniffed, swallowed or injected*	increased heart rate; appetite suppression; reduced tiredness; feeling of alertness	psychological and physical addiction; low resistance to disease; heart failure
D-lysergic acid diethylamide (LSD)	swallowed or dissolved on the tongue as tablets or on pieces of paper	powerful hallucinatory drug; can produce terrifying as well as pleasant visions	psychological damage; increased risks of accidents
ecstasy	swallowed as tablets or impregnated on paper	similar to those of amphetamines and LSD combined; increased dehydration	as for LSD and amphetamines; risk of kidney damage
cocaine and crack cocaine	usually inhaled or can be injected*	a painkiller; similar effects to amphetamines	addictive, particularly crack; damage to nasal linings and bone from inhaling cocaine; other effects as amphetamines
heroin	injected* or smoked	alertness followed by drowsiness	addictive; high doses can lead to coma

* Any drugs that are injected carry an increased risk of HIV and hepatitis infection if needles are shared with other users.

Other dangerous drugs

Prescribed
There are dangers associated with most drugs, although not all drugs are addictive. Many people have become addicted to tranquillisers, such as valium, or to barbiturates. These drugs are prescribed by doctors and have a useful purpose. However, over-prescription and drug misuse means that they have to be included in a list of drugs that are dangerous to health.

Over-the-counter drugs
Some drugs that are commonly available from shops can also be dangerous. Paracetamol is a very useful pain killer, but taking too many paracetamol tablets in a day can be fatal. The drug is normally made safe by the liver but an overdose causes the liver to stop working. Once that happens, other organs in the body stop working one by one; nothing can halt the process and death occurs in a matter of days. Certain other drugs which can be purchased from chemists and supermarkets are dangerous if misused. It is important that you read the label and check with either your doctor or a pharmacist that you understand fully the dose you need to take.

It is equally important to check that the drugs do not create other health hazards. Some drugs cause you to feel sleepy, and so it would be dangerous to drive or operate machinery or do anything else that requires you to be fully alert. Other drugs interact with one another. Alcohol can reduce or increase the activity of some drugs. In some cases it can form a lethal cocktail if taken with other drugs.

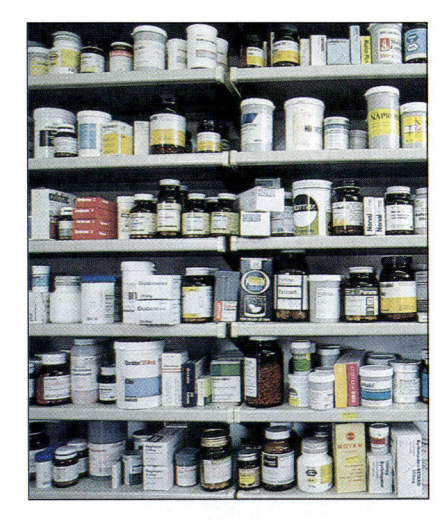

Figure 1.30 Prescribed or over-the-counter drugs can be dangerous if misused

Solvent abuse
Some people, mainly teenagers, inhale solvents to cause hallucinations. These work by reducing oxygen intake and altering body chemistry. Many of the solvents dissolve fatty tissues and so can destroy the insulation around nerve cells (including those in the brain).

Apart from the obvious damage caused by the solvents, there are other serious dangers. The dose taken cannot be determined, nor can the effects. An amount that causes the desired effect in one person may kill another. A person under the influence of solvents may put him- or herself in physical danger. People using solvents often do so in areas hidden from view and anyone requiring medical help may not be noticed.

In recognition of the dangers of solvent abuse, it is now illegal to sell materials containing some solvents to children. It would be impossible to ban the sale of solvents completely, as their use is widespread in normal household products, but many products are now being produced without the solvents where possible.

Promoting health and well-being

▶ Risks and hazards, page 39

▶ Preventing cross infection, page 52

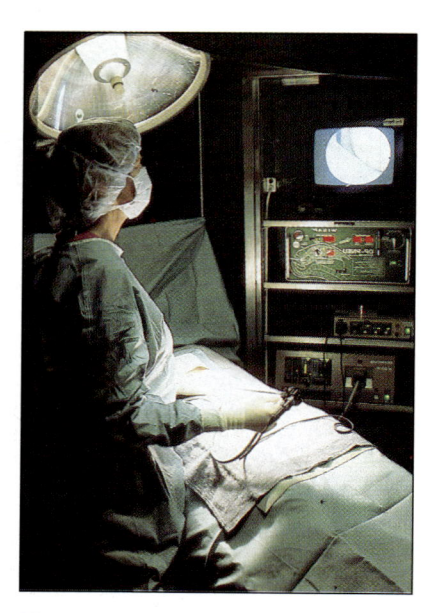

Figure 1.31 A sterile environment – an operating theatre.

FOCUS

Hygiene needs can be:
- personal (teeth, hair, skin)
- public (food preparation, eating, medical treatment).

Sexual behaviour

Sex has evolved as a process for reproduction (having babies) and also to reinforce relationships. It is pleasurable but there are many risks associated with sex.

Risks

One obvious risk is based on becoming pregnant. This should be a planned consequence that has been discussed and agreed by both partners. In many cases this does not happen and girls and women become pregnant without planning.

A second risk is of infection and disease. These include:
- syphilis
- gonorrhoea
- non-specific urethritis (NSU)
- Human Immunodefficiency Virus (HIV) and Acquired Immune Deficiency Syndrome (AIDS).

The simplest way of avoiding the risks is to avoid sex (celibacy). This is certainly an ideal way where a relationship is forming and either partner is unprepared to take risks. If a decision to have sex has been taken then it is important to reduce the risks as much as possible. All of the risks can be reduced by appropriate use of barrier contraceptive methods. These involve the use of a condom before and during any sexual contact. This method, together with other contraceptive measures (e.g. use of a spermicide) is effective in preventing pregnancy in about 97% of cases. The barrier can also prevent infection. Remember, however, those figures indicate that the barrier is not total and so there is still a risk of infection.

Infection can occur when any infected body fluids (blood, semen, vaginal fluids) come into contact with membranes lining parts of the body (e.g. vagina, rectum, mouth) or enter the bloodstream through a cut or puncture (injection). Any sexual activity that increases the risk of infection occurring is an unsafe practice and should be avoided.

The risk of infection from blood also occurs when dealing with a cut.

Hygiene and health

What is good **hygiene**? We would all like to think that we practice good hygiene but none of us works at levels of hygiene like those required in an operating theatre.

A Then and now

Your grandmother's grandmother had no toilet better than a bucket; no toilet paper, toothpaste, soap; no bath, washbasin or underwear.
What advice could you give her in the 1990s about:
(a) personal hygiene
(b) hygiene in the home?
You could discuss this in small groups, share your ideas in the full group and then produce individual responses. These should take the form of:
(a) personal hygiene: a guide to daily and weekly routines, with advice on items to buy (e.g. shampoo, deodorant)
(b) hygiene in the home: as for personal hygiene with an indication as to which rooms need most careful attention and why.
For (a) and (b) use sketches or plans as appropriate to support your information.

Promoting health and well-being

Personal hygiene

Hygiene is about reducing the risk of micro-organisms, such as bacteria, viruses and fungi, breeding and spreading to areas where they are not wanted. Different organisms have different requirements for their growth and spread. Bacteria and fungi are able to survive and grow outside your body while viruses can only grow inside your cells.

In terms of growth, both bacteria and fungi grow best in warm moist areas where there is a supply of food. Your body provides these three things in ample quantities:
- warmth comes from your own body heat
- moisture comes from your sweat
- food comes from dead cells and chemicals in the sweat, particularly in underarm and groin regions.

It is impossible for you to remove safely all the micro-organisms from your body and it would be unwise to try to do so. The simplest way of keeping the population of micro-organisms under control is to wash yourself regularly (daily at least) using warm water and soap. The areas that need particular attention are those areas which sweat a lot: underarms, groin, feet, scalp and hair.

It is also important to wash your hands after using the toilet and before handling food.

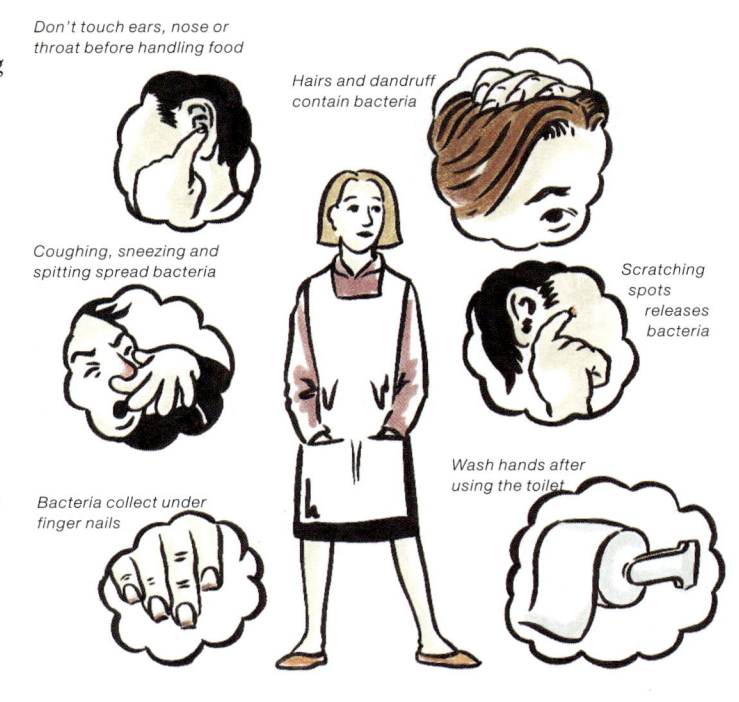

Figure 1.32 Bacteria are often passed from people to food

Hair hygiene

The hair on your head is naturally protected and kept waterproof by a greasy substance called sebum. Bacteria also find the sebum and dead skin cells from the scalp an enjoyable food. Hair falls out naturally, with up to 100 hairs being lost daily. It is important, therefore to try to maintain a balance between cleanliness and protection. Brushing and combing hair spreads the sebum along the individual hairs and helps maintain the protection. This also has a useful side effect in killing adult head-lice.

Washing hair removes the sebum, dead cells and some of the bacteria. Many people counteract the damaging effect of washing by using a conditioner. Many of these contain materials similar to sebum and so provide bacteria with a replacement source of food.

Washing hair frequently can stimulate the glands producing the sebum to produce more sebum. This is particularly so if the shampoo is not thoroughly rinsed off. Not washing the hair for about six weeks would actually enable the hair to reach a natural state of 'good condition'. However, it would require regular brushing/combing and would pass through a state of extreme greasiness. Hair hygiene is, therefore, fairly complex. Finding the right balance in terms of washing, brushing/combing and conditioning can take time. Head-lice like clean hair. If there has been an outbreak of head-lice, a proprietary medical shampoo, e.g. Debac, should be used as a protection against lice. If repeated use is necessary, do not use the same brand of shampoo as lice build up an immunity. Combing with a very fine comb can remove lice from the shaft of a hair. This should not be used as normal procedure as it might cause split ends of hair.

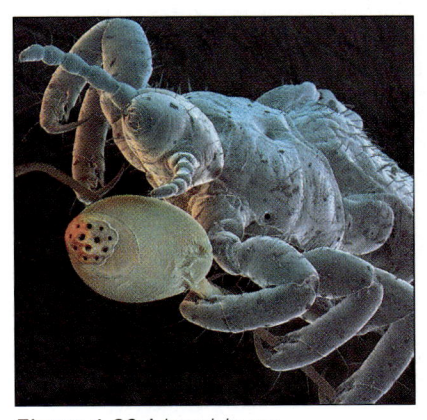

Figure 1.33 A head-louse

▶ Puberty, Table 2.2 page 74

Promoting health and well-being

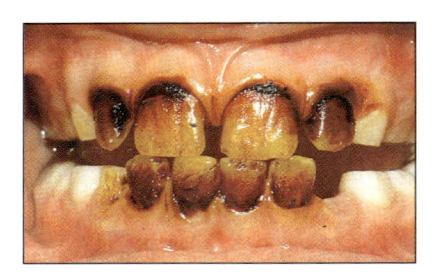

Figure 1.34 The brown areas are patches of bacteria revealed using disclosing tablets

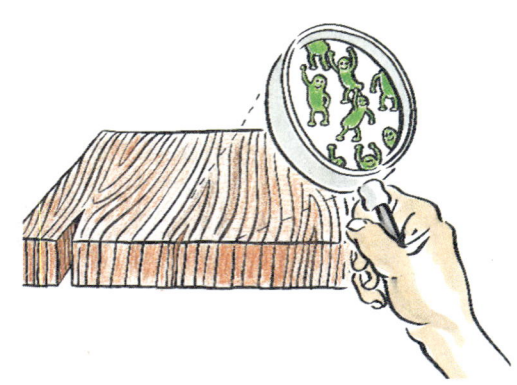

Figure 1.35 Bacteria can lurk in areas that are difficult to clean

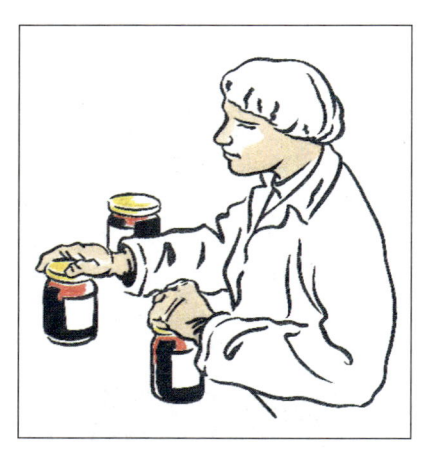

Figure 1.36 Protective clothing is worn to protect the food from contamination

Dental care

Another breeding ground for bacteria is your mouth. In this case the bacteria feed and grow on food residues around the teeth and gums. These bacteria damage your gums and also produce acids that cause tooth decay. Regular cleaning of your teeth after eating reduces the food available and also removes some of the bacteria.

This information is probably not new to you. Most of us are taught as children about personal hygiene by family, friends and at school. Here we shall consider levels of hygiene and the results of failing to establish appropriate hygiene levels.

Levels of hygiene

Look back at the Activity 'Then and now', page 26. You will have identified two or three areas where hygiene is very important. These are:
- toilet areas
- your food preparation area
- your eating area.

Toilet areas

The toilet area is one where there are large quantities of bacteria. Your faeces are made up of up to 30% bacteria. There are great risks of transferring some of these to your hands and thus to anything you touch if you do not wash your hands carefully after using the toilet. You will wash your hands to remove enough bacteria to be reasonably safe.

Food preparation areas

Eating and preparing food can lead to contamination of the food with bacteria. Food, by its very nature, is an ideal medium for growing bacteria. High temperatures (above 63°C) kill most bacteria and so most cooking processes kill almost all bacteria. Figure 1.37 gives a guide to the effect of temperatures on bacterial growth. Unfortunately, some food-poisoning bacteria form spores to protect themselves in conditions that would otherwise damage them. Spores have tough cases and can survive high temperatures, drying and disinfectants. When conditions improve the bacteria are released from the spores and then multiply. Heating food to 120°C and maintaining this temperature for 15 minutes will destroy bacterial spores.

Bacteria on uncooked food may breed. Chilling or freezing does not kill the bacteria, it just slows down breeding. Bacteria can be transferred from raw to cooked food. This is known as cross-contamination.

If the bacteria that are allowed to breed on food happen to be some of the food-poisoning types (*Salmonella*, *Staphyloccocus aureus*, *Clostridium perfringens*, *Bacillus cereus* and *Listeria monocytogenes*) then there is a risk that whoever eats the food will have an attack of food poisoning. This may be something that is of little danger to you, but elderly people, young babies and people with impaired immune systems, i.e. people who have had an operation, or are HIV positive, may easily die from the effects of food poisoning.

Food left out at room temperature for hours uncovered is not only at risk from bacteria, but also from flies which carry bacteria on their legs. Flies also regurgitate matter (e.g. substances absorbed from manure and rubbish previously fed on) onto their next meal, which could be uncovered food. They also defecate (leave droppings) on the food as they eat.

A | The not-too-hot pot

A chef in a residential home for older people once made a Lancashire hotpot for the evening meal. After the meal there was still a lot left in the saucepan so he transferred it to a clean bowl to cool down. Unfortunately, the bowl was not absolutely clean and contained one *Salmonella* bacterium.

The chef left the food to cool down overnight and froze it the next morning. Some days later the evening meal he was preparing burned and so he quickly pulled the hotpot out of the freezer and reheated it in the microwave. Unfortunately, it reached a temperature of only about 50°C. He served the food, and several of the residents died later from *Salmonella* food poisoning. *Salmonella* bacteria are able to double their numbers approximately every half hour, so you can work out how many bacteria were in the pot after the ten hours that the hotpot had stood before being frozen.

Copy and complete the following table:

Hours	Number of Bacteria	Hours	Number of Bacteria	Hours	Number of Bacteria	Hours	Number of Bacteria
0	1	3		6		9	
0.5	2	3.5		6.5		9.5	
1.0	4	4		7		10	
1.5	8	4.5		7.5			
2.0	16	5		8			
2.5	32	5.5		8.5			

Draw a line graph of your results.

If it takes 100 000 bacteria to cause food poisoning in an elderly person, when would there have been that many in the bowl of hotpot? Use your graph to find the answer.

What hygiene mistakes did the chef make?

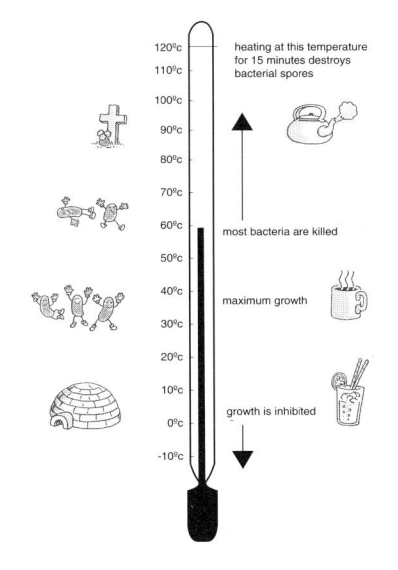

Figure 1.37 Effect of temperatures on bacterial growth. A simple way of remembering this is 'Keep it hot, keep it cold, or don't keep it'

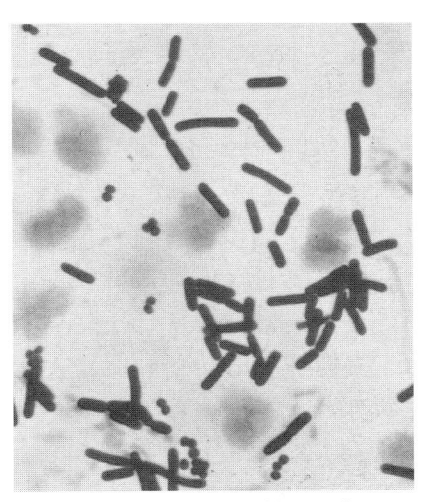

Figure 1.38 Rod-shaped bacteria, seen under a light microscope

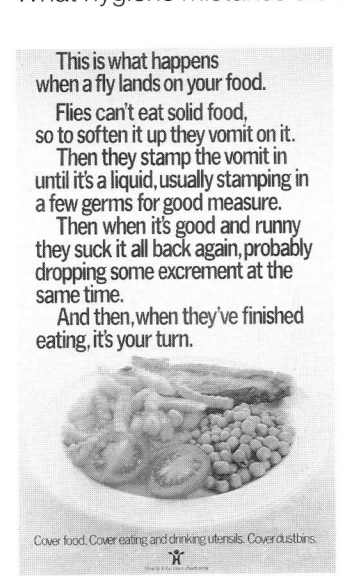

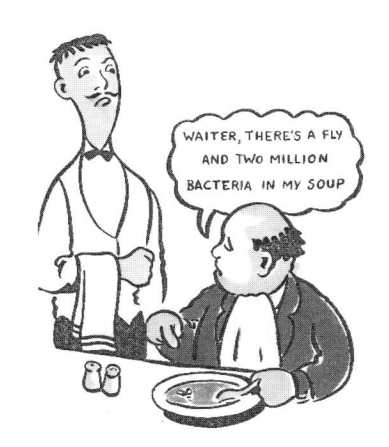

Figure 1.39 Food left out at room temperature for hours uncovered is at risk from flies which carry bacteria

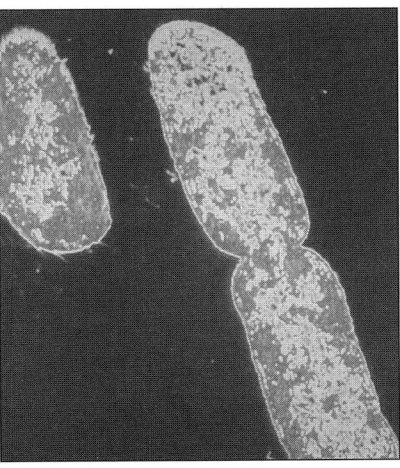

Figure 1.40 *Salmonella* bacteria dividing to increase rapidly in number

Hygiene requirements

It is clear that:
- different levels of hygiene are appropriate in different circumstances
- some groups of people are more vulnerable to food poisoning than others
- where there is a risk of infection, hygiene levels need to be high
- hygiene levels need to be high where individuals are particularly vulnerable to infection.

A surgeon who is scrubbing-up to operate on somebody may go through twenty steps in washing to try to remove the maximum number of bacteria. In the surgeon's case the risk is of infecting a wound. In your case, the risk of catching or passing on a disease is much lower.

Hygiene levels need to be high where poor hygiene may affect a large number of people. The Activity 'The not too hot pot' indicated one such situation. Other similar places are restaurants and cafes. There is legislation covering hygiene in premises handling food for public consumption. It includes measures designed to prevent cooked and raw foods from coming into contact. Take a look in your fridge: you may find you have raw and cooked foods on the same shelf, or raw food above cooked food. Both of these are arrangements where bacteria from raw food can pass to the relatively bacteria-free cooked food. In restaurants, such storage is forbidden by law and in most cases there are two refrigerators, one for raw and one for cooked foods. How do you think you should keep raw and cooked meats in your fridge?

Use the tick list below to check the contents of your fridge:

- ☐ All items are covered and in separate containers.
- ☐ The fridge is at the correct temperature (1-4°C).
- ☐ Cooked foods are kept above raw foods.
- ☐ Raw meats are on the bottom shelf.
- ☐ No food has passed its 'use by' date.
- ☐ Do you have a fridge thermometer?

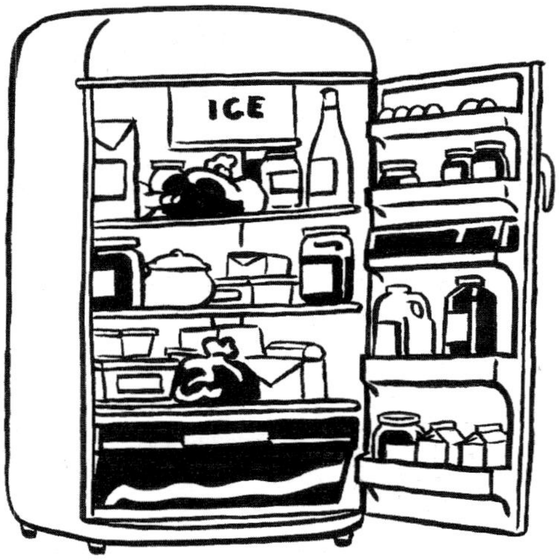

Figure 1.41 Food stored in optimum conditions

How is hygiene maintained?

When considering levels of hygiene it is important to consider levels of risk. Although not washing yourself involves minimal personal risk, the smells produced may reduce your social life! The ideal solution is using soap and water.

Toilet areas

Toilet areas are a danger because of the number of bacteria. The solution is to clean the area regularly using products such as chlorine-based bleaches which kill most bacteria, thus preventing a dangerous build up.

Food preparation areas

Food preparation areas are regularly exposed to bacteria and so need regular cleaning. Bleaches are no longer permitted in food preparation areas. The answer is to wash all utensils in very hot water with detergent. Clean work surfaces with a sanitiser (a chemical that cleans and disinfects, e.g. Dettox).

Prevention of risk is important: make sure that food preparation areas do not have corners and cracks that trap dirt and bacteria. Protective clothing should be for specific use in the kitchen and regularly washed.

Hair, a potential source of contamination should be tied back where necessary and covered.

Food storage should ensure raw and cooked foods are kept apart. Foods should be kept hot at high enough temperatures to kill bacteria (above 63°C) or cold enough to virtually stop bacterial growth (3°C in a fridge or –18°C in a freezer). Other preserving methods can be used, such as drying, pickling, canning, bottling, smoking and jamming. In each case, storage will have to maintain the quality of the hygiene.

Other areas in the home
Living rooms and bedrooms also need to be clean. Disease prevention methods include regular vacuum cleaning and dusting, and maintaining good ventilation to ensure any airborne viruses, fungi and bacteria are diluted with fresh air.

Care establishments
Hygiene levels in care establishments need to be especially high as the people in your care may be more vulnerable. This is particularly important for elderly people but it applies to all care establishments.

The immune system
In spite of all precautions, people will be exposed to disease. We have an immune system which should be able to cope with many infections. In fact, it is our exposure to micro-organisms in small numbers that enables us to develop an immunity that stops infection from causing a disease. Part of a baby's growth has to involve exposure to disease and development of immunity. Without natural exposure and development of immunity many common diseases can be killers. Assessing risk and determining the level of hygiene required, can help to give us all a safer environment in which to live.

A | **Hygiene investigation**

Produce a short report comparing hygiene in your home and a place of work. In a place of work (this may be your school, college or placement) find out how good hygiene is maintained. Are there specific instructions about cleaning, in particular the frequency? Compare the frequency and thoroughness and the methods and materials used, with what happens in your own home. Try to explain why there are differences.

Actions to promote personal health
It is clear that we are not all the same. We have our likes and dislikes and also have different social and financial circumstances. It is not possible to identify any one set of activities or actions to promote personal health that will meet the needs of all of us but some general guidelines are useful.

Action to improve diet and exercise should be possible for most people. It is possible to improve the nutritional value of a diet without increasing the costs too much. Exercise does not have to cost money. A quarter of an hour of brisk walking every day contributes to increased fitness. There is no magic formula – be it a specialist diet or a novel exercise routine – that will take the effort out of staying physically fit and healthy.

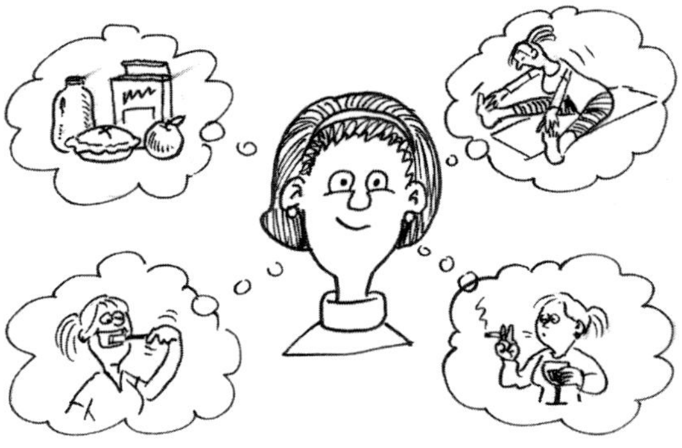

Figure 1.42 Personal health promotion

Promoting health and well-being

▶ Lifestyle profile, page 4

▶ Height and weight table, page 19

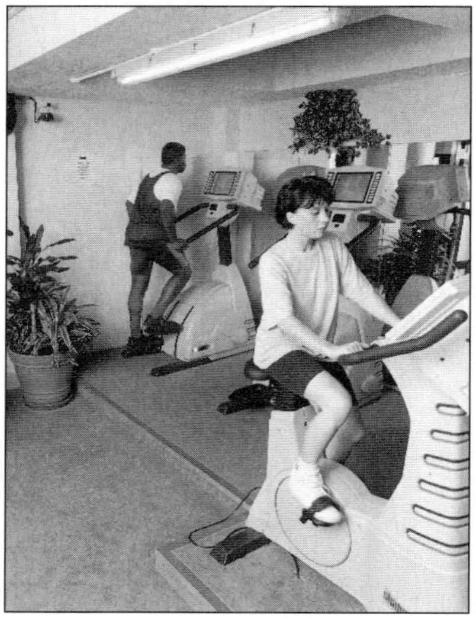

Figure 1.43 Fitness studios have various tests which measure fitness

Personal health assessment

A personal check up

Throughout the first part of this unit we described some health issues and risks. This is the time to pull together all this information and use it to help you review your own lifestyle. As a result of this you will be able to start on the production of a health action plan for yourself.

Review the initial diary of your activities in your Lifestyle profile, and assess how your lifestyle reflects the need for balance in diet, sleep, exercise, work and recreation. Use the height and weight table to determine if you are over-, underweight or neither. Use the Activity 'Checking your own fitness' to find out how fit you are.

A Checking your own fitness

Fitness clinics in sports centres can use many different tests to measure your fitness. A very crude measure of fitness is to undertake some moderate exercise and record how long it takes to recover from it by timing how long it takes for the heartbeat to return to its resting rate.

With a partner decide what you consider to be moderate exercise. Try to find something that makes you slightly breathless. It could be walking upstairs and downstairs several times.

Try to relax totally for five minutes. Ask your partner to check your pulse and count the number of beats in 15 seconds. Use this to calculate the beats per minute.

Now exercise for about two minutes. Check your pulse immediately after exercise to see how much it has increased over your resting pulse. Take the pulse every minute. Record how long it takes to come back to the resting rate. The longer it takes to return to the resting rate the more unfit you are. You can monitor your return to fitness whilst following a general exercise routine by repeating this activity exactly every week.

The time taken to return to resting rate should decrease as your fitness increases. You may also note that your resting pulse rate decreases as your fitness increases.

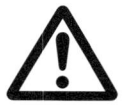

⚠️ Do not attempt to carry out this activity if you know you have any breathing difficulties or heart disease. The activities are not dangerous in themselves but it would be best to get medical advice about exercise routines.

Looking at your diet

Use the Activity 'Monitoring your diet' to look at your diet. Remember that if you need to lose weight, exercise and diet go together well.

A Monitoring your diet

Keep a diary for two or three days of what you eat and drink. Compare this with The Balance of Good Health (page 15). Are there any food groups that are missing? If there are, look at the Five Food Groups to see what nutrients you may be missing – this table can also help you to select foods to balance your diet.

Notice how many of the fatty and sugary foods you are eating, particularly if you have a problem with being overweight. How does your overall diet match

the proportions suggested in The Balance of Good Health? Do you eat larger quantities of fruit, vegetables and cereals than the other groups?
Check that any changes you plan are practical and achievable for you in your life.

Extension

For a further two or three days, keep a more detailed diary. Try to be honest about it! Many people ignore the between-meal snacks or underestimate the amount of various foods they have eaten.

Where the food or snack has nutritional information on the pack, cut it out and use the figures given to help calculate your nutritional intake. Wherever possible weigh the food that you eat. If you cannot do this then estimate the weight that you eat.

Within your class spend some time weighing different foods to find out what a typical portion weighs. Produce a chart of some of the more commonly-eaten foods. An example is given here.

Food	Portion	Weight
peas	2 tablespoons	
rice (uncooked)	¼ mug	
potato	1 medium size	
sugar	10 teaspoons	

Knowing the weight of ten teaspoons of sugar means that you can work out the weight of one teaspoon of sugar. Your measurement of the weight of ten teaspoons of sugar may be easier than one teaspoon on kitchen scales.
Use standard food composition tables to determine your energy intake and the total amount of fat. If you have time, analyse your diet for imbalances in other nutrients, e.g. protein and fibre.

Developing your plan to improve your health

If you have followed the activities you should now have information about your diet, your fitness and your general lifestyle. It may confirm your excellent state of health or it could indicate that there are areas for improvement which need further monitoring.

Short and long term targets

You should make use of all of the information available to you to start on your personal health promotion action **plan**. This may be one that means changing your lifestyle. In this case have short, medium and long term targets which include the rewards for success, for example, a glossy magazine when you have lost 2 kg, a new CD when your pulse recovery time after exercise reduces by 2 minutes, or a meal with a friend after you have not smoked for a month.

FOCUS

Plan:
- priorities for action
- personal targets (short term/long term)
- reassessment of targets.

Making a personal health promotion action plan

The action plan may be one of monitoring and maintaining your current status. In this case still have short (up to two weeks), medium (three months) and long term (six months or more) aims, in terms of monitoring, and think again about personal rewards.

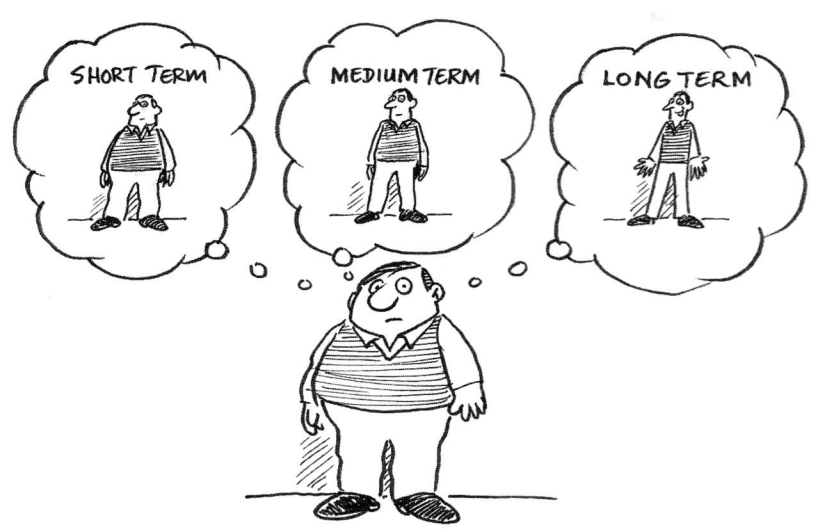

Figure 1.44 Set yourself targets that are realistic

A   A personal health action plan

Make a personal plan such as this:

Goals		Week 2	Week 4	Week 6	Week 8	Week 10
Weight loss	target					
	actual					
Smoking reduction (max. smoked)	target					
	actual					
Fitness	target					
	actual					

Reward: e.g. cassette each time target and actual agree!

Set realistic targets

In your plan be realistic in your targets. Make them achievable and within your own control. This may well mean looking at any costs (e.g. entrance charges to the swimming pool), and making agreements with other members of your family who may be affected. If you do not buy and prepare your own food, then you need to negotiate (come to an agreement) with whoever does.

Simply making a personal health promotion action plan is not sufficient. It is important to try to make it achievable as part of your normal daily routine. To plan to run for one mile a day to get fitter may be reasonable, but not if you know that you will never stick to it. You know your weaknesses and so make sure your plan recognises them and is realistic.

The structure of your health promotion action plan
Ask yourself these questions:
- what is my current health state: weight, height, etc.?
- do I want to change my health state?
- what am I prepared to do about it?
- what are my short, medium and long-term aims?
- how will I know when I have reached the improved health state? (This may be when you reach your target weight or have stopped smoking for three months, and hopefully for ever.)
- what benefits do I expect to feel from changing my state of health?

Those people who wish to maintain their health status can use the questions to identify what they are doing to maintain their current health state.

By answering the questions honestly and prioritising your health needs you stand a better chance of success if you carry out the plan. If you do undertake the plan then spend some time evaluating why it was a success or failure. If you do not undertake the plan then reflect on whether it might succeed or fail, and why.

In both cases the success or failure is largely determined by your real desire for it to succeed and the way it can be achieved with the minimum disruption to your current lifestyle.

Health promotion advice

It does little good to tell substance abusers to stop taking the drug. Most people will recognise activities that potentially damage their health. What they may not be prepared to do is undertake the change that is necessary.

If you are targeting a group that is already involved in bad health practices then your advice may help them decide that they no longer wish to take the risks involved with those particular practices.

Your strategy needs to be flexible enough to take account of the composition of your target group. If you wish to promote the message 'Don't start smoking' to young children, then you are looking to educate them into good habits.

If, on the other hand, your client group is people who already smoke, then simply telling them to stop will have little effect. They may already be addicted and may almost certainly have accepted that in their case the pleasure they gain outweighs the risk. The health promotion you undertake needs to appeal to them in different ways. Health promotion may focus on the harm they do others, and how others see smokers, rather than the risk to their own health.

Producing health advice

As workers in a health and caring environment you will be called upon to give advice about a number of issues. In some cases you will need to refer the person on to someone with more specialist knowledge.

The following activities will help you to gain experience of providing advice, and making a presentation.

Promoting health and well-being

> **FOCUS**
> Presenting advice:
> • what?
> • who?
> • how – written?
>   – diagrams?
>   – pictures?
>   – audio-visual?

> **FOCUS**
> Target group:
> • active
> • sedentary
> • children
> • elderly people
> • people with disabilities.

A What advice do people need?

Here you need to do some research. It is not enough to assume that everybody needs **advice**.

Identify a group

You should first identify the group of people you are intending to make a presentation to. This could be:
- children
- pregnant women
- elderly people
- active people
- sedentary people
- people with disabilities.

Identify a topic

Take some time to identify a topic for your presentation. Write out a list of possible topics and discuss them with your lecturer.
   The list could be built up by:
- asking the members of your chosen group about health-related issues and identifying areas that they know little about. This could be done using questionnaires. If you find out what your target group understands before your presentation, it will be easier to work out how effective your promotion has been
- looking at health promotion material aimed at your target group. This tells you what the professional health educators have identified as important issues
- reading magazines aimed at your target group – many of these have articles, stories and advertisements about health-related issues of interest to your target group.

Plan to spend some time on this initial investigation, as good planning now, together with obtaining information, will make the next parts easier.

Pulling the information together

Giving advice about health maintenance is a major role for health educators. Make use of their expertise. Once you have chosen your topic and **target group** pick up leaflets and posters from a doctor's surgery, a chemist, your local health promotion unit. In fact gather as much material together as you can. You may be able to use the posters and leaflets in your health promotion or they may give you ideas for your own material.

Planning what advice you want to give

1 Identify the key points you want to make. Try to limit them to three. Start writing your plan for the presentation with the sentence 'At the end of this activity my target group will:
      know ...
      understand ...
      be able to ...'
   In other words why does your target group need the presentation and how will they benefit?

2 Decide what advice you need to give and how it will be presented: written information? pictures? videos? audiotapes? Be very careful about producing your own videos or audio tapes, as it takes much time and skill to make good ones. Whatever you decide, use at least two different methods.

3 Plan your presentation. It should include details of all the materials and equipment you need. Make sure that what you need is available. If necessary, book it well in advance or arrange to borrow it. Health promotion units may be willing to help you. Most of them have a list of available resources. Check if your school or college has a copy.

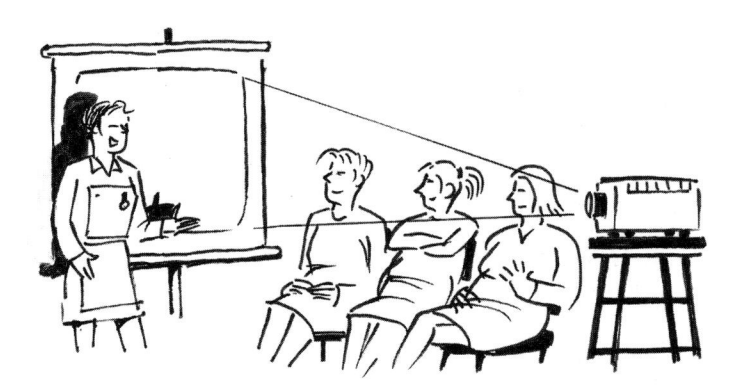

Figure 1.45 Visual aids can enhance your presentation

Preparing the presentation

What you need to do here varies according to the type of presentation you are planning. You must identify what information you are giving and put it into a suitable form. This may be a written leaflet or hand-out. It may be prompt cards with notes of the main points you want to make. It may be in the form of a poster or overhead projection transparencies or a combination of all of these. Whatever you do, make sure it is clear and easy to follow. If you intend to read from your material make sure that you can find where you are very quickly.

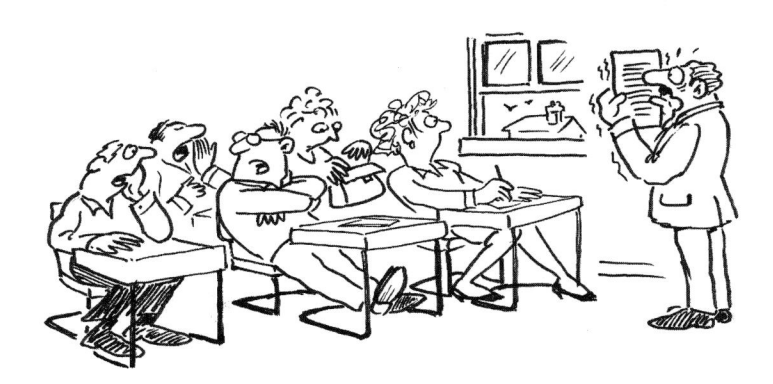

Figure 1.46 You must look at your audience – don't read your talk

> ### Using prompt cards to give a talk
> **Don't:** try to read a talk to your audience – you will tend to forget to look at your audience and to read very rapidly (especially if you are nervous).
> **Do:** write down the key points that you want to make on separate cards in large, easy-to-read writing. Use each card in turn to remind you what you want to say. Under each key point add a small number of important words that will jog your memory or major facts and figures that you need to get right.
> Using this method means:
> - understanding clearly what you are talking about. If you don't then you will lose the thread of what you are saying
> - practising your presentation several times before you 'go live'. This helps you learn how to use the cards!

Checking your information

When you have worked out the information you want to pass on you must check it:
- for accuracy
- for language appropriate to your target group's understanding, e.g. don't talk down to children, but do make sure you use language they understand.

FOCUS

Impact:
- feedback on presentation
- response to advice.

Assessing the impact

The final aspect of planning is identifying how you will determine the **impact** of your presentation on the target audience. For this you need to look back at the start of your plan. You wrote the sentence: 'At the end of this activity my target group will …'. How will you know that your target group can do what you planned?

There are many ways of checking that your information has been taken in and understood. You could:
- ask questions at the end of a talk to check understanding
- produce a questionnaire to find out if the group understood and if they intend to respond in any way
- observe your target group about two weeks later to see what use they make of the information and if or how they have responded to your advice.

If you investigated your topic well you should also be able to compare the group's understanding of the information before and after your presentation.

Examples of topics you might choose:

- **Agony Aunt advice**
  presenting information about a topic as a series of questions with the answers prepared by you

- **It's good for you**
  explaining to children about a current programme of immunisation

- **Why does it always change?**
  nutritional guidance based on the latest reports – plan a menu to introduce dietary guidelines

- **Fitness for living**
  different types of exercise and their benefits to your target group

- **Beware of the sport**
  the need for warming up before strenuous exercise

There are many others you could choose.

We have not given examples relating to smoking, drinking and drug abuse. These are areas where special care needs to be taken to make it suitable for the target audience. It may be difficult to assess the impact of your advice on your audience. However, this should not stop you from thinking about what you could tackle on these topics. There is a great deal of material published about these areas and you should look very carefully at these to see how the 'experts' present advice.

Health and safety

'The environment is so dangerous we are sometimes surprised that anybody manages to survive.' This may seem an odd statement, but if you look around you, you will see all sorts of dangers:

- people are killed by electricity and fires caused by faulty electrical equipment
- kitchen knives can cut skin and even cut through bone
- your home will contain hazardous chemicals like bleach or medicines
- fires can be caused by cigarettes
- burning fabrics produce poisonous smoke
- people trip and fall downstairs
- people drown in garden pools
- garden tools can be lethal weapons
- cars and lorries are accidents waiting to injure people
- many common plants are poisonous.

The list is endless. It is also an indication of real risks. There are many other examples. You might like to think of some more.

Risks and hazards

A **hazard** *is something that is dangerous (drowning in a garden pond and electrocution by a badly wired appliance are hazards associated with having a garden pond or electrical equipment, respectively). A risk is an assessment of the likelihood of a hazardous incident taking place.*

In considering health and safety issues you need to balance risk against the benefit, e.g. of having medicines, bleach, garden ponds, etc.

Example of hazard and risk

Household bleach
Household bleach is a hazardous material. Undiluted on skin it can cause chemical burns. If drunk it can kill. If mixed with other cleaning agents it can produce a toxic gas.

Imagine a room containing a bottle of bleach
Imagine the following people in the room and see how the risk of injury varies even though the hazard is the same:

- **new born baby** – unable to move around the room, so there is little risk to the baby from the bleach
- **a toddler** – able to move around the room, the bleach presents a high risk. The risk is reduced if the bottle has a childproof cap.
- **an adult** – the adult understands the hazards and is able to read the warnings on the bottle. The risk of injury is low, but only if people read and act on the warnings.
- **confused arthritic elder** – the understanding of the hazard may be limited. Difficulty with childproof tops may mean the bleach is transferred to a container which is easier to use. The risk of injury is increased by this.

These four separate cases have the **same** hazard, but **different** risks.

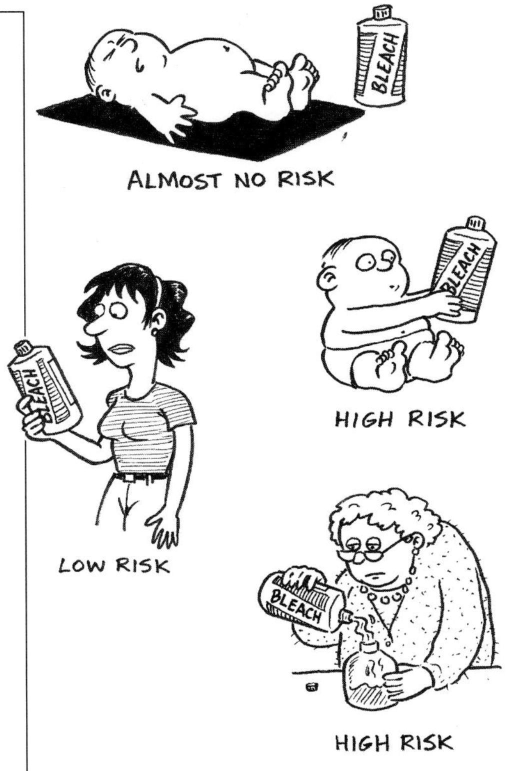

Figure 1.47 A comparison of risk levels

Promoting health and well-being

A | Hazards to personal safety

Study the pictures and identify the **hazards**. Write them down in the first column of a table; next to each hazard identify the risk to the people in the picture; and say how the risk could be reduced.

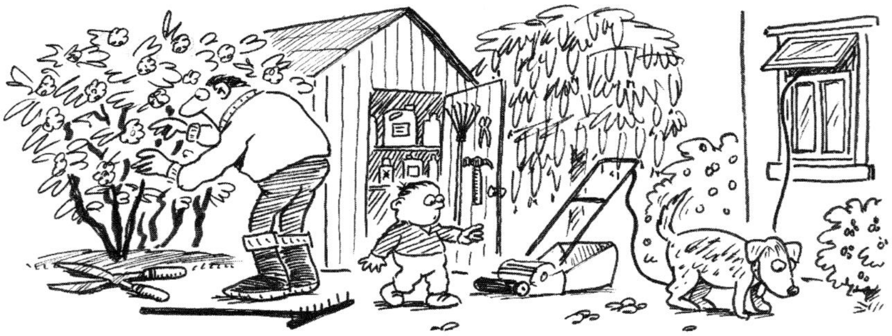

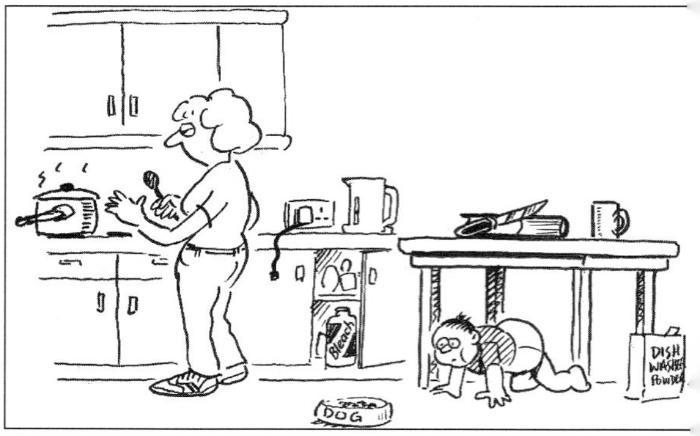

Figure 1.48 Hazards in and around the home

FOCUS

Hazards to individual in the:
- home
- garden
- road
- local environment
- social settings.

Hazard	Risk	Reduced by
sharp knives	low for adult high for child as within reach	store in knife block place at back of work surface
kettle		

FOCUS

Risks depend upon the individual's:
- age
- health (degree of infirmity)
- level of understanding.

To determine the **risk** you need to know the abilities of the people involved to understand that risk. For example you may be quite happy crossing a busy road because you are able to judge the speed of approaching vehicles. You may also be quick enough to respond if you have made a mistake. A child under the age of eight or nine is unable to judge the speed of an approaching car reliably and so needs assistance crossing a road. The Green Cross Code attempts to recognise this and encourages a very safe approach. Table 1.8 shows some of the abilities of babies and toddlers with associated increased risks.

Table 1.8 Development stages and potential risks

Developmental age and abilities	Risk
3 months: wriggles and waves limbs	Can move sufficiently to fall from raised surfaces Head can be trapped in badly-designed cot
5 months: puts objects in mouth	Choking from small objects, e.g. buttons and pins
8 months: crawling	Falling down steps Cuts from contact with and grasping sharp objects Climbing/falling out of buggies and high chairs
12 months: opens lids	Choking and poisoning from things put in boxes and tins
18 months: imitates, climbs and explores	Climbing onto window sills May be able to open medicines without child resistant containers May be able to undo child restraint in cars
2 years: turns on taps	Risk of scalding from hot water system

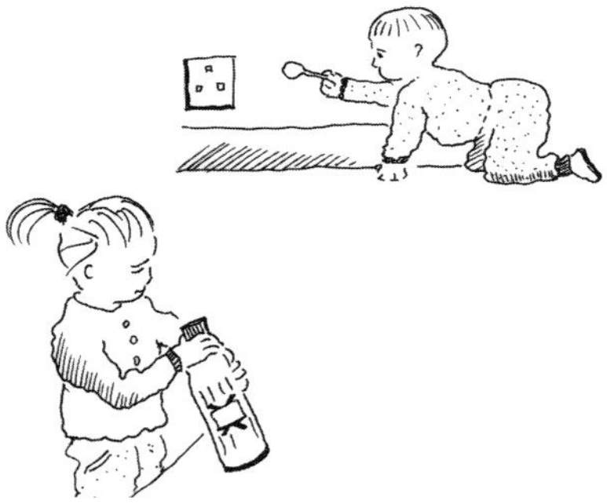

Figure 1.49 Potential risk at different ages

Source: Taken from *GNVQ Advanced Health and Social Care* by Clarke, Sachs and Waltham, published by Stanley Thornes Publishers.

A Areas of hazard

Working in a group with a few others, identify areas of hazard in and around your home and college and/or school. These should include:

- **in the home**
  mechanical and electrical appliances
  dangerous substances
  knives and tools
  furnishing fabrics

- **in the garden**
  water hazards such as ponds
  garden equipment such as electrical lawnmowers
  garden chemicals such as weed-killers, pesticides, fertilisers
  poisonous plants

- **on the road**
  as a pedestrian, cyclist, driver or passenger

- **in your locality**
  playgrounds
  railways
  rivers and canals
  dangerous plants

- **in social settings**
  recreation, e.g. sports injuries, hill walking
  work and school, e.g. passive smoking, back problems caused by lifting, chemical cleaners.

▶ Hazchem symbols, page 56

For each of these hazards identify the people most at risk and say why they are most at risk. You should consider groups of people such as children, teenagers, adults and elders.
Identify the measures taken by you, your college or other people in authority to reduce the risks. These measures may include storage conditions, warning notices or safety equipment. You may find sketches and photographs (for instance) helpful.

A Designed for safety

You are asked by your supervisor to plan a room for an elderly person who needs to use a wheelchair.
The room must contain a bed, a small table, a chair for visitors, a wardrobe, a small chest of drawers and a bedside table. The room measures 3 metres by 4 metres with two doors, one to the corridor and one to the bathroom on the adjacent wall. It also has a glass double door (like a French window) leading outside which acts both as a window and a fire exit. This is opposite the door to the corridor. The fourth wall has no doors or windows.
By taking appropriate measurements (of single beds, wheelchairs, door widths, furniture, etc) draw a plan to scale of an appropriate room.
Produce a report for your supervisor indicating the measurements you have used and highlighting the important safety aspects to minimise risks.

Promoting health and well-being

> **FOCUS**
>
> **Your roles in an emergency:**
> - **assess**
> - **make safe**
> - **contact emergency services**
> - **provide support**
> - **transfer to services.**

Dealing with health emergencies

In the street, at home, at college, at work, you never know when an emergency will arise. You need to think through how you will cope and you have to consider the whole situation, not just a casualty. For you it may be a frightening experience; for the casualty it may be fatal.

It is important for you to know what to do in an **emergency.** You need to know your own roles and responsibilities. To provide first aid you should be able to:

- assess the emergency
- maintain your own safety
- contact the emergency services
- support the casualty physically
- support the casualty emotionally
- understand your own limitations
- transfer the casualty to emergency services
- provide information to the emergency services.

This section will help you identify First Aid Emergencies and give the appropriate help to the ill or injured person until skilled help arrives. Much of First Aid is common sense but people often do not take any action at an accident because they are frightened of doing something 'wrong'. Developing the skills described here will help to give you the confidence to act, as you will know the appropriate action to take.

Assessing an emergency

Keep calm, use your common sense. Don't try to do too much. As you approach the casualty think 'safety': are you safe? See if there is any danger – to you, to the casualties, to the bystanders:

- what help do you need?
- can bystanders help?
- is anyone's life in danger?

You might be able to send someone for help straight-away if it is obvious you need it.

Make the area safe

You will need to act quickly as the casualties need your help. Bystanders can help if they are at the scene. Ask/tell a bystander what to do, for example:

- turn off a car's ignition and put the hand brake on
- disconnect the battery of a damaged car
- use the hazard warning lights or move a bystander's car to warn oncoming traffic (but not to create danger)
- warn oncoming traffic.

You should beware of spilt petrol and leaking chemicals.
Do not enter smoke filled buildings or use a lifeline.
Do not jump into lakes/canals unless specially trained.

Assessing a casualty

Order of priority
When dealing with any casualty it is important to deal with the injuries that they have in the right order.

Your aims are:
1 to preserve life
2 to prevent deterioration
3 to promote recovery.

To help achieve these aims each can be broken down:

1 to preserve life:
- check for consciousness
- open airway
- check for breathing
- check for a pulse
- control any serious bleeding.

2 to prevent deterioration:
- look for illness or injury by thorough examination
- treat wounds
- cover burns
- support fractures
- place in recovery position if appropriate.

3 to promote recovery:
- reassure
- relieve pain
- keep warm.

The approach
A casualty who is sitting or standing and perhaps talking is obviously a conscious casualty. Consider a casualty lying quietly on the ground.

Any ill or injured person must be quickly checked to find out whether their life is in danger. You need to do these five checks which should take about 30 seconds in all to complete.

> **The five checks**
> Safety
> Shake and shout – don't be rough
> Airway – can air get to the lungs?
> Breathing – check for five seconds
> Circulation (pulse) – check for five seconds

Each of the techniques needed is explained in the following sections.

FOCUS

Physiological basis:
- circulation
- breathing.

FOCUS

Basic life-saving techniques:
- opening and maintaining airway
- placing in recovery position
- cardio-pulmonary resuscitation
- controlling haemorrhage.

Promoting health and well-being

Notes:
Casualties may get worse, e.g. change from route (ii) to route (i)
You need to change the treatment.
Sending for help. There is usually a bystander you can send to the telephone. He's called LIONEL, as the message should contain the following:

L for Location – where you are
I for Incident – what's happened
O for Other services – Fire or Police
N for Number of casualties
E for Extent of their injuries
L for Location – as it's so important it's mentioned twice

If working alone, but quite close to a telephone
- in route (i) go immediately after you've done the five checks – before starting 2 breaths and 15 compressions routine
- in route (ii) go after one cycle of 10 breaths.

It is best to put the casualty in the Recovery position while you telephone.
Modifying the Recovery position. Depending on the Casualty's condition, you may have to adjust your technique to avoid making things worse (for example, if there are spinal injuries).

Figure 1.50 First aid flow chart

Figure 1.51 Opening the airway

▶ Circulation, page 51

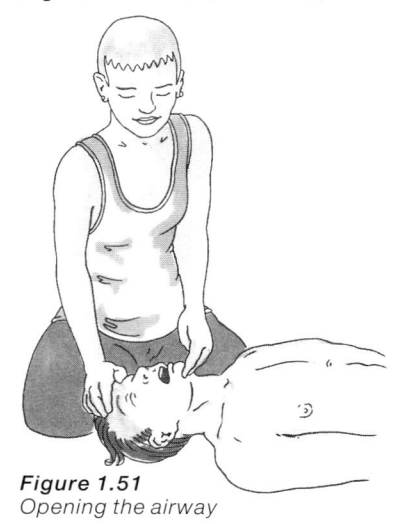

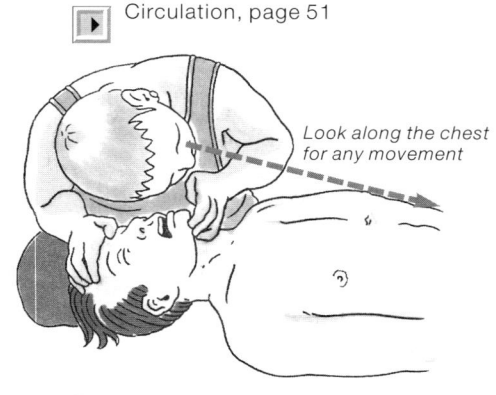

Figure 1.52 Checking for breathing

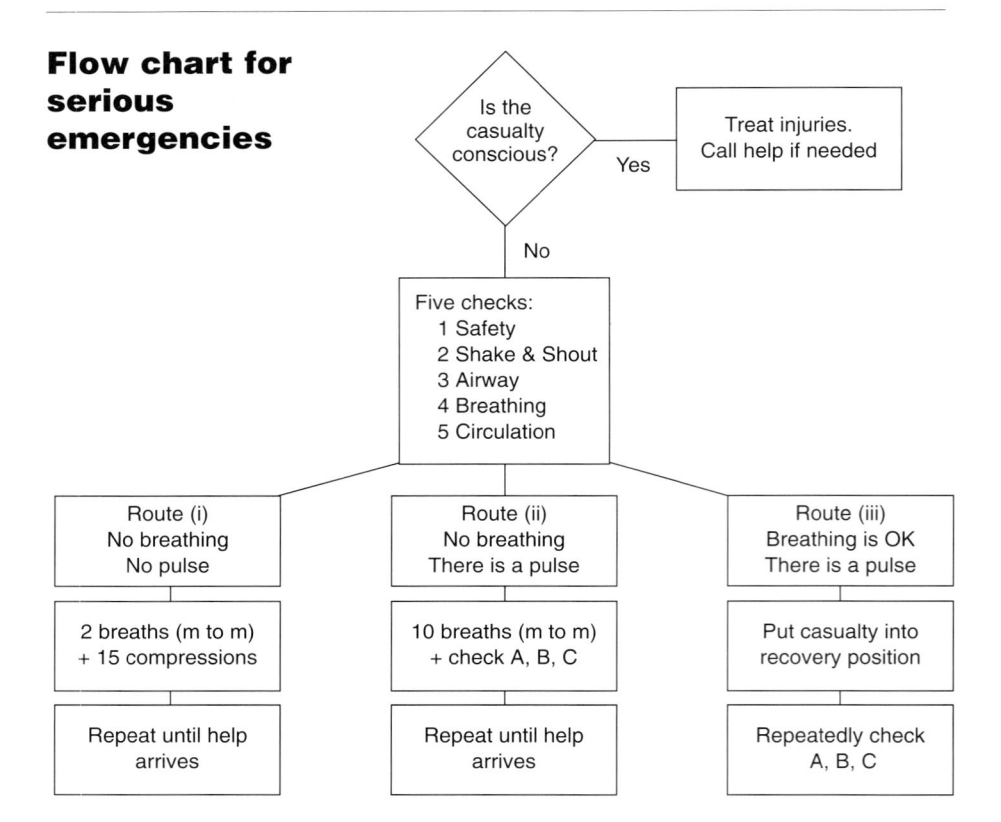

Flow chart for serious emergencies

```
                    Is the
                    casualty          Yes      Treat injuries.
                    conscious?     ────────▶   Call help if needed
                        │
                        │ No
                        ▼
                   Five checks:
                   1 Safety
                   2 Shake & Shout
                   3 Airway
                   4 Breathing
                   5 Circulation
         ┌──────────────┼──────────────┐
         ▼              ▼              ▼
    Route (i)      Route (ii)      Route (iii)
    No breathing   No breathing    Breathing is OK
    No pulse       There is a pulse  There is a pulse
         │              │              │
         ▼              ▼              ▼
    2 breaths (m to m)  10 breaths (m to m)  Put casualty into
    + 15 compressions   + check A, B, C      recovery position
         │              │              │
         ▼              ▼              ▼
    Repeat until help   Repeat until help    Repeatedly check
    arrives             arrives              A, B, C
```

The five checks (Safety, Shake and shout, A, B, C)

1 Safety
As you approach the casualty think 'safety'. Are you safe?

2 Shake and shout
Kneel down, gently shake the shoulder and ask loudly, 'Are you OK?'.

3 Airway
Open the airway - remove any obvious obstruction from the mouth. Place two fingers under the jaw and lift. At the same time, put your other hand on the forehead and tilt the head back. This will prevent the tongue from sagging back and blocking the throat.

4 Breathing
Lean down and look and listen for breathing. Do this for at least 5 seconds.

5 Circulation
If the heart is beating it will generate a pulse in the neck where the carotid artery runs up either side of the larynx (voice box).

Find the right place to check the carotid pulse in the neck and feel for it for at least 5 seconds.

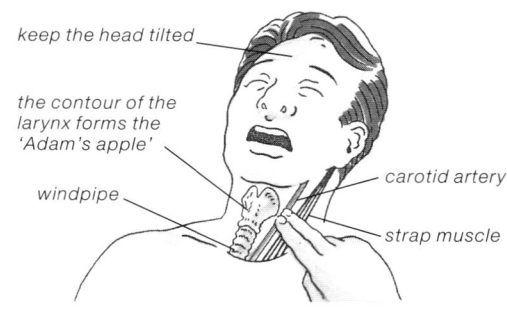

Figure 1.53 Locating the carotid artery

A | **The five checks**

44

Promoting health and well-being

A Order of actions

Using the first aid flow chart on page 44, state the correct order of actions in each of the following cases:
- a casualty who is conscious with a broken leg
- an unconscious casualty who is bleeding
- a casualty who has stopped breathing but whose heart is beating
- a casualty who is not breathing and has no pulse.

Mouth-to-mouth resuscitation

Do not carry out mouth to mouth resuscitation on a person who is breathing normally. It can be dangerous. You will need to practise this on a specially-made dummy person.

Breathing, and why mouth-to-mouth resuscitation works

Breathing involves the chest volume increasing. This reduces the pressure inside the lungs and air is pushed into the lungs by atmospheric pressure. The chest volume is increased by the diaphragm (sheet of membrane and muscle separating the chest from the abdomen) being pulled downwards and at the same time the ribs moving upwards and outwards.

When you breathe in, oxygen in the air (about 20% of air) passes across the lining cells of the alveoli (air sacs) and into the blood. Carbon dioxide passes from the blood to the lungs. The air breathed out has less oxygen than the atmosphere and more carbon dioxide.

Even so, the air you breathe out still contains 16% oxygen, which is enough to keep a casualty alive. You can breathe for a casualty by blowing into his/her lungs. The act of breathing into the casualty's lungs causes them to inflate (fill with air). The movement caused by inflating the lungs can trigger the person to start breathing naturally.

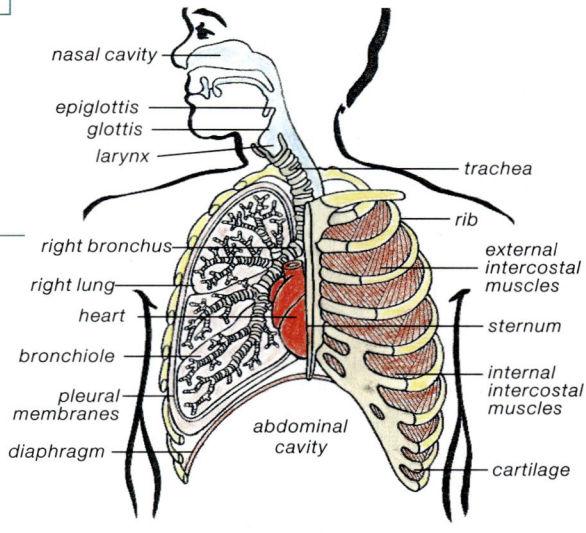

Figure 1.54 The respiratory system

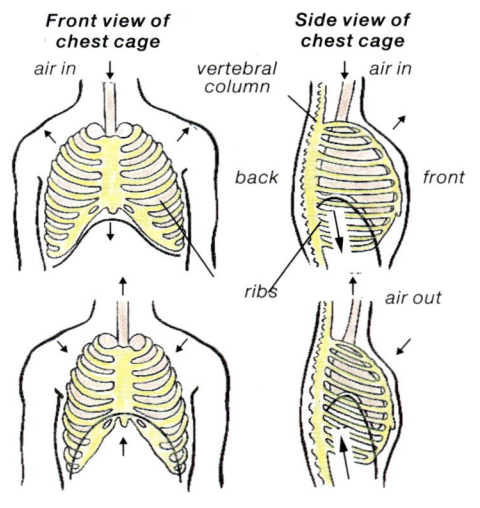

Figure 1.55 Breathing movements

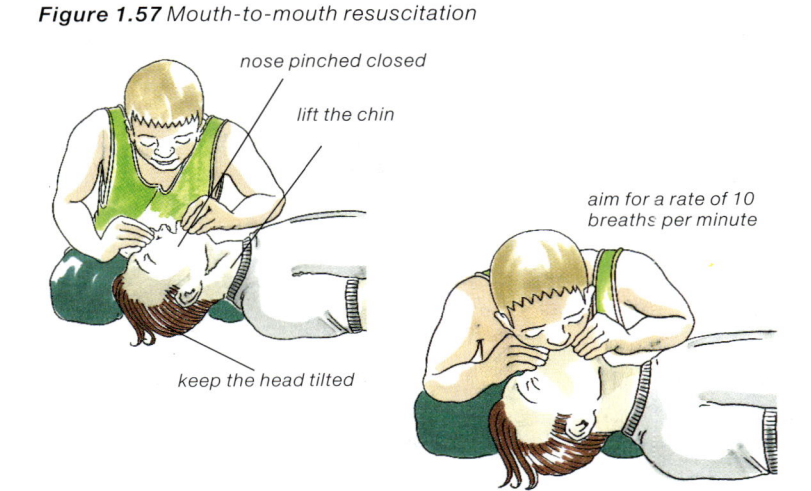

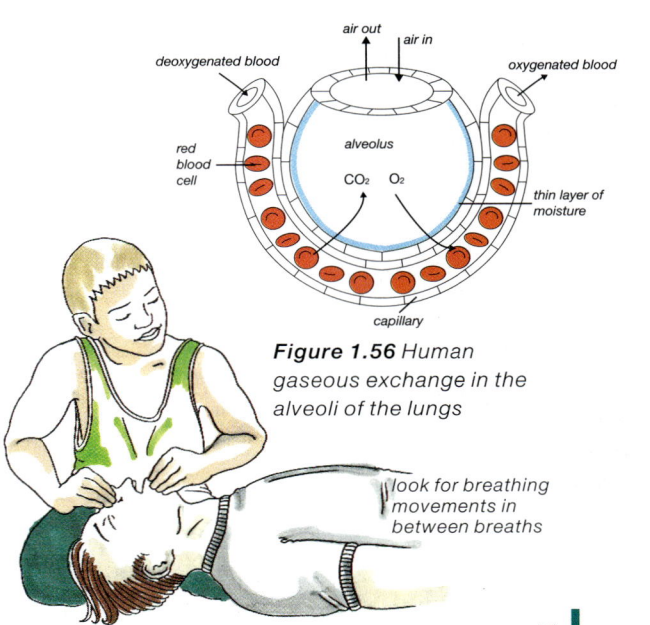

Figure 1.56 Human gaseous exchange in the alveoli of the lungs

Figure 1.57 Mouth-to-mouth resuscitation

Promoting health and well-being

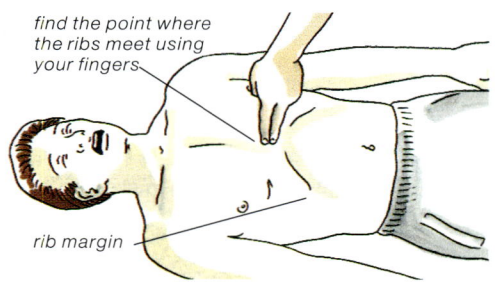

find the point where the ribs meet using your fingers

rib margin

Figure 1.58 *Finding the bottom of the breastbone*

slide the heel of your hand onto the breastbone to meet the fingers

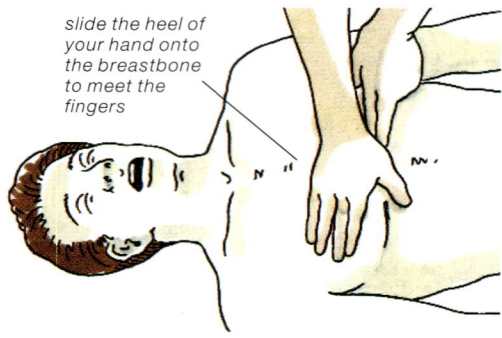

Figure 1.59 *Finding the correct hand position*

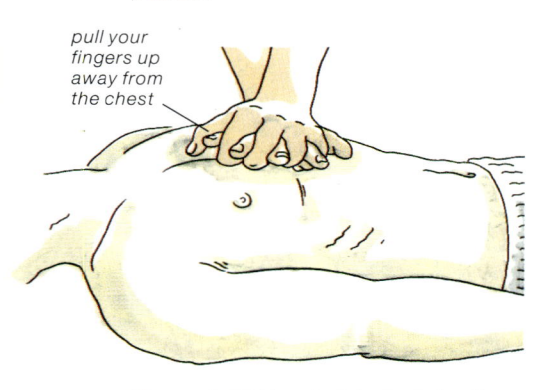

pull your fingers up away from the chest

Figure 1.60 *How to interlock the fingers*

you may find it useful to count 'one and two and...' to keep time

press straight down with the heel of your hands

keep the fingers clear of the chest

Figure 1.61 *Timing the compressions*

Do the five checks first and then follow either route (i), (ii), or (iii).

Check 1
Think 'Is it safe for me to approach?'
Approach the casualty and kneel down

Check 2
Use 'Shake and shout'

Check 3
Lay the casualty on his/her back.
Check the mouth and remove obvious obstructions or loose dentures.
Tilt the head back to open the airway (two fingers under chin, other hand on the forehead).

Check 4
Lean down to listen and look for breathing for 5 seconds.

Check 5
Check for a carotid pulse for 5 seconds.

Route (i)

If the casualty is not breathing and has no pulse
Go for help, even if you are on your own. Ideally send someone else to get help, and then:
- give two breaths as quickly as you sensibly can
- lie the casualty on a firm surface (not a bed)
- find the bottom of the breastbone
- put 2 fingers on the bottom end of the breastbone
- place the heel of your other hand onto the breastbone next to your fingers
- interlock your first hand on top of your other hand and lift the fingers up from the chest
- lean over the casualty so that your shoulders are over your hands
- straighten your arms
- push straight down to depress the breastbone by about 2" (5 cm)
- do 15 compressions in a rhythmic manner (aiming at a rate of 80 a minute) then two breaths
- repeat compressions and breaths until help arrives.

Route (ii)

Casualty is not breathing but there is a pulse
This is the situation where a good first aider saves many lives:
- pinch the nose
- take a good breath and seal your mouth over theirs
- blow in steadily for about 2 seconds, watch for chest rising
- count 4 seconds
- repeat 9 more times – aim for 10 breaths in a minute
- get help – if on your own leave the casualty. If possible send a helper
- return to the casualty and repeat checks on breathing and pulse
- continue mouth-to-mouth and continue pulse and breathing checks.

Promoting health and well-being

A Mouth-to-mouth resuscitation

Practise mouth-to-mouth resuscitation on a Resusci-anna-type dummy.

Chest compression

How does it work?
Pushing down on the breastbone increases pressure in the chest which pushes blood out of the heart. As the breastbone is released the chest rises and blood re-enters the heart.

This has to be done in connection with mouth-mouth, the oxygen you blow into the lungs needs to be pumped around the body by your chest compressions.

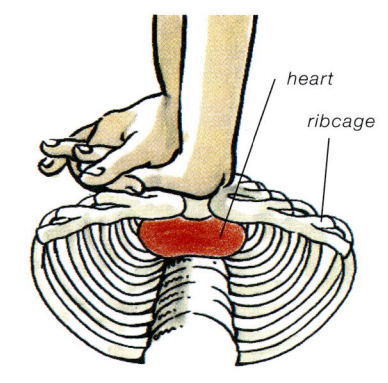

Figure 1.62 How chest compression works

A Cardiac compression

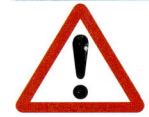

Practise cardiac compression on a Resusci-anna-type dummy.
Do not try it on your partner – it is very dangerous to do this if the heart is beating!

Route (iii)

The casualty is breathing and has a pulse
This is less serious but can get worse, so put the casualty into the recovery position.

The recovery position

The recovery position prevents the tongue from blocking the airway and allows fluids to drain out of the mouth so the casualty won't choke on his/her vomit.

Any unconscious casualty should be put into this position. First you will have checked their breathing and pulse and made a brief examination for other injuries; you may need to modify the position to take account of other injuries. Remove glasses if the casualty is wearing them and check pockets for lumpy objects.

- Open the airway using the chin-lift and head-tilt.
- Bend the nearer elbow so the hand is in line with the head.
- Bring the further arm across the body placing the back of the hand against the cheeks, and hold it there.
- Lean down and grab the further leg at the knee and bend it so that the foot rests on the floor.
- Pull the knee towards you and roll the casualty towards you holding the casualty's hand against their cheek.
- Tilt the head back to keep the airway open. Check that the hand under the cheek helps keep the head tilted back.
- Check that the knee is bent at a right angle.
- Dial 999 if you haven't already done so.
- Keep checking pulse and breathing.

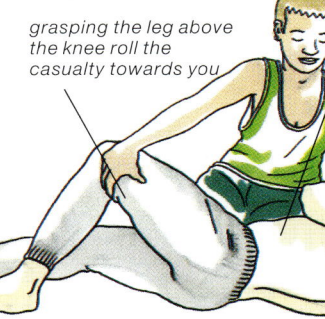

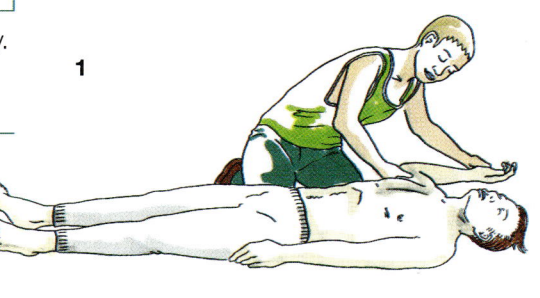

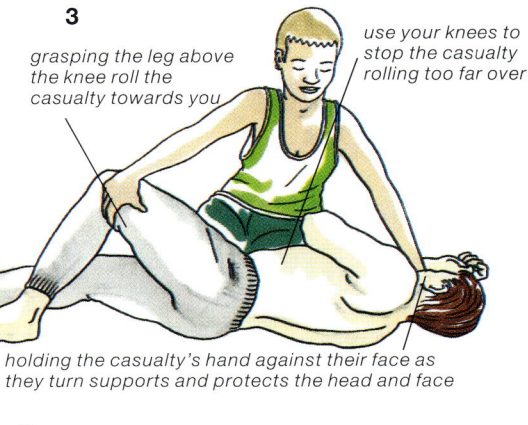

1

2

3
grasping the leg above the knee roll the casualty towards you

use your knees to stop the casualty rolling too far over

holding the casualty's hand against their face as they turn supports and protects the head and face

Figure 1.63 Putting the casualty into the recovery position (1–4)

47

Promoting health and well-being

A — The recovery position

1. Practise putting a partner into the recovery position.
2. **(a)** You find a casualty lying on the ground who is apparently unconscious: someone else says that the person is breathing. Demonstrate how you would approach, assess and position this casualty.
   (b) You find a casualty who you discover is not breathing, but has a pulse. Demonstrate you assessment of this casualty and take the appropriate action.
   (c) You find a casualty who you discover is not breathing and whose heart has stopped. Demonstrate your assessment of this casualty and take the appropriate action.
3. Write a short report (1–1 ½ sides of A4) of one of the incidents role-played in 2, as required under the Health and Safety Regulations of the institution.
   Make sure you give all relevant information, identifying people and places, as well as the condition of the casualty and actions taken by you. It should be clear who will receive the report. Remember to date it.

How to examine a casualty

Once you have dealt with the five checks of first aid and followed routes (i), (ii), or (iii) you can than go on to examine the casualty in detail.

Recognition

There are 3 things to help you to recognise the problem:
1. history – of the incident/illness, i.e. what has happened. You might obtain this from a witness.
2. signs – what you find out using your senses of touch, sight, smell and hearing.
3. symptoms – what the casualty can tell you about their own feelings.

A — What's happened?

In pairs discuss:
1. what clues bystanders might give you at, for instance, a road accident (history)
2. what each of your senses (touch, sight, smell, hearing) might tell you about the casualty (signs)
3. what sort of things a casualty might tell you that they feel (symptoms).

Move into a larger group and share your ideas. Check with the checklists that follow – what did you miss?

History

Did they bang their head?
Did a car run over them? Where (legs, arm, chest, etc)?
Were they knocked out?
Which side was hit?

48

Promoting health and well-being

Signs
Table 1.9 Signs to find out using the senses

Sight	Touch	Hear	Smell
wounds	wetness	breathing	alcohol
bleeding	sweat	groaning	solvents/glue
sweating	skin temperature	their response to your touch	chemicals
vomit	swelling		burning
bruises	deformity		gas
swelling	tender to touch		incontinence
deformity	irregularity		
needle marks	pulse		
medic alerts			
containers			
breathing problems			
skin colour - flushed red - pale - blueness			

Symptoms
- pain
- unable to move some part as normal
- a limb or an area feeling 'funny' or 'numb' or 'tingly'
- thirst
- sickness, dizziness or weakness
- faint
- hot or cold
- anxious, scared.

Priority
Remember with any casualty to use the correct order of priority:
- deal with serious conditions using the five checks and routes (i), (ii) or (iii) first
- deal with any obvious injury
- examine the casualty thoroughly from head to toe, move clothing if necessary but don't 'strip' them, and take care not to offend
- compare each side as you work (arm to arm) and use both hands.

Flow chart of serious emergencies, page 44

Promoting health and well-being

Examining the casualty
- always talk to the casualty and reassure them
- explain simply what you are doing
- ask for guidance, for example: 'Does this hurt?'.

1 Keep the head still, look for and feel for any bumps or dents, or blood. It may also be possible to check the neck section of the spine at this stage (see point 9).
2 If closed, gently open the eyes. Do the pupils shrink in size? Are they the same size as each other? Is there any injury to the eye?
3 Can the casualty hear normally? Is there blood or fluid coming from the ear?
4 Is there blood or fluid coming out of the nose?
5 Look inside the mouth, is there a wound? Is there any obstruction (e.g. loose dentures)? Are there broken teeth? Is there any swelling or blueness of the lips? Is there any smell (alcohol, bleach)? Check the rate, depth and ease of breathing.
6 Feel the skin, temperature and state (cold/warm/hot – dry/sweaty).
7 Check the carotid pulse, rate, rhythm, strength. Look for a medic-alert necklace.
8 Check the collar bones, breastbone and ribs. Check for tenderness and deformity. Is the ribcage moving normally as the casualty breathes?
9 Very carefully feel along the back and spine for swelling and tenderness. Remember not to move the casualty if you have any doubts about back injury.
10 Gently feel the tummy for injury or tenderness. Hardness means that there could be internal bleeding.
11 Find the hip bone on each side. Gently 'rock' the pelvis to check for pelvic fracture.
12 Check one arm against the other – look for swelling, tenderness, deformity and ask if the casualty can move them normally. Check the circulation in the fingers.
13 Can the casualty move their legs normally, do they feel normal? Check for tenderness, swelling or deformity.

You may also need to check a pocket or bag for external clues such as an appointment card or medicine card, or tablets.

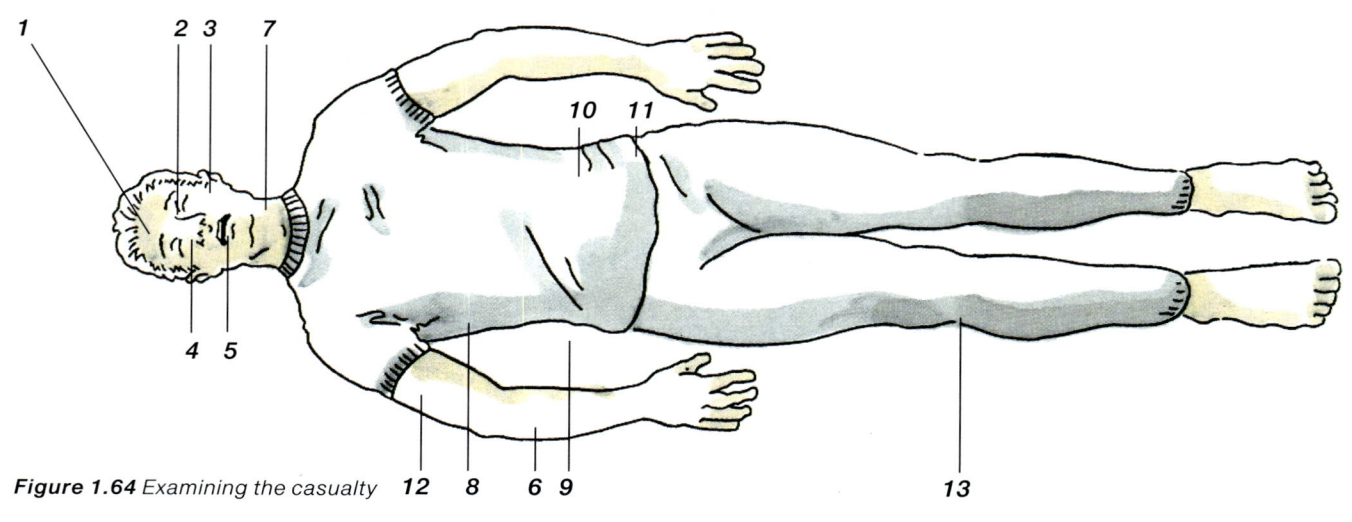

Figure 1.64 Examining the casualty

Promoting health and well-being

A Examining a casualty

In pairs, examine your partner gently and carefully. You could choose whether your partner is unconscious or conscious. As you practise you may find it helpful to say out loud what it is you are looking for. Alternatively, practise talking in a calm and reassuring manner as you examine a conscious casualty.

Wounds and the treatment of bleeding

Any abnormal break in the skin is known as a wound. Through the wound blood can be lost and germs enter. Bleeding is classified by the type of blood vessel that is damaged, whether it is an artery, a vein or a capillary.

The circulatory system consists of the heart, arteries, veins and capillaries. The heart pumps blood from its right side through the pulmonary artery to the lungs. The blood then passes through a network of capillaries, picking up oxygen and giving up carbon dioxide. The blood then passes through the pulmonary vein to the left side of the heart. From the left side of the heart the blood is pumped to the rest of the body, passing through capillary networks until it returns to the right side of the heart through the veins.

The heart pumps about 70 cm^3 of blood from each side every time it beats. It beats about 70 times a minute. Cardiac compression as a first aid treatment uses external pressure to compress the heart and so pump the blood around the body.

> A cut artery spurts blood in time with the heart beat.
> A cut vein may pour blood profusely but steadily.
> A cut capillary only oozes blood.

Bleeding from an artery or a vein can be very serious and needs quick action. As some casualties may carry an infection in their blood it is important to maintain a high standard of hygiene to protect yourself. This also protects the casualty from any risk.

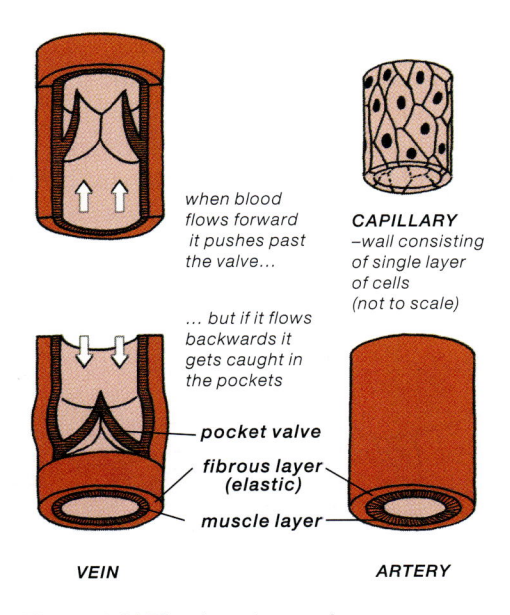

Figure 1.66 The three types of blood vessel

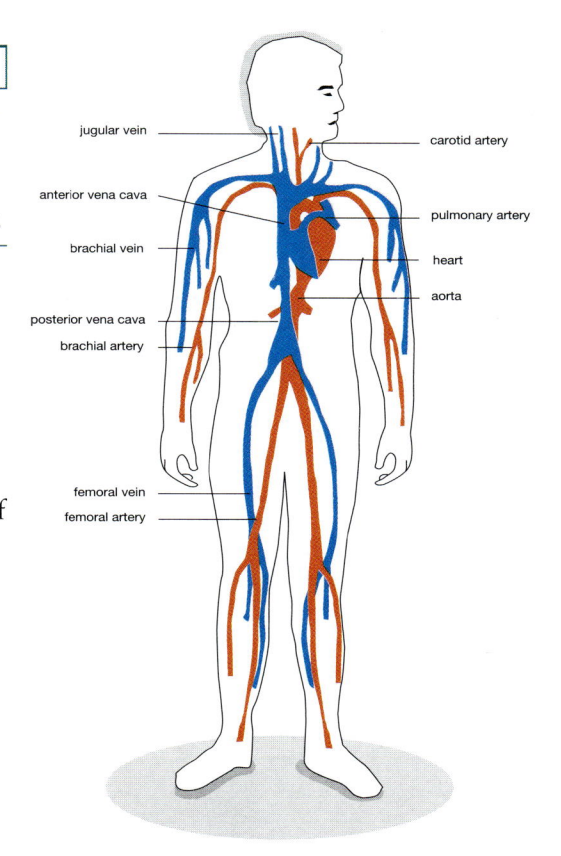

The main blood vessels
Oxygenated blood = red, deoxygenated blood = blue.

Oxygenated blood = red, deoxygenated blood = blue

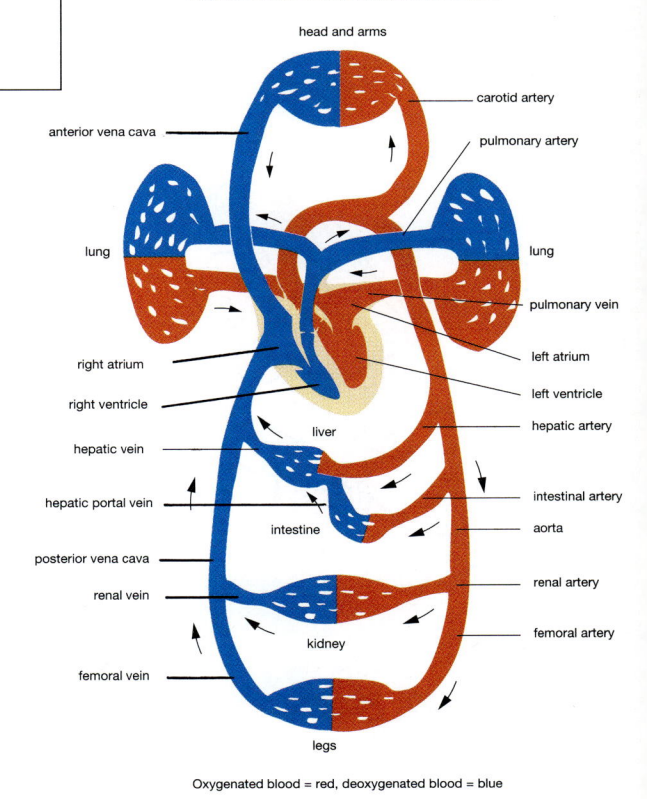

Figure 1.65 The human circulatory system

51

Promoting health and well-being

Preventing cross infection
Follow these simple rules:
1 Cover any cut or grazes on your own hands with a waterproof dressing.
2 Use disposable gloves or improvise with plastic bags.
3 Ask the casualty to dress his or her own wounds with your guidance.
4 If you are unable to use gloves wash your hands very thoroughly immediately afterwards.
5 Do not cough or sneeze over the wound and make sure that your hands are clean.
6 Use a solution of 1 part bleach:10 parts water to mop up blood or other body fluids.
7 Make sure all used dressings are disposed of in a sealed plastic bag and incinerated.

Treating severe bleeding
This is an obvious problem and can be frightening. Don't forget the Priorities of Treatment and the five checks first.

The two most important rules when dealing with bleeding are:
1 Pressure – to stop the blood flow.
2 Elevate – to raise the injured part above the level of the heart, to help slow blood flow.

To control bleeding
1 Check the wound for anything stuck in it, but don't pull it out.
2 If there is nothing in the wound apply direct pressure over the wound. If you have a clean pad or sterile dressing put it over the wound and press down tightly with your hands/fingers. The casualty may be able to do this for herself/himself.
3 Lay the casualty down.
4 Raise the injured part (if possible) above the level of the heart. If a leg is involved rest it on your shoulder.
5 Put a sterile dressing over the pad and bandage firmly to put pressure on the wound.
6 Call 999 if you have not already done so.
7 Check that blood is still circulating in the limb beyond the bandage. Look for colour changes and ask about numbness.
8 If blood is still being lost, put another bandage on top of the first one, but do not take the first one off (it would dislodge any clot that was forming).

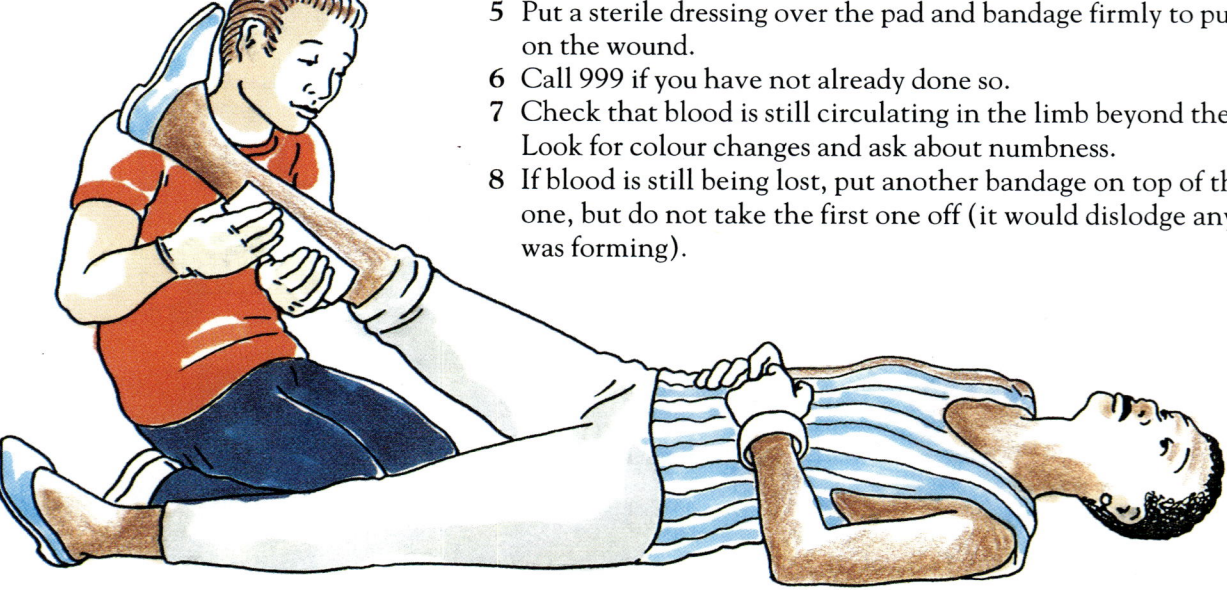

Figure 1.67 Apply direct pressure over the wound

52

Promoting health and well-being

A   Severe bleeding

Practise this in pairs. One person acts as a casualty with severe bleeding from the arm, the other acts as the first-aider.
Then you change over but this time the casualty should have severe bleeding from the shin.
Remember to talk to and reassure your casualty, explaining what you are doing.

If something is stuck in the wound

1. Do not try to pull it out.
2. Apply pressure by pushing down firmly on each side of the object or squeeze the sides of the wound together.

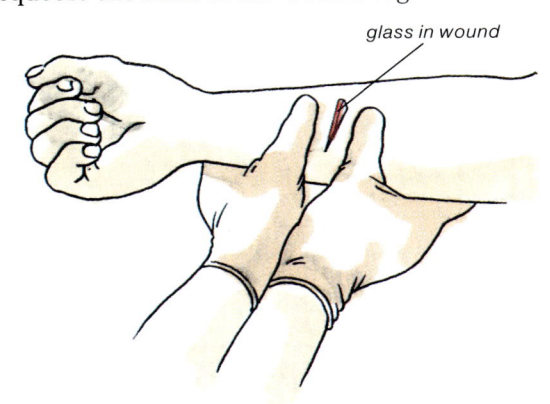

Figure 1.68 Squeeze the sides of the wound together

3. Put pads on each side of the object and if possible build them up high enough to bandage over the object without pushing it further in.
4. Bandage firmly over the pads. Use a figure of eight if the object protrudes above the pads.
5. Remember to elevate the injury if it involves a limb.

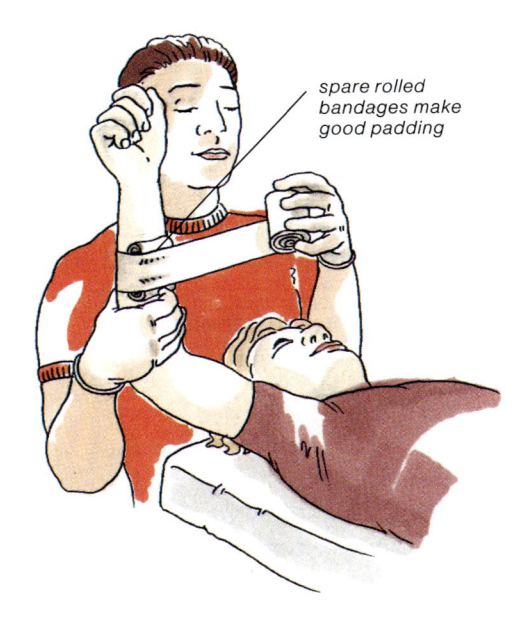

Figure 1.69 Pad the wound on either side before bandaging

53

Promoting health and well-being

> **A** — **Practise stopping bleeding**
>
> Practise this in pairs – draw a 'wound' with a washable felt tip colour and use a pen cap or screw lying on the skin as the foreign body.

Stopping bleeding using indirect pressure

Sometimes it is not possible to control bleeding using direct pressure. To stop the casualty from getting rapidly worse use a pressure point to stop the blood flowing into the injured limb.

Pressure point: where an artery can be compressed against a bone to cut off the blood supply to the limb.

However you can only use one for 10 minutes after which you must let the blood flow through the arm/leg before reapplying it.

- To stop bleeding from the arm – use the brachial pressure point.

The artery runs along the inner side of the upper arm. Press your first 3 fingers between the muscles (to compress the artery against the bone). You should find a pulse – push hard on it.

- To stop bleeding from the leg – use the femoral pressure point.

The artery crosses the pelvic bone in the centre of the groin crease. Bend the leg outwards on the injured side and find the pulse. Then push on it very firmly with both thumbs.

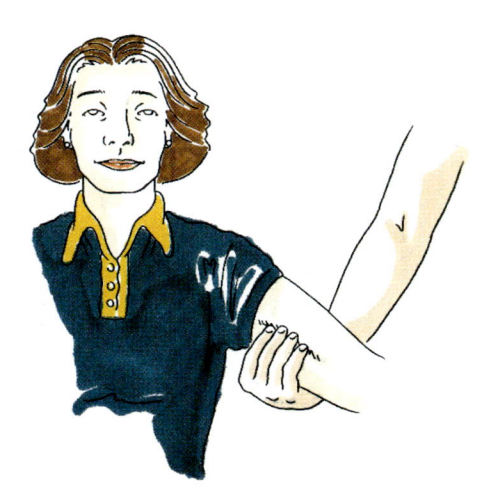

Figure 1.70 Using the brachial pressure point

> **A** — **Finding pressure points**
>
> Find each of the pressure points on yourself. Apply the brachial one for a minute or two *(no longer!)* to see how it feels. To find the femoral one you have to lie on the floor and bend the knee outwards, feel in the middle of the leg along the line where the bottom of a pair of briefs would come to (Figure 1.71).

Dealing with minor bleeding

'Minor' bleeding is that which is easily controlled using direct pressure and elevation. Medical aid is only needed if there is something stuck in it, if it is likely to become infected (a dirty puncture wound or dog bite) or if it is not healing.

1. Wash your hands – put gloves on if available.
2. If the wound is dirty rinse it under the tap if practicable.
3. Dry gently with a swab or tissue.
4. Put a piece of sterile gauze over the wound and then clean around it using soap and water. Always wipe away from the wound and use a new swab for each wipe.
5. Pat dry and then apply a plaster or dressing and bandage.

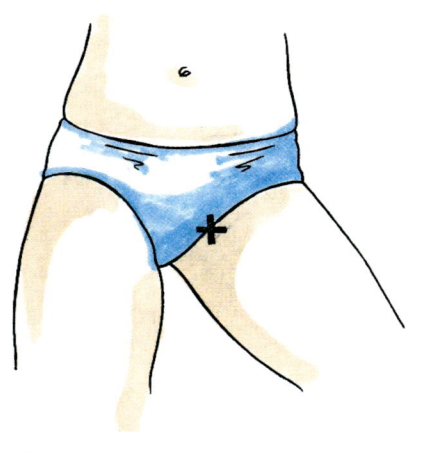

Figure 1.71 The femoral pressure point – marked with a cross

Shock

Blood is pumped around the body by the heart so that oxygen and nutrients can reach all of the body's tissues. In the average adult there are about 6 litres of blood. If the circulatory system starts to fail then the tissues do not get all of the oxygen that they need and 'shock' develops. Shock can kill so it must be recognised and treated.

The causes of shock

1 Loss of volume of the circulating fluid as in:
 - bleeding
 - severe diarrhoea and vomiting
 - burns.
2 The pump failing, i.e. heart attacks.

How to recognise shock
- pale, grey skin – especially inside the lips
- skin cold and clammy to the touch
- a rapid pulse which may feel 'weak' at the wrist and become irregular
- feelings of weakness and giddiness
- feelings of thirst
- may become restless, talkative or anxious
- may lapse into unconsciousness.

How to deal with shock
Treat any obvious cause (e.g. severe external bleeding).
Place the casualty as shown in Figure 1.72 (if injuries allow for movement).

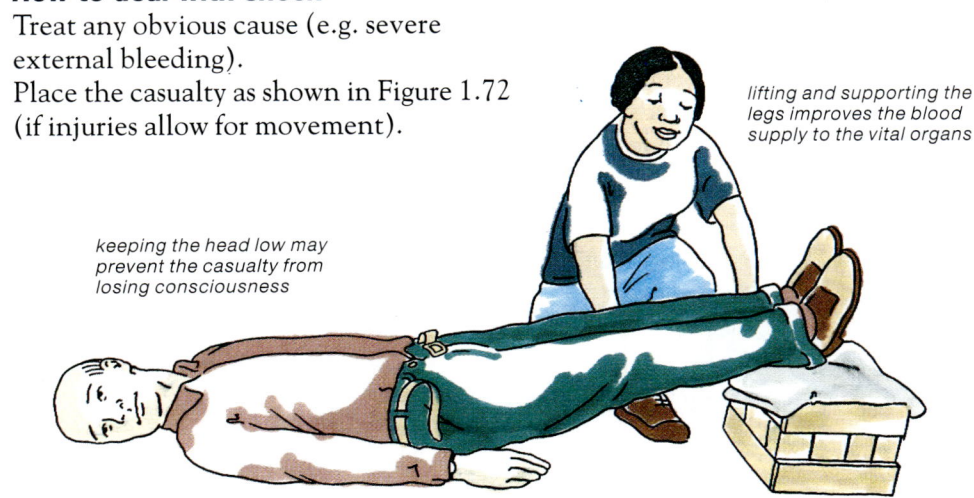

keeping the head low may prevent the casualty from losing consciousness

lifting and supporting the legs improves the blood supply to the vital organs

Figure 1.72 *Positioning a casualty who is in shock*

Do:
- keep the head low
- reassure
- check and record breathing/pulse, level of responsiveness
- raise and support the legs
- protect from cold above and below
- loosen tight clothing.

Do not:
- allow casualty to eat, drink or smoke
- allow casualty to move
- put hot water bottles anywhere near the casualty or place casualty by a radiator or in front of a fire.

Contacting the emergency services
In the procedures for the various different situations you have been told to contact the emergency services. If you were dealing with an emergency you would probably send someone to do this. If you do ask somebody to contact the emergency services, tell the person to come back and report to you. If you are on your own or if you are the person asked to contact the emergency services then you need to know what to do.

Promoting health and well-being

To contact the emergency services you:
- pick up the receiver of the phone
- wait for a dialling tone
- dial 999.

You do not need to put money into a pay phone to dial 999. If you are phoning from a school or office you may need to dial a code for an outside line first. Details are normally on the telephone or on a notice by the side. The operator answers and asks which service you require.

By dialling 999 you can alert:
- Fire Brigade
- Ambulance
- Mine/Mountain/Cave Rescue
- HM Coastguards
- Police (they may have to control a dangerous situation).

Say which service you require and be prepared to give as much information as you can. You may need to:
- give the number of the telephone you are phoning from
- give the exact location of the incident or injured person
- say what has happened
- say how many are injured, their sex and age
- say what you think is wrong (heart attack, childbirth, burns, drowning, broken leg, etc.)
- warn of any dangers (spilt chemicals, gas leaks, fog on motorway, broken power lines). If the incident involves a lorry which has a Hazchem symbol, quote the numbers.

Don't put the receiver down until told to do so.

Figure 1.73 Hazchem symbols

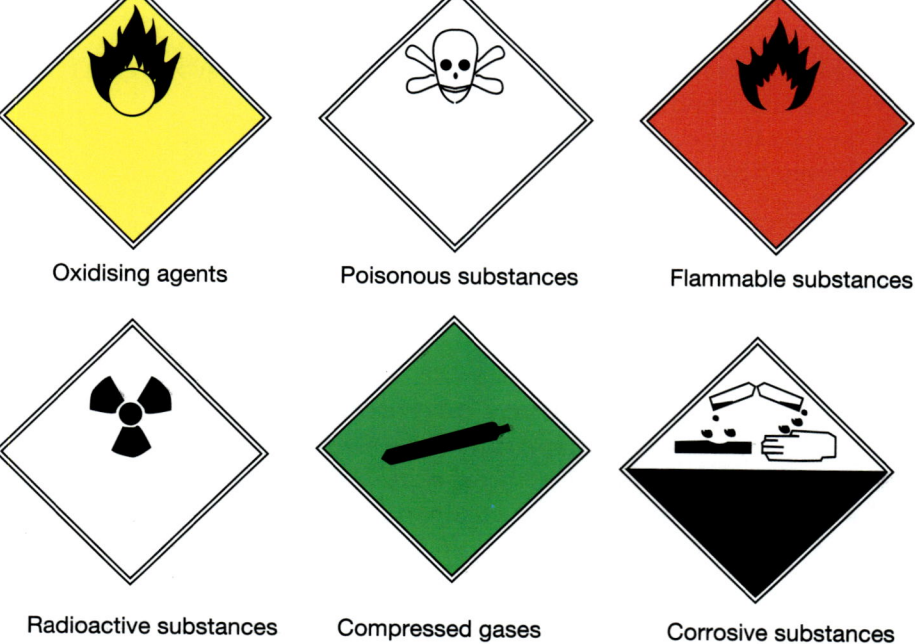

Code information for the emergency services: 2WE
United Nations number for the substance: 2447
Telephone number for further information: (0123) 45678
Nature of potential danger

- Oxidising agents
- Poisonous substances
- Flammable substances
- Radioactive substances
- Compressed gases
- Corrosive substances

56

What to do when the emergency services arrive
This is the time when you need to tell the services exactly what you found out in assessing the casualty. You will need to report:
- any changes in responsiveness
- the pulse rate and any changes to it
- any action you have taken
- any information you have about the casualty (name, age, address)
- the time the accident happened and the times of anything you observed or did (for example, how long ago the casualty became unconscious).

Above all, you will need to be as accurate as possible and as precise as possible. The information you give may help the experts diagnose a problem that you are unable to recognise or treat.

A final note
Reading this book does not qualify you in First Aid. It only describes some of the basic emergency treatments. You should not try to carry out any First Aid that you are unsure about. The ideal thing for you to do is train with one of the organisations that offers First Aid training and assessment. In becoming qualified you will have demonstrated the skills of First Aid and should be competent to deal with an emergency situation.

Promoting health and well-being

Assignment

PROMOTING BALANCED LIFESTYLES

Setting the scene

Your school or college is holding a Health 2000 day for which you are to prepare some materials. These will be in the form of booklets, posters and possibly audio visual displays. You will also have to present information to individuals or small groups.

Some of this assignment will require teacher input but you should be able to do a lot of the work in the library, with computers and at home.

Note: If it is not possible to arrange for people to visit your Health 2000 day then you might (individually or in small groups) arrange to take the display to them.

Although most of the activities can be carried out in a group, you must prepare your own materials.

Task 1

The theme of the Health 2000 day is 'Maintaining balanced lifestyles'. Produce a piece of written work that explains:
- what a balanced lifestyle is
- the importance of a balanced lifestyle
- risks and benefits associated with aspects of lifestyle.

The written work should be displayed and supported by a poster or diagram that identifies risks and benefits of a balanced lifestyle for an individual.

Task 2

Part of your display is to be about balanced diets.

Prepare a display that shows what constitutes a balanced diet for each of:
- a child
- an elderly person
- a pregnant woman.

In doing this choose one of the people to have an active lifestyle and one other to have a sedentary one. Explain why the needs of the people are not the same.

Within the display indicate what each of the components of the balanced diet is used for. (Remember that we all use the components for the same things, so you will only need to do this part once.)

Task 3

Identify a target group of people from:
- people with disabilities
- children
- elderly people (active or sedentary)
- pregnant women

and invite them to your Health 2000 day.

Discuss in your group the main health risks for your target group. Identify ways that you can use to check an individual's health against a measure of the risk. (You might for example check height against weight or units of alcohol drunk in a week.)

Task 4
Within your own group carry out assessments of health against the measures that you identified. You do not need to do this for all the members of your group. Some may prefer not to undertake the health check.

Use the information that you have gained from the activity to prepare an action plan for a 'typical' member of your target group. Decide short, medium and long term targets and how and when their achievement will be assessed.

Task 5
Produce a booklet of health advice for your selected target group of people who will attend the Health 2000 day. The booklet should include ways in which your target group might check their health, and advice on how health can be improved.

Individually, devise 'pre Health 2000' and 'post Health 2000' questionnaires to identify what members of your target group already know about the area of health that you are addressing and what they have gained from your Health 2000 day.

Task 6
Produce a booklet setting out guidelines for good practice in maintaining personal hygiene. Choose any one public area and include a description of the possible harmful effects of the introduction of micro-organisms into that area by poor hygiene levels.

Task 7
Run the Health 2000 day. During the day approach members of your target group and ask them to complete a 'pre Health 2000' questionnaire. Introduce them to the display. Then, after they have looked at the display, ask them to complete the 'post Health 2000' questionnaire.

Task 8
Using the information from your two questionnaires produce an evaluative report on the impact of your health promotion display.

Task 9
Write a summary to show the key difference in the way the advice would be presented for the other possible target groups.

Promoting health and well-being

Opportunities to collect evidence
On completing these tasks you will have the opportunity to meet the following requirements for Intermediate GNVQ Health and Social Care.
Unit 1
Element 1.1 PCs 1, 2, 3, 4, 5, 6
Element 1.2 PCs 1, 2, 3, 4, 5

Core skills
The tasks support core skills development in communication, both written and oral.

The booklets produced could be word processed and/or desk top published which would support the information technology core skill. Analysis of the questionnaires could involve production of graphs. The display from Task 2 could involve using pie charts. Both of these support the application of number core skill.

Grading
All grading themes are supported within this assignment. To bring the activities together on a given day will involve careful action planning. Information seeking is essential to achieve task 2.

The final task involves evaluation and so helps to develop the skill. You should always evaluate any activity and use your conclusions to assist future action planning. In particular you should evaluate how you worked to your action plan to meet the deadline set by the date of the Health 2000 day.

Quality of outcomes will be assessable for parts of the assignment (e.g. Tasks 1 and 2). It will also be a theme for the whole of the assignment.

HAZARDS AROUND THE SCHOOL/COLLEGE

Setting the scene
Your college has decided to make the dining area open to the public. In doing this it expects to attract many parents with young children and babies, and older people.

Task 1
You have been asked to identify the hazards in the dining area, the nearby toilets and the route from the street to these areas. You should also consider the hazards on the street outside, which they have to cross to reach the entrance.

For each of the hazards identified describe the potential risks for:
- children
- teenagers
- adults
- elderly people.

Produce a chart that describes the hazard, identifies the risk for each of the groups listed above and proposes ways to reduce the risk.

Task 2
For this part you will need to arrange for a resuscitation dummy to be available.

Having opened up the dining area to the public you are sitting eating a meal when you hear a crash in the kitchen. You look inside to find that one of the staff has slipped on a patch of spilled custard. In doing so she has fallen and is lying motionless on the floor. She may be bleeding from a wound on her leg, you cannot see.

Use role play, using a dummy when necessary, to demonstrate how you would deal with the situation and summon help in the following situations.

> ⚠️ *Safety: Only do mouth-to-mouth and cardiac massage on a dummy.*

Situation 1
The person is breathing and has a pulse. The cut is bleeding freely and steadily.

Situation 2
The person is breathing and has a pulse. The cut has a piece of glass in it.

Situation 3
The person is not breathing but has a pulse. The cut does not appear to be serious.

Situation 4
The person is not breathing and has no pulse. The cut does not appear serious.

Task 3
Write a report to your health and safety officer describing:
- the four situations
- your actions in each situation
- the physiological basis behind the life-saving techniques you used.

Opportunities to collect evidence
On completing these tasks you will have the opportunity to meet the following requirements for Itermediate GNVQ Health and Social Care.
Unit 1
Element 1.3 PCs 1, 2, 3, 4, 5

Core skills
The major core skill developed will be communication. There may be opportunity to use information technology in producing the table (Task 1) and the report (Task 3).

Grading
Task 1 involves planning, information seeking and evaluation.
Task 2, with its practical setting, will provide evidence for demonstration of basic life-saving techniques.

Questions

Each question shows more than one possible answer, **a, b, c** and **d**; only **one** is correct

1. Which one of the following food components is part of a healthy diet? Foods which are:
   a high in fat
   b high in salt
   c high in sugar
   d high in fibre.

2. Which one of the following groups of foods is the main source of carbohydrates?
   a oil, butter, cheese
   b cereals and sugar
   c meat, fish and eggs
   d oil, butter, meat and fish.

3. In the five checks for first aid, the last three are 'A', 'B' and 'C'. These stand for:
   a always be careful
   b airway, bleeding, compression
   c airway, breathing, circulation
   d all bleeding checked.

4. Blood travels away from the heart in:
   a arteries
   b veins
   c capillaries
   d lymph vessels.

5. Which one of the following foods provides the best source of fibre?
   a brown bread
   b brown sugar
   c wholemeal bread
   d free range eggs.

6. Which one of the following activities will increase risk to health?
   a having a balanced diet
   b celibacy
   c smoking
   d avoiding alcohol.

7. Which one of the following activities could be classed as unsafe sexual behaviour?
   a unprotected sex
   b protected sex
   c massage
   d celibacy.

8. When presenting a health education topic to a group of young children, which one of the following would be the best format?
   a a written text
   b an audio-visual presentation
   c a flow chart
   d a diagrammatic representation of figures.

9. The components of a balanced diet are:
   a proteins, carbohydrates, fats, vitamins, minerals, water, fibre
   b proteins, carbohydrates, fats, vitamins
   c proteins, carbohydrates, vitamins, minerals
   d proteins, carbohydrates, fats, vitamins, minerals.

10. A sedentary life is characterised by:
    a increased physical activity
    b inactivity
    c lack of sleep
    d recreation.

11. When talking about components of a healthy diet, we often use the terms 'saturated' and 'unsaturated'. These refer to:
    a proteins
    b carbohydrates
    c fats
    d vitamins.

12. Care workers must be aware of good hygiene practices. Care of teeth, skin and hair is referred to as:
    a public hygiene
    b personal hygiene
    c public health
    d medical hygiene.

13. You are asked to prepare a booklet offering healthy eating tips to parents of young children. In this context, these parents are:
    a your peer group
    b your topic group
    c your family group
    d your target group.

14. When giving health advice to groups, participants may be asked to complete a questionnaire. This is one method of:
    a giving advice
    b presenting information
    c obtaining feedback
    d keeping the group healthy.

15 A chair against an open upstairs window would present the greatest hazard to:
  a a toddler
  b an adult
  c a teenager
  d a newborn baby.

16 In a first aid emergency which of the following is the correct order of procedure:
  a give emergency aid, get help, make the area safe, assess the situation
  b get help, give emergency aid, assess the situation, make the area safe
  c gake the area safe, assess the situation, get help, give emergency aid
  d Assess the situation, make the area safe, give emergency aid, get help.

17 Bleeding or loss of blood is referred to as:
  a herpes
  b haemophilia
  c a haemorrhage
  d a hepatoma.

18 The heart, arteries, veins and capillaries form:
  a the circulatory system
  b the respiratory system
  c the nervous system
  d the renal system.

19 The NACNE and COMA guidelines on diet in the UK say that in general people should eat:
  a less sugar, more salt, less fat and more fibre
  b less salt, less sugar, more fibre and less fat
  c less fibre, less salt, less fat and less sugar
  d more sugar, less fat, less salt and more fibre.

20 Which one of the following is the best example of a solvent?
  a cocaine
  b cannabis
  c lighter fluid
  d heroin.

21 Some people find it difficult to stop using drugs and have become dependant on them. This is referred to as:
  a tolerance
  b withdrawal
  c classification
  d addiction.

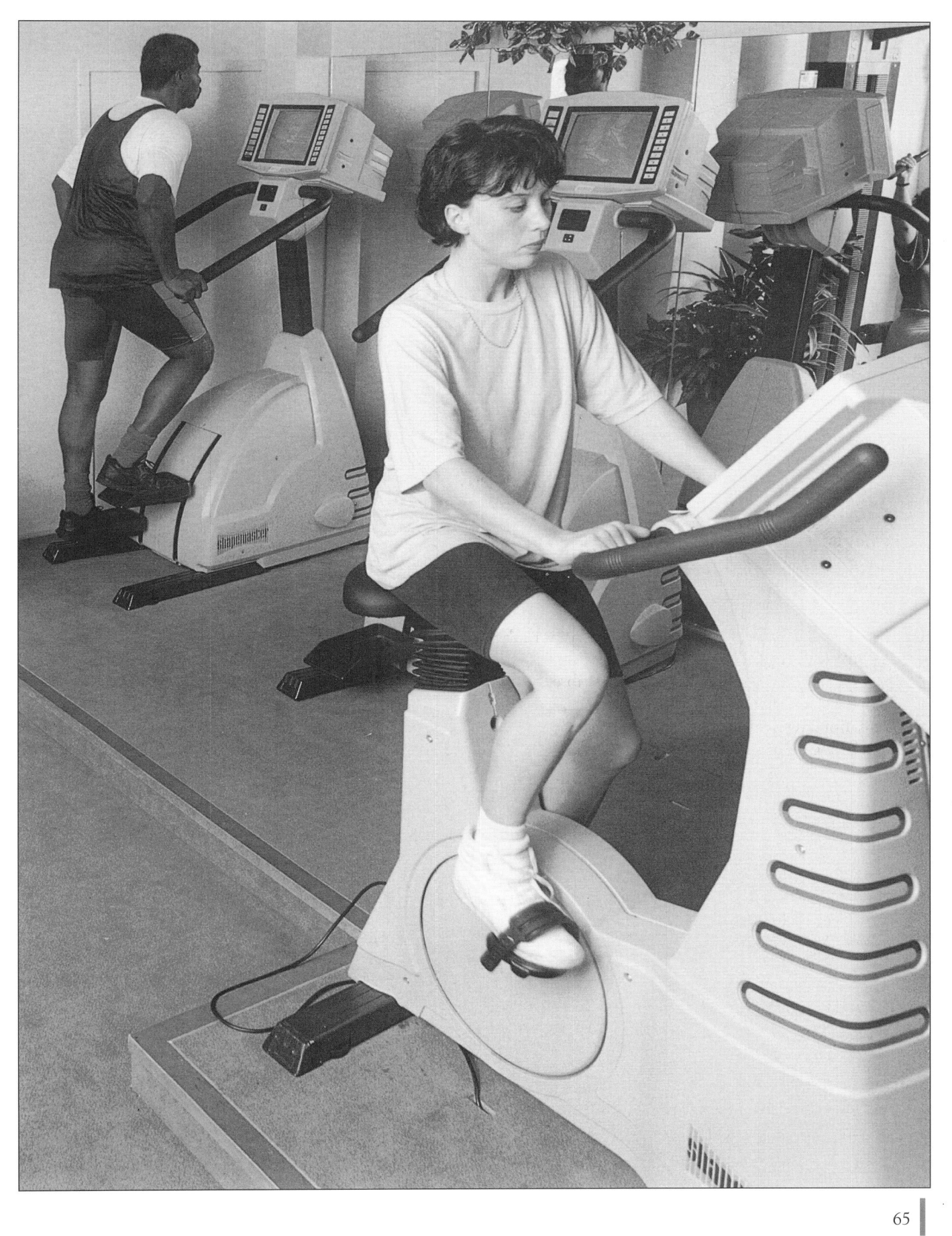

Promoting health and well-being

2 | Health and social well-being

Everybody is an individual. Each of us has a biological, cultural and social inheritance that helps to shape who we are and what we become. We are also part of a family within which we develop as individuals. At the same time, we also form groups with people who share similar beliefs, ideals and objectives.

This unit looks at the way individuals develop from biological, intellectual, social and emotional viewpoints. It looks at issues within society which affect an individual's health and social well-being by considering interpersonal relationships and broader groupings within society. This will help you to understand the many features and complexities of health and social well-being.

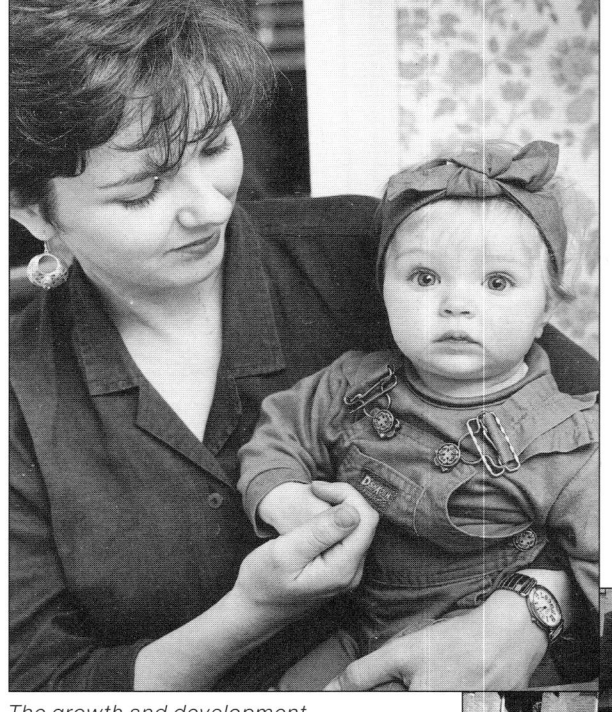

The growth and development of a new individual causes many changes for the parents

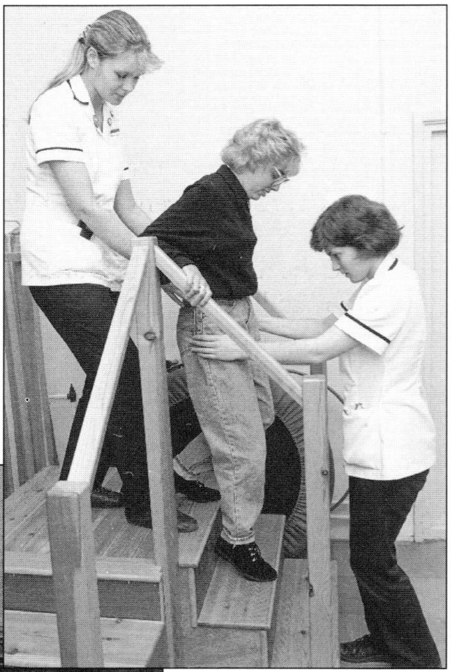

Figure 2.1 Issues which affect health and social well-being

Interpersonal relationships in work and social life contribute to well-being

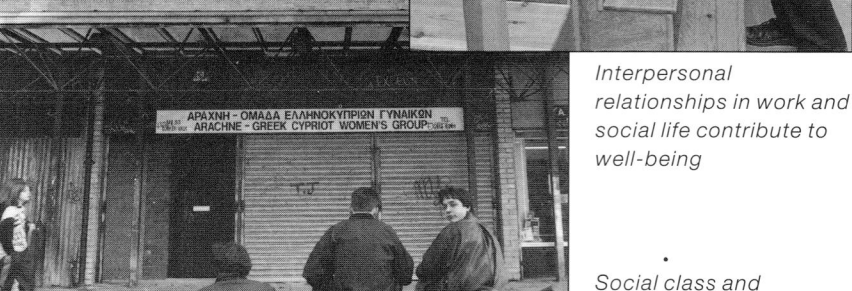

Social class and divisions in society affect children's health

Health and social well-being

The Elements

Explore the development of individuals and how they manage change
- describe the main characteristics of development in the different life stages
- explain the factors which influence an individual's self concept
- describe the impact on people of changes caused by major events
- describe ways in which people manage change caused by major events.

In this first element you will explore the characteristics of the different life stages and some of the major events that may affect individuals. You will also look at how their view of themselves influences their health and well-being.

▶ Key life stages, page 68

Explore the nature of inter-personal relationships and their influence on health and well-being
- describe relationships formed in the contexts of daily life
- describe causes of changes in relationships
- describe reasons why people form relationships
- explain the role of the family in the development of individuals
- identify the consequences of breakdown in relationships on health and well-being.

In the second element, you will focus on the nature of inter-personal relationships. You will also look at their influence on health and well-being; in particular, the role of the family.

▶ Relationships and their influence on health and well-being, page 92

Explore the interaction of individuals within society and how they may influence health and well-being
- identify the different roles which individuals take within different group settings
- describe how laws, rules and social conventions affect the roles of individuals
- compare the characteristics of different social and economic groups using a standard classification system
- identify the possible impact of the characteristics on individual choices which affect health and well-being
- assess the classification used.

In the third element you will investigate relationships in society and the different roles individuals adopt. You will also need to consider the impact of socio-economic factors on the choices which individuals can make, which may influence their health and well-being.

▶ Group roles, page 97

Health and social well-being

Life stages

Shakespeare's summary of the seven ages of man starts with the infant 'mewling and puking' and ends with second childishness, 'sans (without) eyes, sans teeth, sans taste, sans everything'. Even in the fifteenth century, life stages were identified and described.

Whilst Shakespeare identified seven life stages, we would now include development in the womb and birth in the list. An outline of the key life stages is listed below. In later sections we will consider the modern versions of the seven ages.

Key life stages

- **conception, pregnancy and foetal development** – a period of total dependence on the mother
- **birth** – a traumatic time when many physical functions come under control of the child. Dependence on parents for almost everything
- **infancy (0–5)** – a period of rapid growth and development. It is a time when a young child develops the physical skills that take it from being totally dependent on an adult to being able to practice many skills including walking, talking and socialising
- **childhood (5–11)** – a time of learning, particularly in the UK, learning through play. A period of very rapid intellectual development; developing socially and emotionally. Learning to relate to other people socially and emotionally. Still very reliant on adults for role models
- **adolescence (11–18)** – a period of rapid physical growth and associated hormonal changes. The time during which the individual becomes sexually mature. A time of great social change when parental roles are challenged and new social relationships develop. Emotional development very strongly affected by changes in hormone balance
- **adulthood (18/21–45)** – the period of greatest physical maturity. Social development associated with forming of strong emotional relationships, reproduction and child rearing
- **mid-life (45–65)** – often associated with social and emotional stability. Children no longer dependent. This may create its own tensions as roles change. Often a period of financial stability
- **old age (65+)** – emotional and social changes associated with retirement. Physiological processes, particularly repair, are reduced. Increasing need for support from others. This period may also be associated with increasing ill health.

Adulthood, mid-life and old age are not easily defined in terms of chronological age. The ages given are approximate and reflect times of social and biological change.

> **FOCUS**
> Life stages:
> - infancy to childhood
> - adolescence
> - early adulthood
> - mid-life
> - old age.

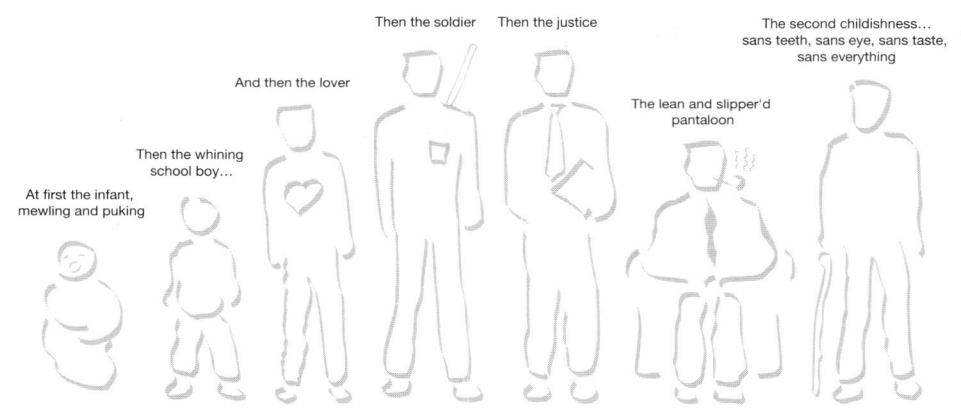

Figure 2.2 'And one man in his time plays many parts'

Health and social well-being

Personal development

The development of a human being is an amazing event. Starting as one cell you have developed into a complex, thinking organism that even the best machines and computers cannot replicate. Although we may be able to produce machines that are faster, stronger and more able to calculate, we have not yet been able to reproduce one with the range of skills and ability to learn that we all possess.

In order to understand the influences on an individual's development we can look at them from a variety of viewpoints. Traditionally, four main themes for development have been identified:
- physical
- intellectual
- emotional
- social.

These aspects are easy to remember, as the first letters spell out the word PIES. Many people would add a fifth aspect, spiritual, to reflect some of the psychological and 'feel good' features. We will use the outline given us by (s)PIES to consider personal development.

Physical development

One of the easiest ways of studying **physical development** is to look at growth. Professional health workers use the increase in size as a simple measure of how development is progressing in children. The rate of growth follows common patterns and is seen as a useful way of determining the age and stage of development of a child. The size of a foetus can be determined by ultrasound imaging and so a more accurate prediction of the birth date can be given.

Growth has three forms:
- increase in cell numbers
- increase in cell size
- increase in complexity.

In the first three months of pregnancy rapid growth of all forms occurs as the foetus develops from a single cell to a miniature version of an adult. By the end of three months all the different tissues and structures have developed. After three months the growth is mainly in cell number and cell size.

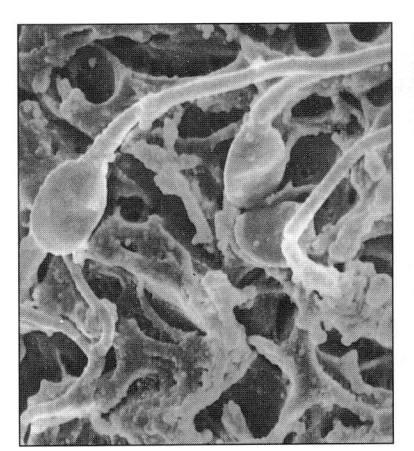

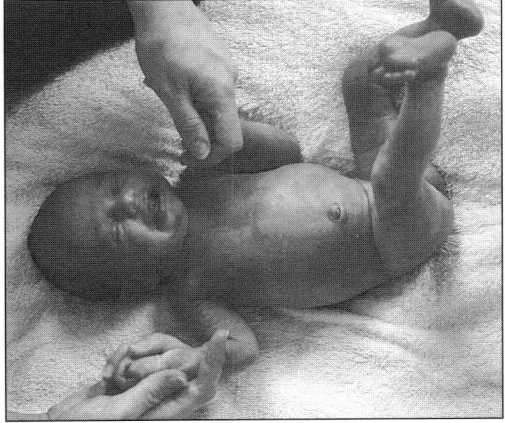

> **FOCUS**
> **Physical development and growth are related to:**
> - hormonal changes, e.g. puberty
> - age, e.g. maturity and ageing of tissues.

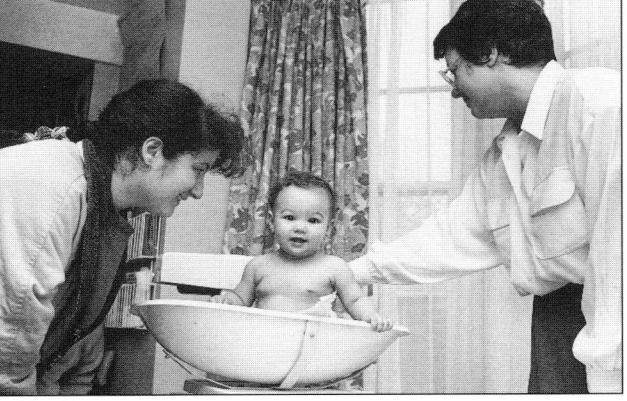

Figure 2.3 Monitoring growth is an important way of looking at child development

Figure 2.4 To grow from (**a**) an ovum (egg) to (**b**) a new-born baby requires:
- an increase in cell numbers – there is one ovum (here being fertilised), yet one drop of blood in the newborn baby contains 5 000 000 cells
- an increase in cell size – cells vary in size, with some in the nervous system stretching the length of a limb
- increase in complexity – the fertilised ovum is spherical; a neuron (single nerve cell) may have many projections that contact other nerve cells. Millions of such cells form the brain

a *b*

Growth in infancy and childhood

A Using growth data

The table gives the average changes in height and weight for boys and girls between birth and sixteen years old.

Age (years)	Boys Length/Height(cm)	Boys Annual Increase	Girls Length/Height(cm)	Girls Annual Increase	Boys Weight (kg)	Boys Annual Increase	Girls Weight (kg)	Girls Annual Increase
0	50	0	50.0	0	3.5	0	3.4	0
1	76.5	26.5	77.0	27	10.1	6.6	9.7	6.3
2	86.0	9.5	85.0	8	12.6	2.5	12.5	2.8
3	94.0	8	93.0	8	14.5	1.9	15	2.5
4	102.0	8	100.0	7	16.5	2	16.5	1.5
5	108.0	6	107.0	7	18.5	2	18.5	2
6	114.5	6.5	113.0	6	20.5	2	20.5	2
7	120.5	6	119.0	6	22.5	2	23	2.5
8	126.0	5.5	125.0	6	25	2.5	25	2
9	131.5	5.5	130.0	5	27.5	2.5	27.5	2.5
10	137.0	5.5	136.0	6	30.5	3	31	3.5
11	142.0	5	142.0	6	33.5	3	34	3
12	147.0	5	149.0	7	37	3.5	40	6
13	152.0	5	157.0	8	41	4	47.5	7.5
14	161.0	9	160.5	3.5	48.5	7.5	53	5.5
15	168.5	7.5	162.0	1.5	56.5	8	55	2
16	172.5	4	162.0	0	60.5	4	56	1

Use the growth data to plot graphs of boys' and girls' growth. Plot one pair of graphs of height against age for boys and girls on the same sheet of paper. Plot a second pair showing annual increase in height against age.
When is growth fastest?
What other changes are occurring during the periods of rapid growth?

In the activity above you were asked to plot heights and weights for both boys and girls throughout infancy and childhood. More complex versions of the graphs you have drawn are used by health professionals to monitor growth in children. Centile charts show not only the averages but also the ranges within which 94% of children fall.

Centile charts: *graphs that show the average pattern of growth (height, weight, head circumference, etc.). Each chart has statistical details of the normal ranges for the growth pattern displayed. The second graphs you drew make the periods of rapid growth easier to see.*

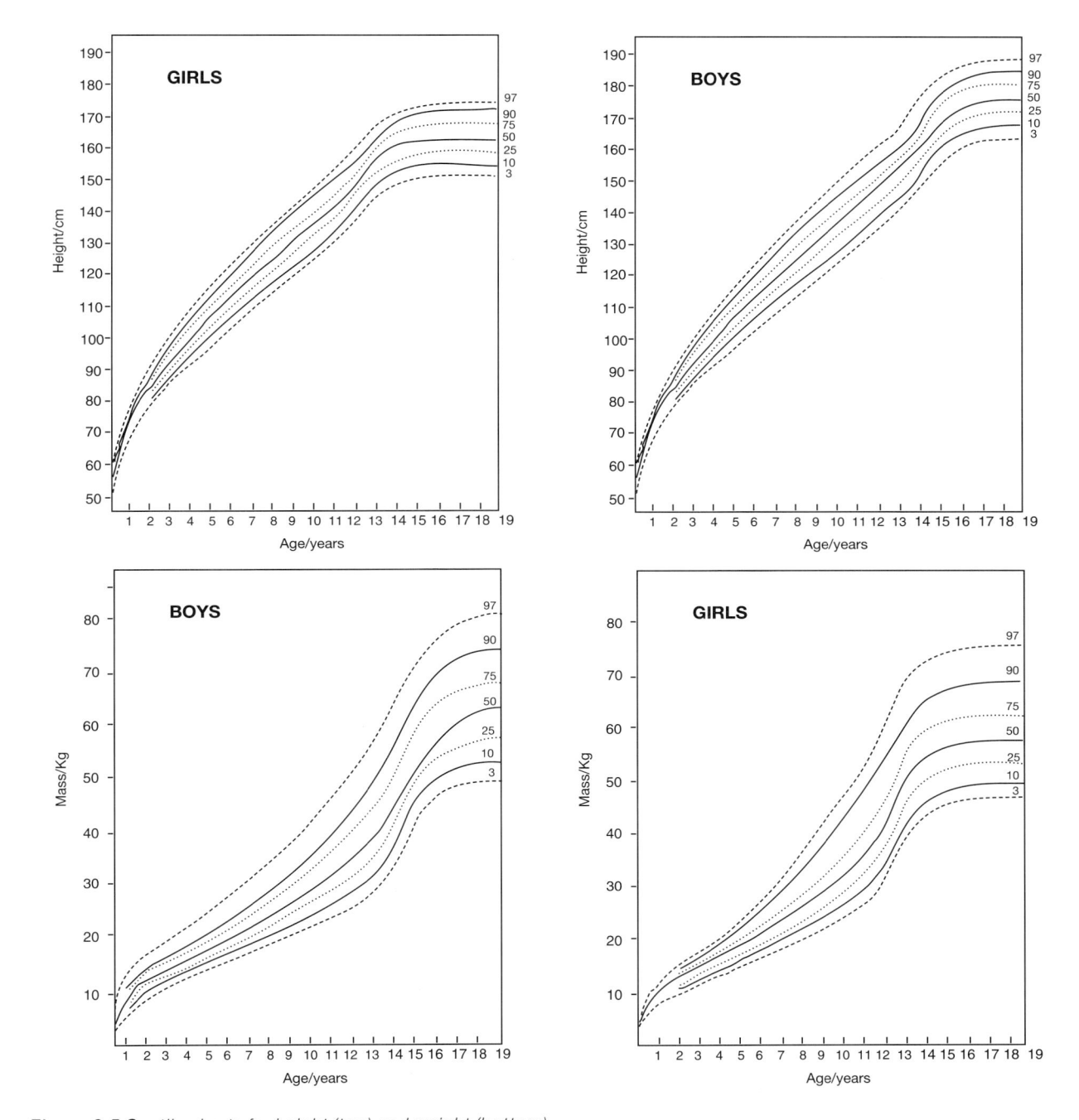

Figure 2.5 Centile charts for height (top) and weight (bottom)

The early period of rapid growth after birth is slower than the growth in the womb. However, it is a period of great physical development. The development is related to the changes in co-ordination. New-born babies are unable to do much independently. By the age of five, children are able to exercise control of the large movements (gross motor control) and delicate controlled movements (fine motor control) associated with walking and feeding themselves.

After the early period of rapid growth, the rate of growth levels out: growth continues but by about the same amount each month. It is an important time for physical development, as many physical skills are being developed and refined. Table 2.1 summarises some of these developments in the first five years.

Health and social well-being

Table 2.1 Aspects of physical development

MOTOR DEVELOPMENT — THIS DESCRIBES THE CHANGES IN THE CHILD'S ABILITY TO MOVE, FOR EXAMPLE CRAWLING, WALKING AND RUNNING.

Age	Motor development
1 month	Large jerky movements of limbs. When held in sitting position, head falls forward. Makes reflex stepping movements when held in standing position.
3 months	Limb movements smoother. Kicks vigorously. If placed downwards on face, lifts head and upper chest using forearms as support. When held in standing position, sags at knees.
6 months	Lifts legs and grasps foot. Sits with support. Holds up arms to be lifted. Can roll over, front to back. If held in sitting position, head is firmly erect and back straight. When held in standing position, baby bears weight on feet and bounces up and down.
9 months	Sits alone. Can turn body to look sideways. Attempts to crawl. Pulls self to standing position with support. If held in standing position, steps purposefully on alternate feet.
12 months	Can rise to sitting position from lying down. Walks with one or both hands held. May walk alone.
15 months	Walks unevenly, feet wide apart and arms held out to balance. Bumps into furniture. Crawls upstairs. Kneels. Stoops to pick up toys from floor.
18 months	Walks well and starts and stops safely. Runs. Pushes and pulls large toys round floor. Walks upstairs with help. Creeps backwards downstairs. Can carry a large toy while walking.
2 years	Runs safely. Walks backwards pulling a large toy. Climbs on furniture to reach things and can get down again. Walks up and down stairs holding on to rail. Throws small ball. Sits astride large wheeled toys and propels them forward with feet on the ground.
3 years	Walks upstairs alone with alternating feet usually jumps from the bottom step when coming downstairs. Can turn round obstacles and corners whilst running and pushing large toys. Rides tricycle. Can walk on tiptoe. Sits with feet crossed at ankles.
4 years	Climbs ladders and trees. Can run on tiptoe. Hops on one foot. Expert tricycle rider.
5 years	Runs lightly on toes. Skips on alternate feet. Dances to music. Can stand on one foot and hop. Active and skilful in climbing, sliding, swinging, digging and various 'stunts'.

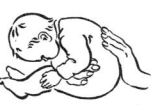

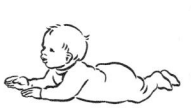

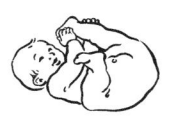

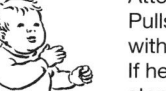

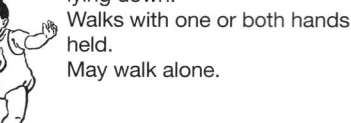

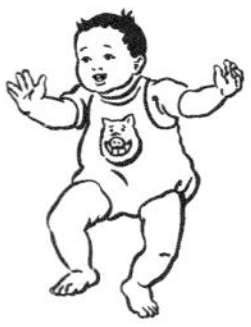

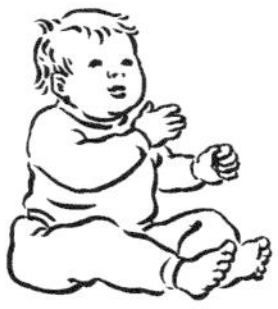

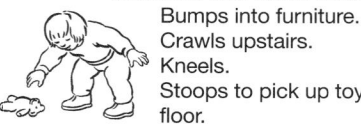

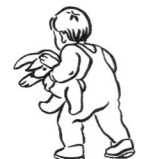

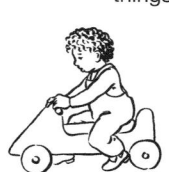

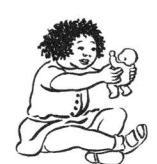

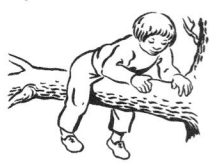

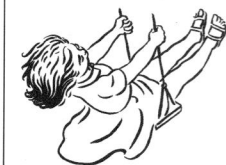

HAND-EYE CO-ORDINATION — THE SKILLS OF SIGHT AND MANIPULATION. WORKING TOGETHER, FOR EXAMPLE SEEING AN OBJECT AND GRASPING IT WITH THE HAND.

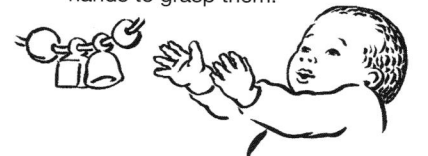

Age	Hand-eye co-ordination
1 month	Not yet able to control hands.
3 months	Watches own hands moving.
6 months	Fixates eyes on interesting small objects within 15 to 30 cm and stretches out both hands to grasp them.
9 months	Stretches out, one hand leading, to grasp small objects immediately on catching sight of them. Has learnt to co-ordinate hand-eye movements to pick up objects. 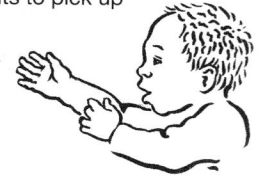

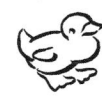

Health and social well-being

SENSORY DEVELOPMENT — THE DEVELOPMENT OF THE SENSES OF SIGHT, HEARING, SMELL AND TASTE.

Age	Sensory development
1 month	Turns head and eyes towards light. Follows light briefly with eyes. Shuts eyes tightly when light is shone directly into them. Eyes follow a dangling toy. Looks at mother's face while feeding. Startled by sudden loud noises. Stops whimpering at sound of human voice or when picked up.
3 months	Visually very alert. Very interested in human faces. Follows adults' movements with head and eyes. Watches movements of own hands. Sudden loud noises still cause distress. Turns head and eyes towards sound, brows wrinkle and pupils dilate. Shows excitement at sound of approaching footsteps.
6 months	Moves head and eyes eagerly in every direction to see objects and people. Eyes move in unison. Forgets toys that move out of sight. Turns immediately to mother's voice. Responds to baby hearing tests. Takes everything to mouth.

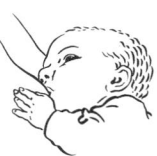

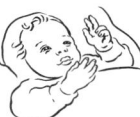

Age	Sensory development
9 months	Very observant. Watches activities of adults, children and animals within 2 or 3 metres with eager interest. Immediate response to baby hearing tests. Enjoys peek-a-boo games. Finds hidden toys.
12 months	Looks in correct places for toys which roll out of sight. Finds hidden toys quickly. Throws toys deliberately and watches them fall to the ground. Watches movements with interest. Recognises familiar people approaching from far away. Knows and immediately responds to own name. Listens with obvious pleasure to percussion sounds.
15 months	Looks with interest at pictures in books. Stands at window and watches events outside for several minutes.
18 months	Touches and recognises own nose, eyes, ears.

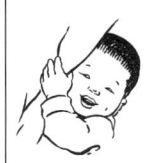

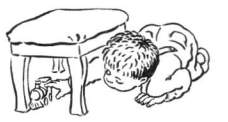

Age	Sensory development
2 years	Enjoys picture books, recognising favourite pictures and turns pages singly. Recognises familiar adults in photographs.
3 years	Matches 2 or 3 primary colours. Listens eagerly to stories and demands favourites over and over again. Recognises minute details in picture books. Recognises self in photographs.
4 years	Matches 4 primary colours correctly.
5 years	Matches 10 to 12 colours correctly. Loves stories.

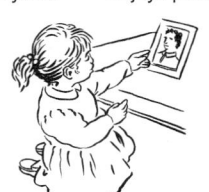

MANIPULATIVE SKILLS — LEARNING HOW TO USE THE HANDS.

Age	Manipulative skills
1 month	Hands tightly clenched and will only open when touched. Grasps finger.
3 months	Begins to clasp and unclasp hands together in finger play.
6 months	Uses whole hand to grasp objects.
9 months	Pokes at small objects with index finger. Grasps sweets, string between finger and thumb in scissors fashion. Passes objects from hand to hand.
12 months	Picks up small objects such as sweets and string with precise pincer grasp of thumb and index finger. Points with index finger at objects which interest. Uses both hands.

Age	Manipulative skills
15 months	Picks up string, small sweets and crumbs neatly with thumb and finger. Builds a tower of 2 cubes. Grasps crayon and imitates scribble.
18 months	Picks up beads, pins, threads immediately on sight with delicate pincer grasp. When given paper and crayon scribbles immediately using preferred hand. Builds a tower of 3 cubes.
2 years	Removes wrapping paper from small sweets. Builds a tower of 6 or more cubes. Hand preference becoming evident. May be left- or right-handed.

Age	Manipulative skills
3 years	Builds a tower of 9 cubes also a bridge of 3 bricks if shown how. Can close fist and wiggle thumb in imitation. Cuts with scissors.
4 years	Builds a tower of 10 or more cubes and bridges of 3 bricks on request. Builds 3 steps with 6 cubes after demonstration. Imitates spreading of hand and bringing thumb to each finger in turn.
5 years	Builds 3 steps with cubes. Counts fingers on one hand with index finger of other.

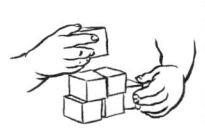

73

Health and social well-being

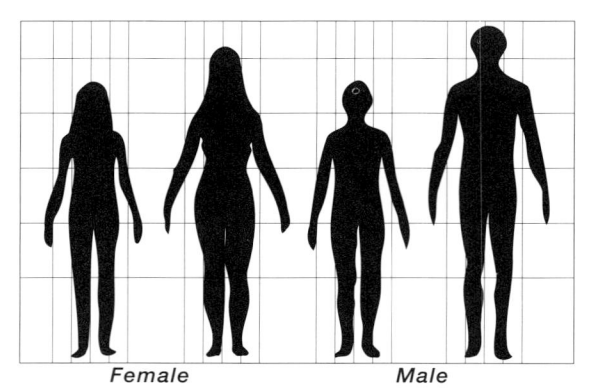

Figure 2.6 Changes in body shape and proportion, of boys and girls before and after puberty

Growth in puberty

The second period of rapid growth occurs during puberty. This is the period of physiological transition from childhood to adulthood. During this period four important physical changes occur:
- changes in body size
- changes in hip and shoulder proportions
- maturing of reproductive organs
- development of secondary sexual characteristics.

Some of these changes are shown here.

Table 2.2 Changes occurring at puberty

BOYS	GIRLS
Hair Pubic hair appears followed by underarm hair and beard and body hair.	**Hair** Pubic hair appears after hips and breasts start to develop (see below). Underarm hair appears after menarche (first menstruation).
Skin The skin becomes coarser, less transparent, and sallow in colour, and the pores enlarge.	**Skin** The skin becomes coarser, thicker, and slightly sallow, and the pores enlarge.
Glands Oil-producing (sebaceous) glands in the skin become active. Sweat glands under arms and in the groin produce nutrient rich sweat. Bacterial growth can cause body odour.	**Glands** Oil producing (sebaceous) glands become active. Sweat glands under arms and in the groin produce nutrient rich sweat. Bacterial growth can cause body odour. Sweat levels follow the menstrual cycle.
Muscles The muscles increase markedly in size and strength, thus giving shape to the arms, legs, and shoulders.	**Muscles** The muscles increase in size and strength, especially in the middle of puberty and towards the end, thus giving shape to the shoulders, arms, and legs.
Voice Voice changes begin after pubic hair has grown. The voice deepens. Breaking (uncontrolled shifts between high to deep voice) occurs during this period.	**Voice** The voice becomes rounded. Breaking rarely occurs.
	Hips The hips become wider and rounder. Under skin (subcutaneous) fat deposits contribute to rounding.
	Breasts Breasts enlarge as the mammary (milk producing) glands develop. Nipples also become larger.

The maturing of the sex organs means that boys start to produce sperm and girls release eggs. This normally occurs in the early teens, although it has become earlier over the last century. In girls this is marked by menarche, the first menstruation.

Menarche: *the first menstruation. The first time that the lining of the uterus is shed with some blood loss.*

It normally takes time for the menstrual cycle to settle down and so egg release and subsequent menstruation do not initially follow a regular pattern.

The control of the developments during puberty is by hormones. In boys the major sex hormone is testosterone. In girls the controlling hormones are oestrogen and progesterone. The levels of these two hormones control the timing of the release of the egg in each 'monthly' cycle. In both sexes the growth in height is controlled by the growth hormone somatotropin.

Early adulthood

After rapid growth during puberty, the bones continue to grow slowly until the growing points turn from cartilage to bone. This normally happens in the early twenties. It is slightly earlier for women than men. At this point the growth function winds down to one of repair and restoration. In particular, the bones can still be remodelled and change shape to support changes in physical activity. Where a form of regular exercise puts stresses and strains on the bone, it changes shape to compensate.

Early adulthood is a period of peak function for many body systems. The circulatory system, respiratory system and muscles are working at maximum efficiency. The repair functions work well and injuries heal rapidly.

Mid-life adult

In mid-life and beyond, the repair function becomes less effective and the time taken for broken bones to mend becomes greater. This is linked to the turn-over time for replacing tissues. This begins to show as ageing of skin and the formation of wrinkles. Muscle function reduces and the speed of nerve transmission decreases. The flexibility of joints reduces, elasticity of tissues reduces, causing the efficiency of the respiratory and circulatory systems to come down from their peaks. The amount of change and the rate of change depends to a large extent on how active and fit a person has been. These changes, however, cannot be stopped.

▶ Lifestyle profile, page 4

Menopause

One particular event has a major effect on women. At some point in mid-life a woman goes through the menopause.

Menopause: *the time during which the ovaries stop producing eggs. During the menopause egg production becomes irregular and the production of hormones by the ovaries comes to an end.*

This is the time during which the ovaries cease to release their eggs and there are major changes in sex hormone levels. The ovaries cease to produce the hormones oestrogen and progesterone. The small amounts of testosterone produced by the adrenal glands begin to have an effect.

In particular the hormone changes affect the use of calcium. This leads to the loss of some calcium from the skeleton and a consequent loss of height. In extreme cases the calcium loss causes severe weakening of the bones (osteoporosis).

This physiologically traumatic period (time of dramatic alterations in body chemistry) leads to some rapid changes. The effects of the hormonal changes on the skeleton and the elasticity of tissues (particularly the skin) may be controlled by hormone replacement therapy (giving artificial sex hormones to replace those not being produced by the ovaries). This does not stop the menopause but it enables the systems to adjust slowly to the changes brought about by hormonal levels.

A consequence of the menopause is the end of a woman's ability to have children naturally. There is no equivalent of the menopause for men. Although sperm production does reduce with age, men are able to produce viable sperm throughout their life. The changes do not mean that sexual activity stops and both sexes are still able to gain satisfaction from sexual intercourse.

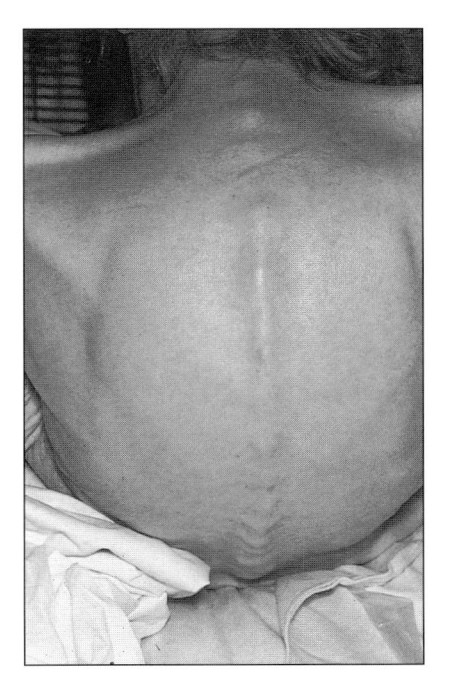

Figure 2.7 'Dowager's hump': the spine of an elderly woman deformed due to osteoporosis, a loss of bony tissue due to lack of calcium salts

Health and social well-being

Old age
Physically, old age demonstrates the gradual deterioration of the processes already described. In simple terms, the tissues become less elastic and repair functions reduce.

Some of the consequences are:

- repair functions
  - cells are not replaced so quickly
  - wounds take longer to heal
  - cell loss does not match cell replacement (men lose 10% of body mass between 65 and 90)
  - kidney efficiency drops to about 50% of its peak
  - the skeleton loses calcium and becomes brittle – this leads to loss in height
  - toxic materials and cholesterol accumulate in cells.
- loss of elasticity
  - skin becomes thinner and wrinkled
  - ligaments and tendons become hard, thus reducing joint flexibility and causing stooping
  - arteries lose flexibility (hardening of the arteries) and blood pressure increases
  - the eyes have a reduced focal range as the lens shape becomes fixed
  - ears have a reduced frequency response and so high notes in particular cannot be heard
  - the biggest breath size drops to half its peak and the speed of breathing out slows (both reduce the ability to supply oxygen during exercise).

Figure 2.8 Old age represents a slowing down of bodily functions

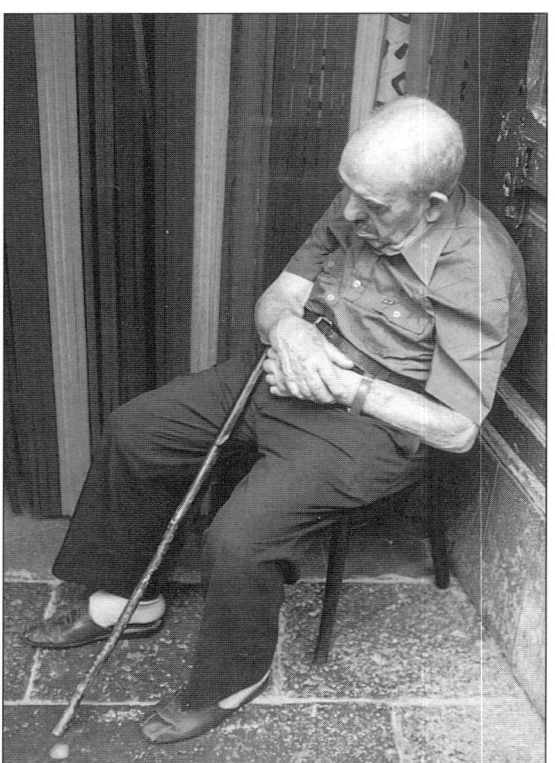

A Growth patterns

The data (left) show the growth pattern for men and women. The heights are expressed as a percentage of maximum height.

Plot the data on a graph with age in years on the x-axis and height (% of maximum) on the y-axis.

Mark these stages on your graph:
- infancy/childhood – bones still contain much cartilage and retain some flexibility. Period of steady growth. Marrow takes on the role of blood cell production.
- puberty – a period of rapid elongation of bone with an associated height increase. Calcium levels increase to almost adult proportions.
- adulthood – bones stop growing, cartilage-based growing points (epiphyses) take in calcium and stop growing. Maximum height attained.
- menopause in women – hormonal changes can cause loss of calcium from bone and consequential fragility and also loss of height. Hormonal treatment and an appropriate diet can reduce and stop this.
- both sexes – loss of elasticity in cartilage and some loss of calcium causes loss of height.

AGE YEARS	HEIGHT %OF MAX MALE	HEIGHT %OF MAX FEMALE
0	29.0	30.7
1	44.4	47.5
2	49.9	52.5
3	55.0	57.4
4	59.1	61.7
5	62.6	66.1
6	65.4	69.8
7	69.9	73.5
8	73.0	77.2
9	76.2	80.3
10	79.4	84.0
11	82.3	87.9
12	85.2	92.0
13	88.1	96.9
14	93.3	99.1
15	97.7	100.0
16	100.0	100.0
20	100.0	100.0
30	100.0	100.0
45	100.0	100.0
50	99.0	98.5
60	98.5	97.0
68	98.0	95.5

Social, emotional and intellectual development

Development in these areas is not so clear-cut and patterns are influenced by other people and the environment. In this section we will briefly describe some key features. The rest of the unit provides links with factors that affect **intellectual, social** and emotional **development.**

Intellectual development is determined by the potential a person is born with (genetic make up) and their experiences during life. It is difficult to determine which factors are most important, although it is a regular subject for debate. What can be said is that although it is not yet possible to control genetic inheritance, it is possible to provide an environment to promote intellectual development. The provision of a supportive environment often depends upon a variety of social and cultural factors.

As these areas (intellectual, social and emotional) are so variable, it is

▶ Socialisation, page 99

FOCUS

Intellectual development:
- knowledge, thinking (cognition)
- language
- memory.

FOCUS

Social development:
- co-operation
- relationships.

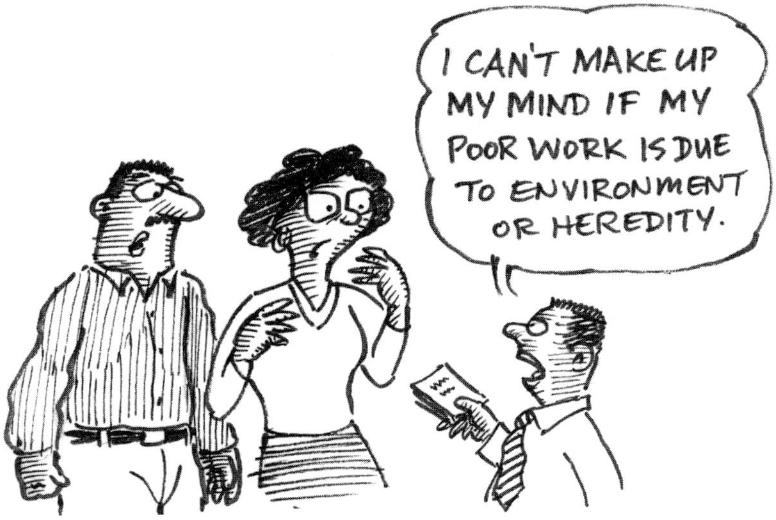

Figure 2.9 Intellectual development is determined by both heredity and environment

not possible to describe development throughout life with any degree of certainty. It is, however, possible to describe development in the early years of an average child. Table 2.3 gives some of the highlights of development across a range of areas in the early years. From the table it is clear this is a period of rapid development.

Bonding

An aspect of **emotional development** that is very important from birth is bonding. This is a process of emotional attachment that occurs between parent and child from birth. When a child is born its eyesight is very weak: it has a very limited ability to focus. The first sensations it would naturally feel are those of the mother holding it. Breastfeeding provides further opportunities for the baby to see, smell and touch its mother. The bonding provided by this early close contact gives the child feelings of security, and the mother develops the protective emotional support that the child needs.

Bonding also occurs with other people who provide a secure comforting environment. Significant people involved in the bonding can be the father and other family members or, where the child has to he cared for in an incubator, the support may be supplied by medical staff. It is important that the child has contact with the parents (or future carers) to help establish the bonds.

FOCUS

Emotional development:
- bonding
- self-confidence
- independence.

Table 2.3 Social, intellectual and emotional development in the early years

Age	Intellectual development	Emotional development	Social development
Birth	Responds to light, sound and touch.	Cries in response to hunger, pain and thirst.	Sleeps much of the time.
1 month	Responds to sounds especially new, simple sounds.	Cries with no differentiation as to cause.	Sleeps up to 20 hours per day. Responds to being picked up.
3 months	Face of carer(s) recognised. Anticipates pleasure, smiles.	Differentiates between carer(s) and strangers. Cries for carer to return.	Positive response to carer. Anticipates pleasure, e.g. feeding.
6 months	Responds to speech. Vocalises and cries differently for hunger. Turns to speaker.	Clear preference for primary carer. Shows anger and frustration, etc.	Explores environment by putting things in mouth.
9 months	Vocalises with some recognisable sounds, e.g. mama, dada. Understands single words, e.g. no.	Recognises familiar people. Likes routine to be maintained.	Plays peek-a-boo. Shakes and squeezes objects. Starts to hold drinking cup.
1 year	Recognises own name. Obeys simple instructions. Uses 5 words with meaning.	Laughs and shows affection. Hugs and kisses familiar people.	Drinks without help from a cup. Holds spoon but cannot use it.
1½ years	Uses up to 20 words consistently. Enjoys repetetive word games and nursery rhymes. Holds crayons in fist. Handedness may show.	Affectionate with familiar people.	Uses spoon to feed self. Holds cup and hands it back. Starts to be able to undress self.
2 years	Uses 50+ words, with understanding of many more. Some simple sentences used.	Awareness of self and own wants. May show temper if crossed. Very demanding for attention of primary carer.	Refers to self by name. Plays in parallel with other children. Asks for drinks and food.
2½ years	Uses 200+ words. Sentences are often questions. A period of enquiry and thirst for information	Still very dependent on adults for emotional cues. Unwilling to share things and people.	Eats with spoon and sometimes fork without spilling.
3 years	Capable of simple conversations. Still constantly asking questions. Likes repetition of favourite stories and recognises change in story.	Begins to be able to share things and people. Can show affection for younger siblings.	Eats with spoon and fork. Some attempts to copy adult use of knife.
4 years	Retells stories heard 3+ times. Repeats familiar nursery rhymes. Pre-writing skills using pretend writing.	Can share things and people. Start of co-operative play.	Able to dress self. Can take turns with other children.
5 years	Writing, reading and number skills developing.	Able to describe own feelings – sad, happy. Early signs of empathy in comforting friends.	Plays games with others and describes rules. Starts compulsory education and develops associated social skills.

Bonding may start at birth, but it also occurs throughout life. Where people establish an emotional relationship, then bonding can occur. This is reinforced with formal ceremonies acknowledging the bond (e.g. marriage, adoption). It is also reinforced by actions. Courtship is a process which helps establish bonding between people. The various expressions of love and giving of presents are open demonstrations of the bonding process. When two people decide they wish to develop a sexual relationship, then making love helps to establish and maintain bonding between the couple (pair bonding).

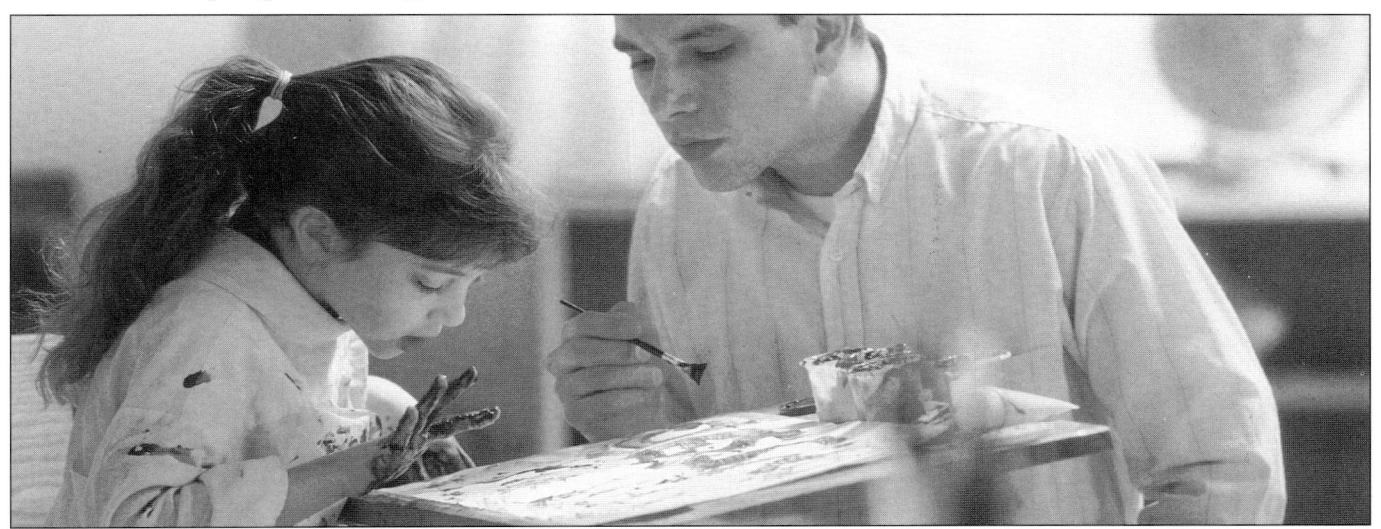

Figure 2.10 Bonding provides both physical and emotional support

Once bonding has been established, it is normally reinforced regularly: a parent continues to provide emotional and physical support for a child. Long periods of separation can alter the relationship and reduce the level of bonding and may lead to feelings of rejection in the people involved. Long stays in hospital should involve regular contact to ensure that feelings of rejection are reduced.

Attachments between the child and its parents (and other close family members) appear to be fully developed by about seven months of age. When a baby is younger than this, they do not show anxiety or distress when the parent leaves. By the age of seven months the infant cries if left with a stanger, or if the parents leave. This shows the child has developed an attachment bond with the parents.

The formation of an attachment bond is a gradual, two-way process. Babies communicate their needs by smiling, crying, making eye-contact and grasping. Parents respond to the needs of their babies by feeding, holding, touching, smiling and comforting. As they interact with each other, a bond is developed.

From the age of two to three years, children become more independent from their parents. By the age of five, when they start school, their peer group (children of the same age) will become important to them and the bonds of friendship will develop. These do not replace the bonds they have with their parents, but are added to them.

When a child leaves home and establishes a life outside the family home, the nature of the bond changes. For many parents this change is a very emotional one. If managed well by both sides, bonding remains. If the change creates conflict, then feelings of anger and rejection can damage the emerging, new relationships.

Language development

In many families the first child relies on adult input to learn a language. Subsequent children have siblings (brothers and/or sisters) as role models. This can lead to rapid speech development. Often it can lead to the youngest child developing successful communication through body language and sounds without developing a formal language.

Stages in acquiring language

C Case study: Adam, Eve and Sarah

In 1973, a detailed study was made of the way children acquire language in their pre-school years. The study was a close look at three children (Adam, Eve and Sarah) and their speech was recorded for four hours every month, throughout their first five years. By getting a set of recordings at regular intervals, in this way, it was possible to see the way the children's speech *gradually* developed, and the stages that the children went through.

It was found that children's language development could be roughly divided into five stages, and that at each stage the children would use different types of sentences, gradually increasing in difficulty. In the first stage, children tend to say only two-word sentences, which might involve possession: 'my ball'; absence: 'all gone ball'; or a simple description of an action: 'Adam hit ball'. The things that they say tend to relate simply to objects around them.

By the second stage, the language is beginning to get more complicated. They might say things like: 'that a book', or use a verb in the past tense: 'Adam walked'. although the sentences are still simple two-word ones for the most part, they have started to use endings on words, instead of just saying the simple word on its own: 'I walking', or 'Adam's ball'.

At the third stage, they have begun to ask the 'why' questions; what. where, why, and so on. They have also started to ask other kinds of questions too, like: 'Does Eve like it?' and 'Where did Sarah hide?'.

The fourth stage is even more complicated: they will tend to use simple sentences involving more than one clause: 'Who is that playing the xylophone?'. Before this stage, if they wanted to ask the same question, they would have probably made two sentences: 'Who that?' 'Play xylophone'. But by this time they can join the two together into one sentence.

In the fifth stage, they have learned to use conjunctions as well, which means that they can join sentences together: 'I did this and I did that too', and they can have more than one subject in a sentence: 'You and I play over here', or 'John and Jay are Boy Scouts'. By this time, they are well on the way to being able to cope with school, with learning to read and the formal kind of language that they will meet there. In short, by this time they have developed the language skills which they will need; they can turn a sentence around if they want to, changing 'that's your cat' to 'is that your cat?', or mix together two sentences which deal with the same thing; 'Mary who lives over there goes to our school', instead of 'Mary lives over there' and 'Mary goes to our school'. They can use their language as they want to.

Questions
1. Draw up a table of the five stages of language development. Write down at what age you think a child reaches each stage. Compare answers and check with your teacher.
2. Discuss in a group why learning language is so important. In your group list all the ways in which you have experienced language today.

The early years are a time when it is easiest to acquire language. It is also a time when a second language can be developed with some ease. Formal teaching of English as a second language has been recognised in the UK, and funding was supplied to support New Commonwealth Immigrants and their families to learn English. Sometimes the formal input needed was minimal.

C Case study: Lee

Lee was the son of two university students from China. His parents spoke Mandarin (a Chinese language) and English. He started in a nursery class when he was three and a half. He was able to speak both Mandarin and English. In the nursery class almost all of the children were learning English as a second language. Most of them spoke Punjabi (a South Asian language) as their first language.

In the nursery few children spoke English and no other child spoke Mandarin. After about four months in the nursery, Lee was observed playing with two friends. One of his friends spoke Punjabi and the other spoke Malay and some English. Lee was speaking English to one friend and Punjabi to the other. In four months he had learned enough of a new language to communicate in it. He had learned three spoken languages before he was four years old.

Lee's acquisition of language was slightly unusual, but almost all of the children in the nursery were learning English as a second language and many started the nursery unable to understand any English at all. It would have been interesting to see if Lee was able to learn to write all three languages, as they all use different characters. Unfortunately, his parents finished their courses at the university and Lee left the country before he learned to write.

Questions
1. Why do you think that Lee was able to learn to speak the different languages?
2. How easy do you think it would be for you to learn to speak these same languages at your age?

Child development

A Child watching

When you watch a pre-school child in a nursery, playgroup or at home, involved in the kind of activities that pre-school children like, how do you make an assessment of how old the child is? What behaviour do you focus on? What skills do you look for? What other evidence do you use to assess the child's development?

1. **(a)** First, on your own, make a list of the kinds of evidence you would look for.
   (b) Share and compare lists with the group and modify your list as appropriate.
   (c) Use your list to create a check list for observing children. Supply key details of the evidence you would use to indicate that a child was two, three, four or five years old.

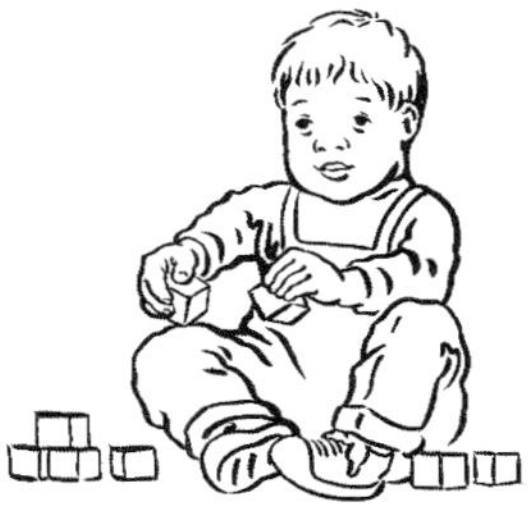

Health and social well-being

Solitary play

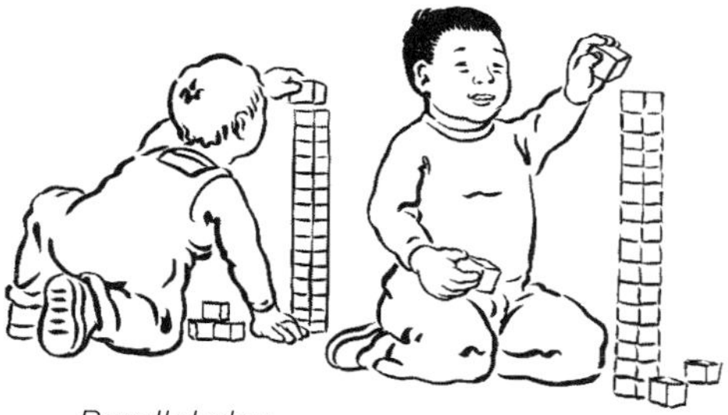

Parallel play

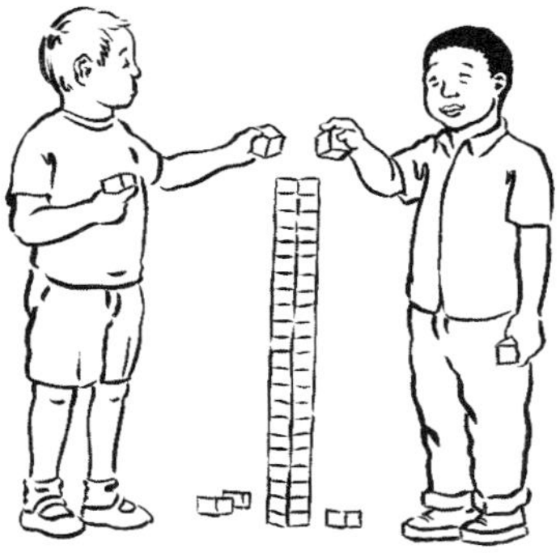

Co-operative play

Figure 2.12 *Developing levels of play*

For example, play develops from playing alone (solitary play) through playing side by side (parallel play) to playing together (co-operative play). The ages at which these types of play typically develop are:
- solitary – up to three years
- parallel – up to four years
- co-operative – four years and over.

2 With your agreed list, observe a young child very carefully for ten minutes (possibly on video). From your observations identify the key developmental stage indicators. Do all the things that you have observed indicate the same developmental stage?

How easy is it to guess the actual age of the child?

Why would it be unfair to determine the developmental age of a child from this single observation session?

A Children's toys

You are asked to design a toy/game to develop in small children the knowledge of shape and colour which also allows them to develop their manual dexterity. It should be fun!

You decide to use foam to produce large, light-weight shapes which you will cover in different coloured materials. The children can use these to build exciting models like houses, cars, ships, etc which they can sit on/in.

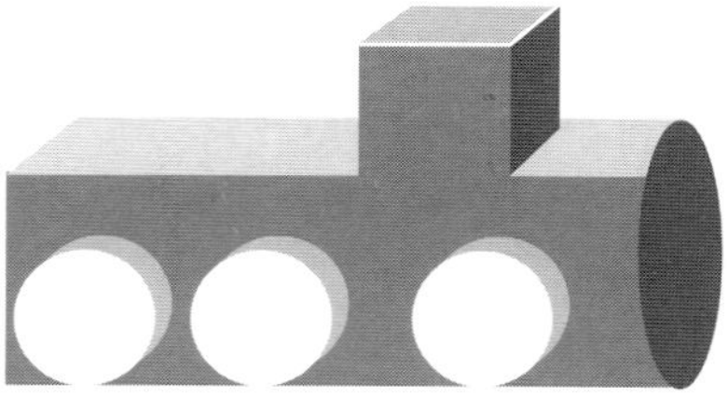

Figure 2.11 *A train?*

Produce drawings (to scale) of the shapes you will use, showing appropriate measurements.

By finding the surface areas of each of your shapes, find the minimum area of material you would need to cover each shape (do not worry about seam allowances!).

Find the volume of foam you would need for each shape.

The table below gives an example of a group of children with their actual (chronological) age, developmental age and the difference between the two. The statistics reflect the wide range of differences to be found amongst children.

Table 2.4 Developmental differences

Child	Actual age (yrs:mths)	Developmental age (yrs:mths)	Difference (yrs:mths)
Richard	4:3	4:6	+0:3
Charles	3:9	3:3	-0:6
Simon	4:2	4:0	-0:2
Ben	2:9	2:8	-0:1
Tessa	3:8	3:0	-0:8
Rachel	5:3	5:7	+0:4
Sarah	4:10	5:0	+0:2
Jo	5:5	5:4	-0:1
Laura	4:11	4:8	-0:3
Chris	5:3	4:7	-0:6

Developmental age: *the developmental age is the age indicated by looking at the developmental stage a child has reached in terms of his/her social, emotional and intellectual behaviour together with physical development.*

It is common for a child to be working at different developmental stages. For example, a very tall 5 years: 0 months child may be physically like an average 6 year old, socially like a 5 year old and intellectually like a 4 year old. Looking at developmental stages may be more useful than trying to determine a single figure for developmental age.

Even within the first five years of life, when it is reasonably easy to predict developmental sequences, there are great variations in timings. This wide variation is recognised, and health professionals (e.g. health visitors) tend to use the extremes (top and bottom 3% of the range) as an indication that further investigation might be in order.

This does not mean that the extremes of development are in any way wrong. It just means that the professionals need to assure themselves that the development is normal for that child and there are no underlying problems.

Case study: Kate

Kate was observed by the health visitor just before she started school. One of the things that she noted was Kate's height. Kate had always been short for her age. The health visitor had measured her regularly throughout her childhood. Each time she looked up her height on a centile chart she found that it was on the 3rd centile. That is, only 3% of children her age were shorter than her. Kate was maintaining a normal growth pattern even though she was small and the health visitor did not investigate further.

Although Kate's height was developmentally up to a year behind her actual age, this was not reflected in her intellectual, social and emotional development. If the health visitor had felt that these, too, were developmentally behind her age then she might have suggested a further investigation.

If Kate's height had moved, for example from the 3rd centile to the 1st, the health visitor would probably have wanted her to be seen by a doctor in case the change in the growth rate indicated that there was something wrong. If it had moved to the 1st centile, her growth rate would have been slowing down.

Centile charts, page 71

Development beyond the early years

Whilst it is relatively easy to predict a child's development in the early years, it is very difficult to be accurate in later life. The environment, in terms of physical, social and emotional factors provides many variables. Food availability, opportunities to be with other people and the amount of love received can all affect development in some way.

The following section identifies some of the important influences on development beyond the early years.

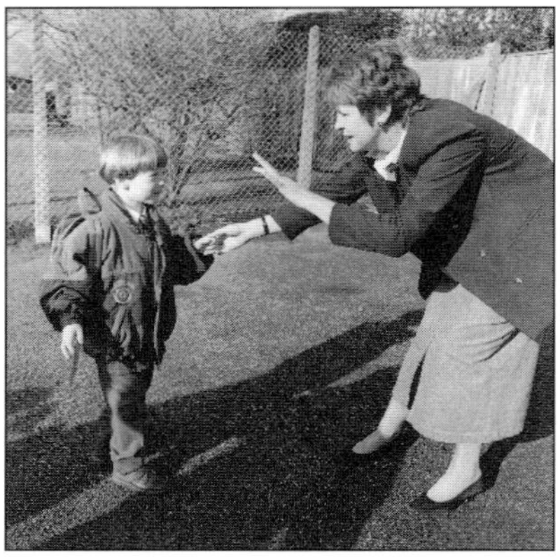

Childhood 5+

Going to school encourages children to focus their learning. Primary school experiences provide a foundation for later development.

Emotionally, starting school can present problems because of the separation from the parents. This stress can be reduced by careful preparation of the child before school. The transition can be supported by sympathetic attitudes from the school staff in their provision of emotional support. The stress is not only for the child but also for the parents.

The opportunities to mix with other children and to experience working with other adults mean that this is a time of rapid social development. The child is able to develop new relationships. This encourages an increased level of self reliance and can be a very positive experience. The staff in the school need to be very aware of the transition, and monitor individuals to provide the emotional support that they may need. Patterns of bullying can develop when children are under stress which lead to poor social development for both the bully and the victim.

Language development continues in school, in the development of reading and writing skills. When children first start learning to read they may pick up a book and 'read' it by telling the story from the pictures. They gradually start to recognise letters and words and finally learn how to sound out unfamiliar words. There are many different reading schemes in schools; can you remember which one you used?

Parents continue to have an important role in helping their children. If they regularly hear their children read, the children will make good progress, and this can be an enjoyable time together for parents and children.

Intellectual development is partly inherited, but is also influenced by schooling.

The National Curriculum provides a framework that describes what skills and knowledge should form part of an individual's learning environment. Even with this control of learning it is not possible to define what each child will be able to do at the end of Year 11. Each child will have been subject to a range of genetic and environmental influences that mean the range of achievement is broad. However, the National Curriculum does try to control one of the variables (the subjects and contents taught) and so increase children's chances of achieving certain learning outcomes.

The primary school years are ones in which the child is introduced to rules and discipline that are different from the home environment. The moral development (understanding of rules and right and wrong) of children at this age can have a significant effect on the later years. The Jesuits (members of a Roman Catholic teaching order) are credited with saying, 'Give me the child until he is seven, and I will give you the man.' This is a recognition of how the early years of a person's life can have a profound effect upon their intellectual, social emotional and spiritual development.

Figure 2.13 Starting school is an emotional time for both parents and children

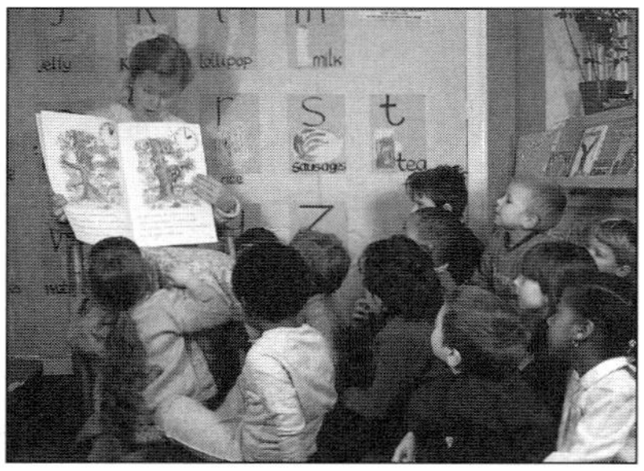

Figure 2.14 School presents a wealth of opportunities and experiences

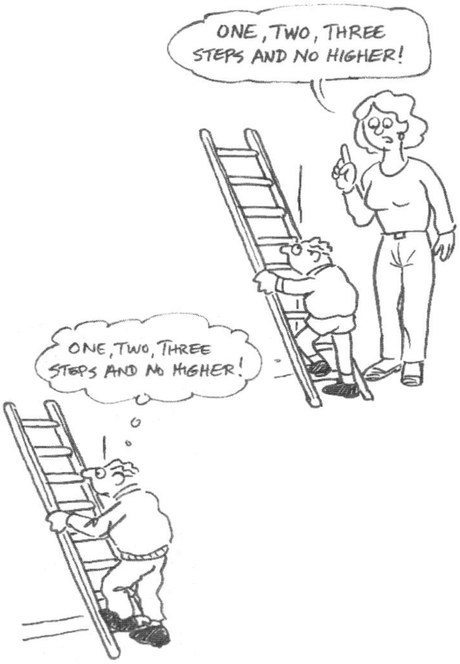

Figure 2.15 Things learned in early life will often stay with us. An instruction about safety is often remembered even when the adult can make their own decisions about safety – a simple example of socialisation

A Starting school

Almost everyone in the UK goes through the experience of starting school twice, usually at the ages of five and on starting secondary school. Some children, for a variety of reasons, attend a series of schools, for varying lengths of time. These may include the children of armed forces personnel, people seeking employment or accepting promotion, for instance.

How far does the experience offer a fresh start, how far is it likely to affect existing contentment? What can it do to self-confidence, relationships and a sense of security?

(a) In small groups decide what you think are the main positive and negative aspects of starting a new school. Distinguish between starting school and changing schools if your group thinks this is important.

(b) In the same group compile a questionnaire that can be used with three different generations, to see if the starting school experience seems to be constant or not. Analyse your questionnaires.

(c) Arrange an interview with one representative of each generation to talk about the experience of starting a new school. You could ask them about the short-term consequences of starting a new school. They may agree to record the interview.

(d) As a group, arrange to interview parents and teachers about the ways they try/tried to prepare children for starting a new school.

Adolescence

Puberty is defined in biological terms as the change to sexual maturity. Adolescence is defined by society. It is the time during which a child becomes an adult. In the UK this is normally said to be between the ages of twelve and eighteen. This transition period is recognised with the different ages of consent (16 to get married, 17 to drive a car, 18 to buy alcohol). In other cultures the transition may be marked by a ceremony determined by the age of the person: after this time the person is considered to be adult, with adult rights and responsibilities.

Emotional changes

Adolescence is associated with emotional changes. The hormonal changes of puberty and the evidence of sexual maturity can create high levels of internal confusion and conflict. It is a period of mood swings that are confusing to the adolescent. The developing sexual maturity also means that friendships can become more intense. This is a time when sexual orientation may be established, even if it is not expressed.

As a transition to adulthood, adolescence is a period during which boundaries are challenged. An adolescent person may well question or reject parental beliefs and standards. This is part of the process of developing personal moral standards and a moral code.

For parents, the challenges and questioning make them justify or review their beliefs. The period of adolescence is a time during which the parents have to acknowledge the developing physical, social and emotional maturity of their children. It can create very strong emotions as many of the primary parental roles recede.

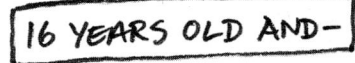

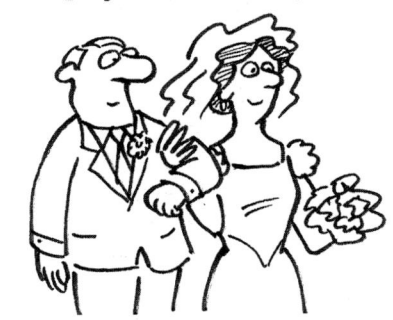

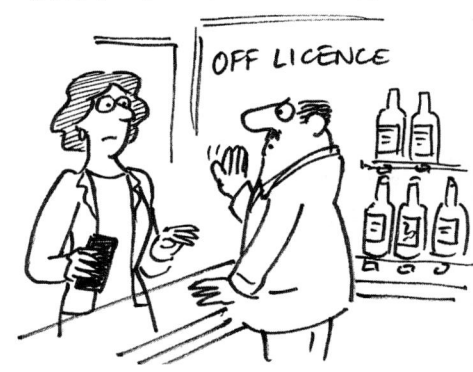

Figure 2.16 Adolescence is defined by society

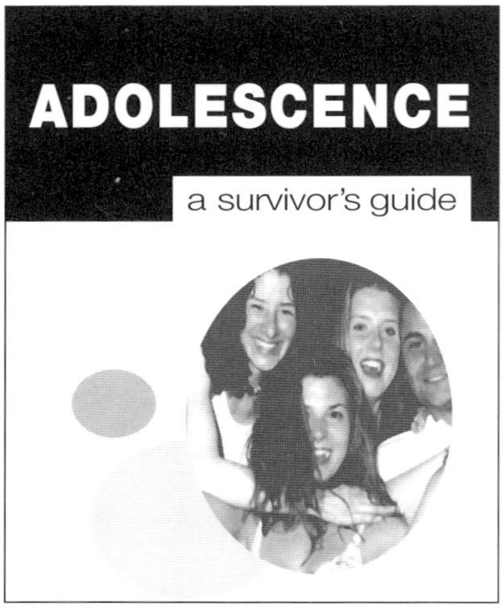

Health and social well-being

Figure 2.17 What would you include in this guide?

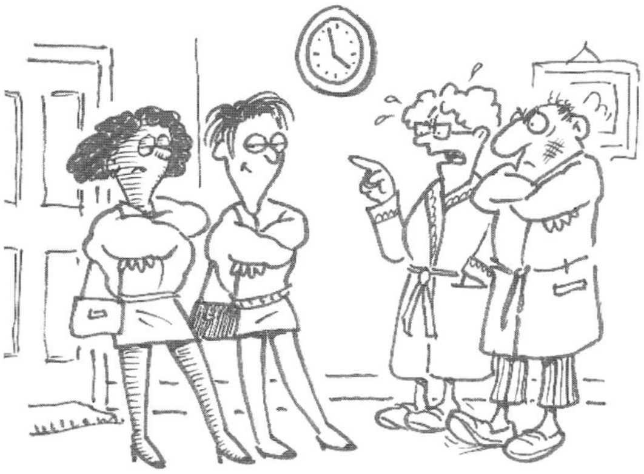

Figure 2.18 Adolescence is a time when rules are challenged and boundaries pushed back

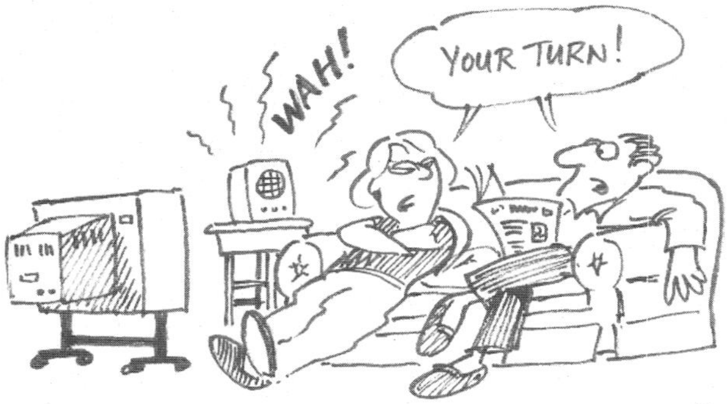

Figure 2.19 Starting a family alters relationships between partners

A Surviving adolescence

If you had to write a guide to surviving adolescence what would you include in it?

This activity can be a very personal one and requires you to review your own adolescence. As such, you are not expected to talk about things which you feel are too intimate, but it could be very useful for you to discuss your general findings with other members of your group.

You should try to review not only your own experiences, but also discuss with parents or carers how they felt about your adolescence, and the issues it raised for them.

Who has had the biggest influence on you during adolescence?

Who has provided you with support? How do you feel about your adolescence now? What are the biggest changes that have happened to you? This could be recorded as a letter to a real or imaginary friend, or as a diary.

A time of challenge

Adolescence is a period when there are opportunities to challenge parental values. This can express itself as experimentation with new experiences (e.g. 'sex 'n' drugs 'n' rock 'n' roll'!). How have you reacted to these situations? What positive things have you gained from the experience of adolescence?

Conflicts with authority figures and identification with peer groups can mean that formal education systems are challenged or rejected. The eagerness to learn that is a characteristic of young children can be replaced by a range of attitudes. These can mean that academic achievement falls away, or improves. Peer–group pressure can mean that there is pressure not to conform to the demands of formal education: it is important to recognise that intellectual development is not confined to school.

Adolescence is a period of experiencing, and learning from, change. It is often important for teenagers to be able to talk to someone outside the home environment. Most schools and colleges make counselling available to students. Other organisations offer similar services to people going through some of the strains of adolescence.

Early adulthood

Social changes in adulthood are associated with moving away from the childhood home to establish a position in a new social group. Traditionally, reasons for moving away have been: getting married, starting work, moving for education. All of these lead to the establishment of new social relationships with relations and colleagues.

Moving away from the parental home also implies financial independence and taking more responsibility for decision making. Financial independence implies a move into employment and the need to follow the disciplines involved in that.

For many people, early adulthood also means starting a family. The changes this involves alter relationships between partners and others. Social and emotional relationships alter, with the added considerations and demands of a child becoming a member of the family. The additional financial implications of taking responsibility for housing and care can affect social and emotional development. Being a parent introduces an individual to membership of another group.

Mid-life

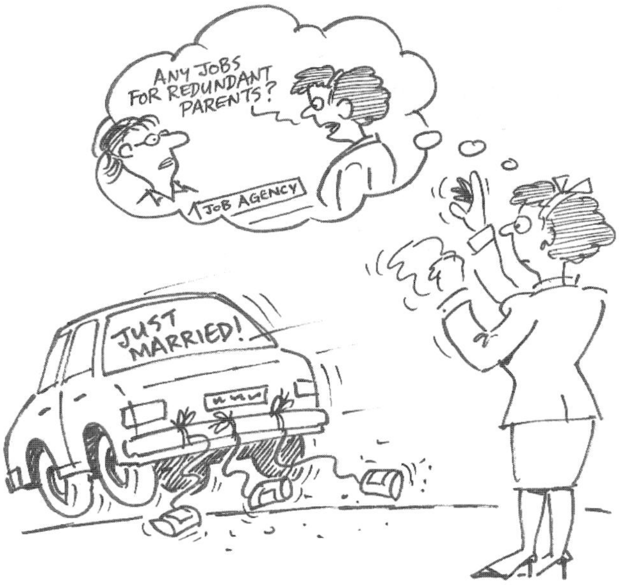

Mid-life is possibly best characterised by the move from being parents looking after children, to being parents of children who have left home. In some respects it is a return to the freedom of the time before children. In others it is a time for grieving. This is particularly true where a parent (most often the mother) has spent many years fully employed bringing up the children. The children leaving home means that the parent is redundant just as much as if s/he had been sacked from paid employment. To be made redundant from a job is usually identified as one deserving the sympathy of others, whereas children leaving home is often seen as a time for happiness.

In developmental terms any person who is made redundant (from paid employment or because a child no longer needs care) is likely to go through a period of grieving. This complex process has to be worked through and affects the emotional state of the person and this can be reflected in social development. There is often a reduction in feeling of self-worth, and depression can result from redundancy. When a company makes people redundant they are sometimes offered counselling. When a parent becomes redundant from child care there is no automatic offer of counselling.

Figure 2.20 There is no counselling for redundant parents

Old age

Many people remain fit, active and mentally agile well into old age and it would be wrong to stereotype what old age means. However, if we define old age as starting at 65, then there are several key features linked to emotional and social issues. Many of these are related to loss. They include:
- loss of status, income and defined role as a result of retirement
- deterioration in bodily function and loss of health leading to loss of mobility and independence
- loss of sexual function
- loss of companions, e.g. spouse, friends
- loss of independence, and home, by admission to residential care or hospital.

A Old age is not only about loss

In the 60's a different view of the aging process was put forward. Those individuals who adjust most successfully to old age are the ones who do not withdraw from society, but keep up their levels of activities, finding new things to do as they give up work.

In particular, it is felt to be important for elderly people to keep up their 'role count' – in other words, to make sure that they always have lots of different social roles. If they lose roles through leaving work, then they should find more through new hobbies and activities which will bring them into contact with other people and interests. The people who do keep up their role count, according to this theory will be the ones who adjust most successfully, and enjoy their retirement years.

(a) Find out what activities are available for elderly people in your area.
(b) In a group, list what activities your grand-parents/elderly neighbours take part in. Which of these would elderly people have taken part in fifty years ago?

Which organisations would provide help and information for elderly individuals?

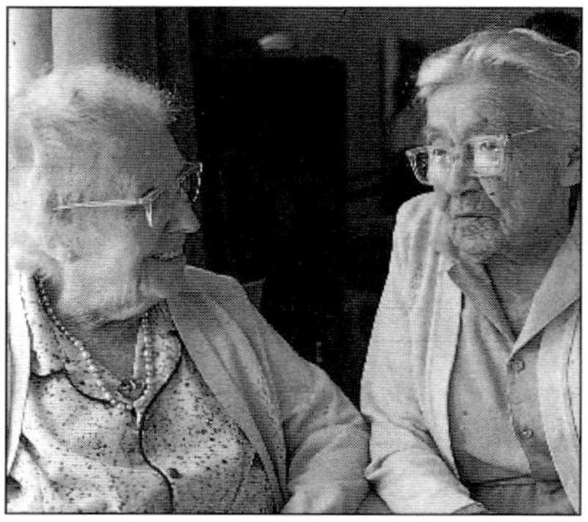

Figure 2.21 Women live longer than men, therefore any gathering of elderly people is likely to have a high proportion of women

FOCUS

Self-concept is based on:
- gender
- education
- maturity (emotional and sexual)
- age
- appearance
- culture
- relationships
- work.

All of these factors affect emotional and social well-being. One issue that is rarely highlighted is the differing average life-spans of men and women and the implications for social development. As people get older, their peers become predominantly female. An implication is that more women than men live alone in old age.

Self-concept

A — Who am I?

Try answering the question:
- Who am I?

Write down the words that you would use to describe yourself.
Now list the characteristics of someone you admire. Select from his/her list of characteristics, those which apply to you.
Now identify contrasts or other differences.
What does the way people treat you say about you? Do they ask you for loans, turn to you for comfort, confide in you, for example?
For one of the characteristics you have listed make a note of the factors you feel may have made you the person you are.
Write a personal statement 'Who am I'. You will need to decide whether you can put it in your portfolio, or keep it completely private.

All of us have a vision of ourselves which may or may not reflect how others see us. If you look back at the last activity you may be able to break down your description of yourself into social roles and personality factors.

Social roles are those which are expected of you by your position in society. Being somebody's brother or sister brings about expectations both from yourself and from others. You are currently a student. This affects how people see you and your position in society. Social roles are also reflected in expectations that we impose upon ourselves.

The personality factors can include being outgoing or inward-looking. Some of the statements may not appear to reflect your personality but, in fact, do so because of the words used. You may describe yourself as fat, overweight, well-built or a bit on the plump side! The words you choose to use reflect to some extent how you view yourself, even though they may all be valid descriptions.

We are continually checking our actions, beliefs and feelings against our own self-concept, and seeing how they 'fit'. Each of us has an idea of our own essential differences from others and relies on the strength of this belief.

This idea of self-concept is important. We often role play in our minds how we would behave in a particular situation. We have confidence in our likes and dislikes in music, clothes and food. All of this adds up to an image of 'self'. This self develops over the years and changes as likes and dislikes change. In particular, during childhood we develop a clearer image of ourselves and how we interact with others and our environment. Gradually, the self-concept develops, and forms a basis for the ways in which we plan and interpret our activities.

A person who has a self-concept that s/he is witty, intelligent and attractive may act by moving into groups to become the centre of attention. A person who believes s/he is unintelligent may try to behave in

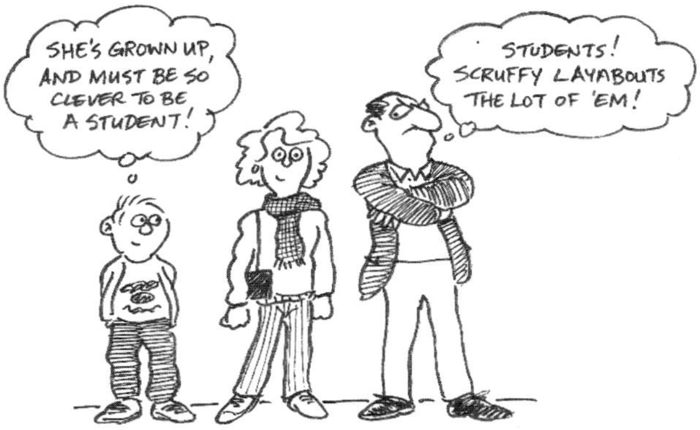

Figure 2.22 Your social role varies according to who is viewing you. A young child may see a student as an adult. An older person may expect stereotypical behaviour. As a student you may not feel either of these things

the way an unintelligent person may react. We think of things from a very personal point of view, with relevance to 'me' and 'my view of the world' being part of any decision making process.

There are four main factors which affect the way we develop our self-concept. They are:
- other people's reactions to us
- comparisons which we make between ourselves and other people
- the roles we play (such as parent, child, being macho)
- identifications we make (comparisons with heroes and villains – I'm as good as ... so I will behave like ...).

A Analysing your own self-concept

Note. This activity is very much a personal exercise: you do not need to share it with others. It asks you to look at yourself, and it can be valuable, but if you feel that you will not benefit from it, then this activity may be left out. Divide a sheet of paper into four sections. Write one of the following headings in each quarter:
- other people's reactions to me
- comparisons which I make between myself and other people that I know well
- the roles I have (such as parent, child, being macho)
- identifications I make (comparisons with heroes and villains – these can be fictional, or people that you do not know well).

In each quarter of the sheet write two things about yourself that fit the heading.

What you have done is started to look at what affects your personal self-concept. This tool can be used to help you change how you feel about yourself, but we would strongly advise you to do nothing more with the information without professional guidance.

Getting to know ourselves is important. We have to be able to plan and make choices. To do this we need to be able to anticipate our behaviour. In some situations we can look back at how we behaved before and either repeat the actions or learn from them. Other situations demand that we develop actions without previous similar experience. In these situations we rely on our self-concept to guide the way we behave.

Any new situation and new activity means that we have to re-evaluate our self-concept. At times activities seem to be forcing us to change. However, we do not lightly abandon our theory of who and what we are, since doing so might threaten our identify. Thus we may destroy a close relationship in order to 'prove' that we are independent. This can occur in the classroom where a student's self-concept of not liking to learn is challenged by a teacher who catches his/her interest. Similarly, teachers have been challenged by intelligent pupils and resort to trying to prove them to be stupid in order to maintain their superiority. It can be very challenging to one's own self-concept to meet a four year old who is more intelligent than oneself!

Health and social well-being

Self-concept and health and well-being

From the description of self-concept it is clear that it is important. If we add to self-concept the feeling of self worth then it becomes easier to see how health and social well-being are linked to self-concept.

I'm O.K., you're O.K.

Within us all there is a core of belief in ourselves that says that we are the best. Built on to this is the belief that what we believe in and what we are is important. As soon as these are challenged then our feelings of self worth can be damaged.

This can lead to self doubt and an increasing decline in feelings of self worth. The cycle continues leading to depression. One consequence of this is increasing ill health and a further cycle of depression. This description is at an extreme end of the scale but is valid to some extent in all situations.

▶ Prejudice, page 190

Often challenges can be based on prejudice and discrimination. Any discriminatory activity can damage an individual's self concept. In particular if the self-concept reflects minority thinking in society, then the pressure to change is going to be great. Wherever people feel pressured to change they tend to group together to support each other. Such groupings may be on the grounds of race, gender, sexuality, religion or ethnicity. They need to have their self-concept and self esteem (feeling of being valued) bolstered by others with similar experiences. Where they are not able to become part of a group, people may be bullied or become bullies themselves.

▶ Discrimination, page 191

An ideal state would seem to be to have a strong self-concept and be happy with it so that you feel happy with yourself, whilst at the same time recognising other people's rights to the same feelings about themselves. This can be summed up in the phrase, 'I'm O.K., you're O.K.' – I'm strong enough in myself to value your strength in yourself.

A Strengthening self-concept

Write down ten things you like and ten things you do not like about yourself. You can destroy the list afterwards without showing it to anybody else.

In a group discuss which list you found easiest to write. Why do you think this was?

We all like to be valued and respected. One way we can help to strengthen a person's self-concept is to pay them a sincere compliment. Turn to a neighbour and tell them something you like about them.

As a recipient of the compliment, accept it. Do not make any comment other than to thank the person for what they said.

In a group discuss how it felt to give and accept compliments. How did the compliments match up to your own self-concept? How would you have reacted to an insult (especially if you felt it was partly true)?

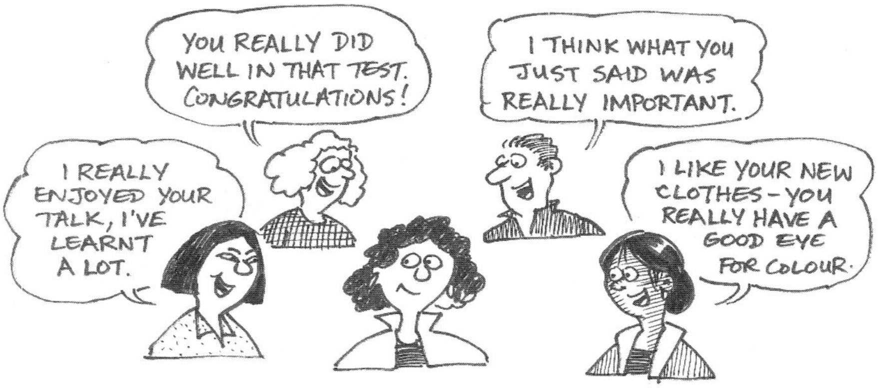

Figure 2.23 How would you respond to compliments like these? We often react by being embarrassed or making a joke. Be prepared to give and receive compliments

Major life events

We have described briefly the different life stages, but within these life stages are **events** that can happen at almost any point in life. These include:
- becoming married (or divorced)
- giving birth/becoming a parent
- becoming unemployed
- becoming retired
- experiencing the loss of someone close
- experiencing a disability
- experiencing a severe illness
- starting a new job
- starting at university or college.

Some of these can be predicted, others are unexpected. Divide the list into predicted and unexpected events.

All of them involve a change of status and involve the individual coming to terms with that status. They can also involve close friends and family members having to recognise and adapt to the changed status. For example, when a woman becomes a mother, her parents become grand-parents.

Almost invariably major life events involve stress and anxiety. These feelings may be less strong where the change is expected and shared with others.

People respond to change in different ways. They may be depressed or happy. They will almost certainly feel some anxiety about the future. Sleep patterns may alter: this often occurs when children are about to start a new school. Although a child may be looking forward to starting at a new school, anxiety can mean that they sleep less well than normal.

Another reaction to change can be alteration of eating habits. Some people 'comfort eat' and increase the amount they eat, often of sweet foods like chocolate. Other people start to eat very little and may lose weight significantly. In both of these cases it is important to encourage the person to maintain a balanced diet, as the reaction to change may be dangerous to health.

How people manage change

When a major life change occurs, people usually need support. In many cases the first group to provide support are members of the family: a death in the family often brings together family members to support each other. Death also has an open acknowledgement of the change: a funeral. This provides a time when people can openly grieve and display their need for comfort and support. It is more difficult for people to cope with death if there is no body (for example, the person was drowned in the sea and the body not recovered).

Many major changes can involve some form of ceremony as the person passes from one stage to another. Becoming a parent often involves a naming ceremony, marriage involves civil and/or religious ceremonies and retiring often involves a presentation.

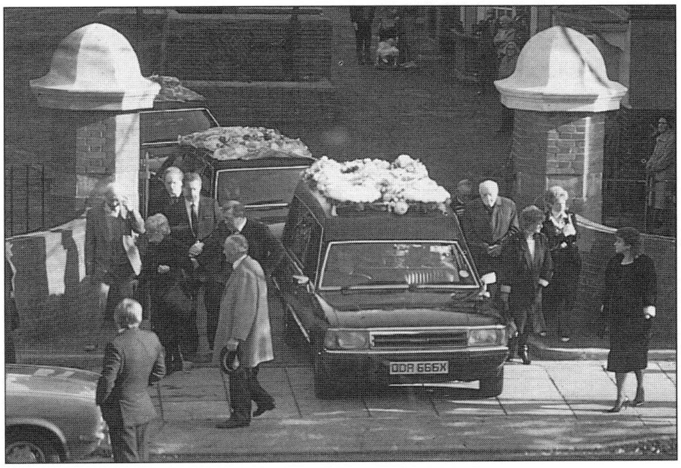

FOCUS

Major life events can be:
- **predictable** – starting school, starting work, changing job, marriage, moving house, having children, retirement
- **unpredictable** – serious illness, disability, divorce, bereavement, redundancy.

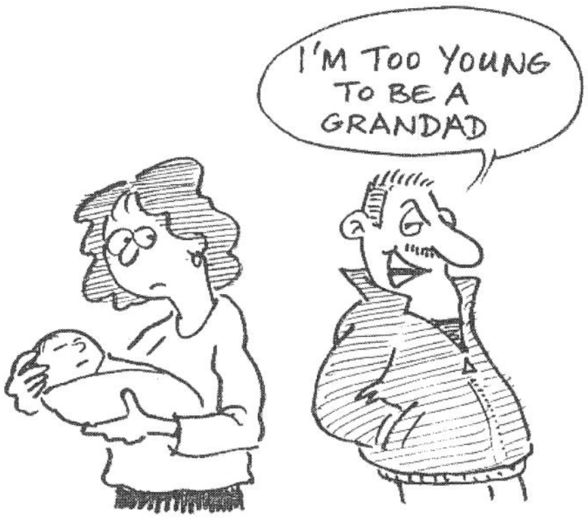

Figure 2.24 Sometimes it is difficult to come to terms with a new status

▶ Eating patterns, page 15

FOCUS

Managing change:
- family support
- social support
- seeking professional help (medical, financial and advisory).

Figure 2.25 The funeral rite provides an opportunity to accept help from family and friends. It also provides a focus that acknowledges the major change in the life of many people

Health and social well-being

A — Marriage ceremonies

Each group should find out about one kind of marriage ceremony.
Make a chart describing the ceremony.
Discuss together what elements the ceremonies have in common, and how and why they are different.

Planning often gives the people involved the opportunity to cope with the stresses of a change. Many cultures have different ceremonies associated with major changes. Funerals can be very quiet, sad affairs or can involve a celebration of the life of the dead person. In some cultures an open display of emotion is seen as a weakness, in others it is expected.

People may need help managing life changes over and above the support provided by family members. Divorce or separation may be made less stressful by conciliation services, or counselling services such as Relate (marriage guidance). Changes caused by job redundancy might be helped by work-seeking advice and financial advice. The financial advice may be important if the redundancy involves a large payment or involves the household having to manage on benefit payments.

Relationships and their influence on health and well-being

Children Learn What They Live

If a child lives with criticism he learns to condemn
If a child lives with hostility he learns to fight
If a child lives with fear he learns to be apprehensive
If a child lives with pity he learns to feel sorry for himself
If a child lives with ridicule he learns to be shy
If a child lives with jealousy he learns what envy is
If a child lives with shame he learns to feel guilty
If a child lives with encouragement he learns to be confident
If a child lives with tolerance he learns to be patient
If a child lives with praise he learns to be appreciative
If a child lives with acceptance he learns to love
If a child lives with approval he learns to like himself
If a child lives with recognition he learns what it is to have a goal
If a child lives with sharing he learns about generosity
If a child lives with honesty and fairness he learns what truth and justice are
If a child lives with security he learns to have faith in himself and in those about him
If a child lives with friendliness he learns that the world is a nice place in which to live
If you live with serenity your child will live with peace of mind

Dorothy Law Nolte

There has long been a debate about the varying influences of nature and nurture on an individual. By 'nature' we mean the biological inheritance. 'Nurture' describes the social and environmental influences. These include the influence of blood relatives (family), friends and colleagues, and marriage or sexual partners. Dorothy Law Nolte's statements provide a clear introduction to the effects of the social environment on a child's social and emotional development. In this section we will look at **relationships** and their influence on health and social well-being.

FOCUS

Relationships in the context of daily life:
- family
- work
- social.

FOCUS

Reasons why people form relationships:
- emotional
- intellectual
- social.

FOCUS

Relationships form:
- within the family
- at work, both formal (with the boss!) and informal
- in social settings.

▶ Social, emotional and intellectual development, page 77

Family

A young person's early experiences are largely within a family setting. In the UK this has generally been portrayed as a nuclear family of a married mother and father with two children. There is the extended family, which is the nuclear family plus relatives such as grandparents, aunts, uncles and cousins who have significant contact with each other.

The model of two parents plus two children may not be common to all people, but families are important. Children learn skills and attitudes from those people who have a great importance in their lives. Members of the family influence social and emotional development significantly. The attitudes and beliefs expressed affect the developing child.

Until the early part of this century people tended to grow up, marry and live in the same geographical area that they were born in. It was not unusual for grandparents to live in the same house as the grandchildren. Extended family members were on hand to provide support for each other. This still happens, but with increased mobility the contact with the extended family has changed. Regular contact has been replaced by telephone calls and occasional visits, with close neighbours and friends taking on some of the traditional family roles.

The nuclear family may be the ideal type portrayed by the media, but families do not always consist of two parents plus two children. Family structures differ. They can involve a single parent, or, because of the increase in divorce and remarriage, reconstituted or step families. This is not a complete list. There are variations around these family types. For example, some couples live together without marrying. This is called cohabiting.

Cohabiting parents: *parents who live together as husband and wife, but are not married.*

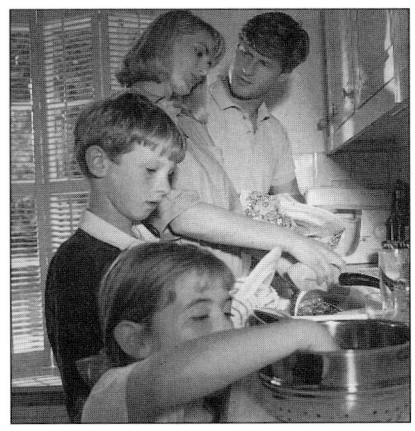

Figure 2.26 A nuclear family

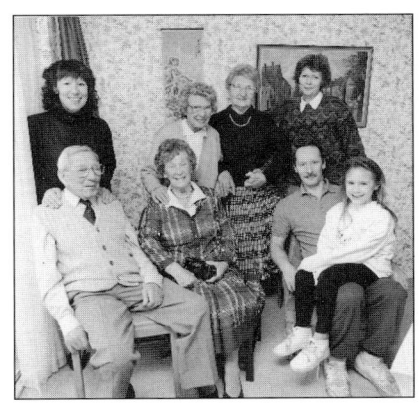

Figure 2.27 An extended family

A Family structures

Within your group discuss the different family structures that you come from: how common is the two plus two model?
Think about the extended families in your group. How close (geographically) are the members of your extended family? With how many relatives do you have frequent contact? Who is the oldest member of your family you talk to on a regular (daily/weekly) basis?

It is important that children have a range of experiences from the different generations in society. This gives them experience of different role models. It also provides an opportunity to experience differing attitudes and hopefully enables them to counter negative experiences with positive ones. The case study below gives an example of the effects of family experience on development.

C Case study: Mark

Mark's parents were not married. His father had two older children in their late teens. Mark was his mother's only child. She had little understanding of how to bring up a child. She cared for him physically. When she held him she did not cuddle him but sat him at arm's length on her knee. She left him in his cot or play pen for long periods while she got on with things that she wanted

Health and social well-being

to do. Mark's father was at work for most of the day but, when he was home, he cuddled and talked to him.

Mark came to the attention of Social Services after his parents split up. His mother handed him to a social worker saying she wanted him adopted. He was 18 months old.

Mark was placed with adoptive parents. His speech was delayed. He made few sounds until he was nearly three years old. He did start to speak, but when upset or challenged he withdrew into himself and did not react to anything that was said to him.

Mark showed affection for his adoptive father and brothers. He would walk over to any man who came into the house but avoided contact with his adoptive mother. His adoptive mother was a keen gardener and on several occasions Mark went round the house pulling the house plants from their pots. He was six years old before he hugged his adoptive mother.

Questions
1. How was Mark demonstrating the limited emotional care from his birth parents?
2. What might have caused his delayed language development?
3. How could his adoptive parents stimulate a more balanced social and emotional development?

The case study of Mark shows something of the effect that his family relationships had on his language development. It also shows some of the effects they had on his social relationships. At eighteen months he would have been expected to be vocalising and beginning to use recognisable sounds. His lack of stimulation from his mother meant that he had not had the opportunity to start to develop his speech patterns. Mark's adoptive parents spent time talking to him and encouraging him to talk to them. It took some time, but with the stimulation from his adoptive parents and the models of speaking from his adoptive brother, Mark's language eventually developed well.

> Social, intellectual and emotional development, table 2.3, page 78

Source: *Davenport G.C. An Introduction to Child Development*

Case study: The twins

Identical twin boys in Czechoslovakia born in September 1960 had suffered severe deprivations. Their mother had died shortly after they were born and their father couldn't really cope. At the age of eleven months they were taken into a children's home where they were found to be normal, healthy children. Their father remarried within a few months, and the twins returned to their father and stepmother when they were 18 months old. They had two older sisters, and a stepsister and stepbrother. The stepmother was a selfish, unpleasant woman who had no idea about bringing up young children. (Her mother had looked after her children when they were young.) The father was of below average intelligence, and his job on the railways took him away from home quite a lot. The family had recently moved to a city suburb where nobody knew them, or knew that the family should have contained six children.

Their stepmother treated them terribly. They were kept in a small unheated room with a sheet of polythene for a bed and very little furniture. They were poorly fed. Sometimes the mother would lock them in the cellar. She would beat them with a wooden kitchen spoon, covering their heads with a mattress in case anyone heard their cries. Their father was also once seen beating them with a rubber hose until they lay unmoving on the ground.

The twins suffered these conditions for five and a half years. When they were finally examined, at the age of seven, they were severely physically and

> Healthy Diet, page 10

mentally retarded. Their bodies were covered in scar tissue from the beatings. They had severe rickets, a disease of the bones caused by lack of vitamin D. They couldn't stand straight, walk, or run, and their co-ordination was poor. They hadn't been taught to speak, had no knowledge of eating habits, and were very frightened of people, and of the dark. It was impossible to give them a standard intelligence test since they couldn't understand the instructions, and they weren't familiar with things like 'pictures' on which some tests are based. It was estimated that their IQ's would be in the 40's. Instead of giving them standard intelligence tests, their abilities were compared to normal children of their age. Their development was equivalent to that of a three year old.

The twins were put in hospital until they were well enough to go to a special school for mentally disadvantaged children. They made good progress at school. When they were sociable enough they were fostered by a particularly kind and loving woman who lived with her sister who also loved children. She seemed to know exactly what the children needed, and there was a happy atmosphere in the whole family, full of mutual understanding. By the age of 11 the twins' speech was normal for their age. They enjoyed some school subjects, such as reading and playing the piano, and were both fairly creative. By 15 the twins' IQ scores were normal, and their emotional state had improved greatly. The atmosphere at home was warm and friendly, and although the boys still remembered their early experiences they rarely talked about them, even to their foster mother.

A Who is close to you?

In the middle of a sheet of paper draw a small circle around your name to represent yourself. Write the names of others who have an influence on your life, using the distance from your name to indicate how close you feel to them. Produce a second diagram, but this time write the names according to how significant their activities are in determining your behaviour. The people need not be the same as in the first exercise. This time the names of the people who have most effect on you should be written closest to your name.
Both lists are likely to contain similar names. The first list may have parents, brothers and sisters, boy/girl friends and pets as being very close to you. The second list may have teachers, religious leaders and other people in authority close to you, as they often have a significant effect on behaviour.

How close I feel

How much they affect my behaviour

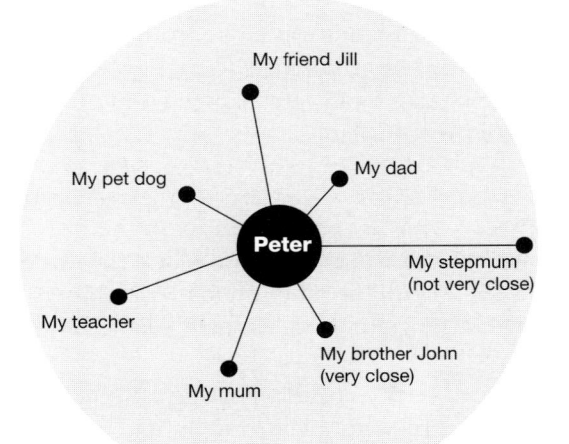

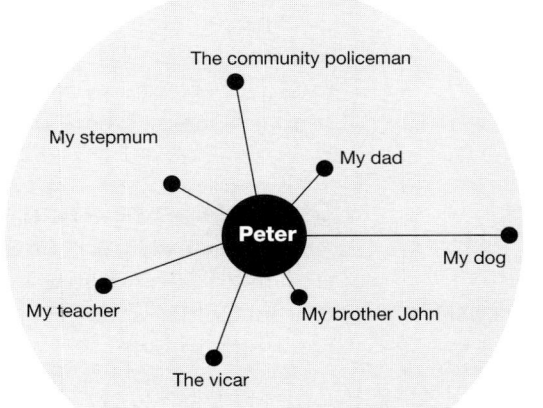

Figure 2.28 Relationship charts

Health and social well-being

Relationships outside the family

You not only form relationships at home but also at work and as part of your social life. Your relationship can be formal (pupil/teacher, employer/worker) or informal (between colleagues at school or work, or in recreational groups). The next activity will help you to explore and understand different types of relationship.

A Relationships

Note. This activity will also contribute to achievement of Element 2.3.

1 **(a)** As a subject group, make a list of the main groups to which you belong. Think about the different situations in which you meet or work with other people.

(b) Individually, identify your relationship with the other people in each group listed. For example:

• one group may be based around where you live. Your roles may be as brother, sister, or parent

• a second group may be in school or college, where your roles include being a student/pupil

• a third group is as a citizen of this country and your role as taxpayer, neighbour or voter (potential or actual depending upon your age)

• broader groupings may be related to social class, race, religion and gender.

2 Ask one or more people of your parent's generation to carry out the same activity and share their list with you. Compare the list with your own, looking for similarities and differences.

For each of the different relationships you identified, write down if it is formal or informal.

How does the nature of the relationship affect the way you speak and the words you use?

When you have completed the activity, retain your lists to help you when you look at social roles and social groups, page 97.

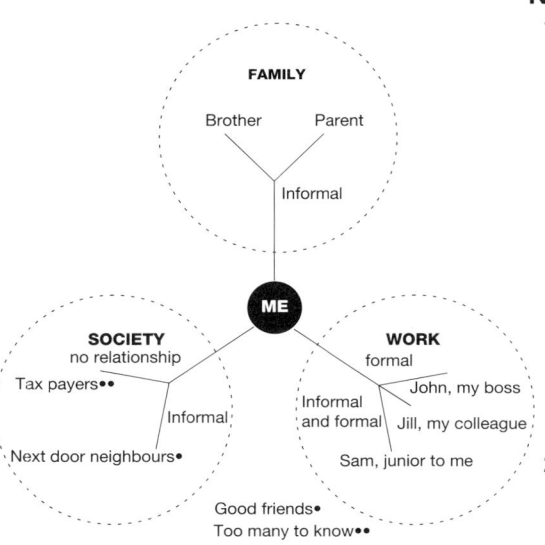

Figure 2.29 A spidergram showing typical group membership

From the activity you will have identified different relationships with people in different groups. Your use of language is often an easy way to identify the nature of a relationship. You do not talk to your teachers in the same way that you talk to your friends, nor do you use the same language with your parents as you do with your friends.

An example of the different use of words comes as a tale from the marines. It was noticed that when marines were talking to each other they used a lot of swear words. When they spoke to an officer they said, 'Sir', in similar places to where they swore with colleagues!

Changes in relationships

As a child grows, **relationships** within the family **change.** When the child is an infant, the family is protective. The infant relies on family members (parents, older siblings and other relatives) for food, warmth, shelter and emotional support.

The first major change experienced by the child is starting school, although some children may have had pre-school learning in, for example, creches or nursery schools. This is a time when some of the emotional,

---

FOCUS

Changes in relationships occur as a result of:
• changes in life stages
• major life events, both predictable and unpredictable.

intellectual and social support for the child comes from teachers. The parents often find handing over responsibility an emotional experience, as it is the first real evidence of the child moving towards independence.

Puberty and adolescence are times of major change in relationships within families. The teenage child challenges parental views and beliefs in an effort to establish independence. The nature of the relationship is both confrontational and protective from both sides.

Adulthood usually involves moving away from home. This change causes emotional stress on all family members. It can also involve financial changes for the child and family. In this stage many relationships are formed away from the family. Some may have started in adolescence or earlier. The adult may marry and form a new family. Work relationships will develop. In all cases new roles and responsibilities will alter the complex pattern of relationships.

A   Effects of change

Look back at the list of major life events or changes.
For each of the major life changes, discuss in a small group the effects the change may have on emotional and social relationships. Also identify how the changes might affect a person's behaviour (physical and intellectual).
An example might be related to losing a job.
The consequences of job loss may be more time at home and less money than before.
How might this affect the person who has lost the job?
What might s/he feel?
How might this affect relationships within the family?
What effects might the job loss have on social life?
(Consider the effects if the social life revolved around the job.)

▶ Major life events, page 91

Group roles

Humans are social animals. Part of this is expressed in the need to be in **groups.** In order to join a group, it is important to understand the values, beliefs and behaviour that govern the group. By adopting those values, beliefs and behaviour, a person can gain the reward of entering the group. By maintaining the group, the values, beliefs and behaviour are reinforced and rewarded. We learn to use the same behaviour again and again to satisfy our need to be in a group.

Accepting a society's culture

In a social context, if we behave in ways that meet with the approval and praise of those around us, we become accepted members of that society. People who are accepted have adapted to the way of life of their society (its culture). The concept of culture is a broad one and includes language, beliefs, eating habits, dress and all the aspects of the lifestyle of a particular society or of a particular group of people. In western societies there may be a mainstream culture, plus a variety of subcultures, each of which differ in some aspects of lifestyle.

FOCUS
Consequences of relationship breakdown on:
- emotional life
- social life
- intellectual activity
- physical habits.

FOCUS
Different roles individuals take in group settings:
- family (wife, husband, parent, child)
- work (employer, employee)
- recreation (organiser, participant)
- community (neighbour, taxpayer, voter).

Health and social well-being

It includes:
- values – the general guidelines for behaviour; beliefs that some things are good and worthwhile. Educational achievement is one example of a value, but values can, and do, vary from culture to culture and from group to group
- norms – the more specific guides to behaviour. They are rules which may be formal and written down, such as the membership rules of a club, or may be informal and unwritten, such as appropriate style of dress for various situations. The clothes that would be appropriate for an interview would be very different from those worn on the beach. Norms vary both within and between cultures
- status – the individual's position in society. For example, a consultant has more prestige than a junior doctor
- role – the behaviour that accompanies your status in society. We all perform a variety of **roles.** You are a student, a son/daughter, perhaps sister/brother, an employee, and you adapt your behaviour to suit each particular role. Each situation combines a set of role expectations: as a care worker, compassion will be required – cruelty will not be tolerated.

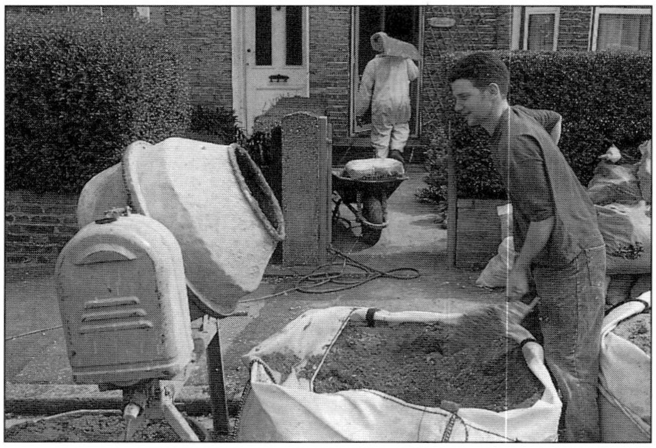

Figure 2.30 Hard work is valued as good and worthwhile. As such, it is a value in many cultures

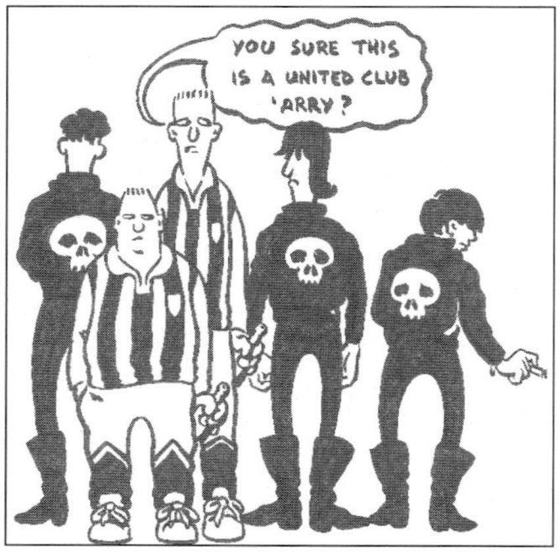

Figure 2.31 Dress often helps identify group members

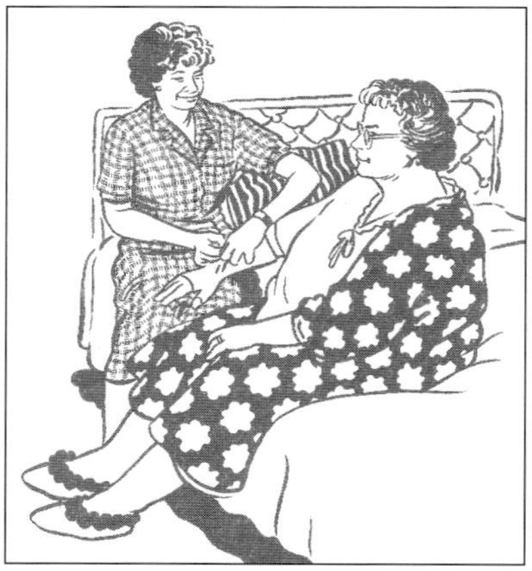

Figure 2.32 Care workers have a caring role

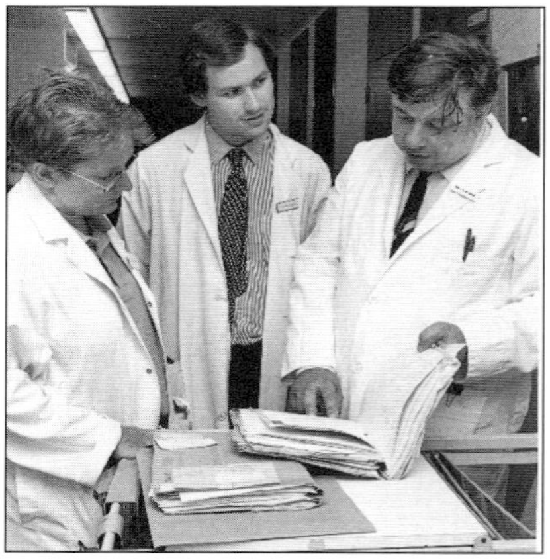

Figure 2.33 A consultant in the health service has a status that commands attention

Rules, laws and conventions

For groups to continue to function there must be rules, laws and conventions. Some of these may be written down, many are not. Your place in a group will be determined, in part at least, by the rules, laws and conventions. To breach any of these invites some form of punishment within the group. In society in general the punishment may be based on the law that was broken. In smaller groups the consequence may be exclusion from the group. If you think of your family there will be many things that are expected of you: pocket money may be lost for failing to tidy your room: you may be 'grounded' for breaches of rules. You will almost certainly have gone through a time when you challenged the norms of your family, and you may have contributed to a change in those norms.

A — Group norms

Note. If role play is used in this activity, read the notes on role play in the introduction first.

In the Relationships Activity you looked at different groups and your roles within those groups (page 96). For each of the groups that you identified write down the norms (rules) of the group. These rules may be written rules for some groups, e.g. school/college rules or unwritten ones such as those that keep a gang of children playing together.

For a placement or job that you are familiar with, write down the codes of practice (rules). What would be the consequence of breaking the rules? Use role play in which a number of group members break the rules of a given group. Select from:

- a family
- a sports group
- a club
- a social group
- a working group.

▶ Role play, page xxi

▶ Relationships Activity, page 96

Within the activity we used the word 'rule', but we could just as easily have talked about laws or conventions. They are similar, and are in many ways interchangeable. Laws tend to be formal and written; conventions are often unwritten 'understandings' within the group. It is often a breach of a convention that is treated more seriously in some groups.

Within society your role and group help to describe your position in society. Your social role and social group are to a large extent determined by your socialisation.

Social role: your position in society defined by what you are and what you do. Roles include parent, sibling, child, employed, unemployed or unpaid worker, neighbour, voter and taxpayer.

Social group: groups of people which can be defined by things such as family ties, living together, place of employment, school or college membership and leisure interests.

Socialisation

A child is born with no knowledge of its parents' culture: it has to be learned. What we learn is shaped by the responses of those around us. Thus, we are likely to adopt the attitudes of the social class to which we belong because we are socially rewarded by the approval of others for holding those attitudes. This lifelong process of learning is called socialisation.

▶ Accepting a society's culture, page 97

Socialisation: the process by which social contacts with other people develop and shape our personalities, values, norms and roles. Because the process takes place throughout our lives, we come to behave, feel and think in similar ways to those around us.

Society tends to maintain a social pattern from generation to generation. The process is complex, and social change can only be brought about by people breaking the pattern. Although members of a group share the same culture, they still remain individuals and are able to make choices on the degree to which they conform to the group's culture.

Those who choose not to behave as society expects them to are said to be deviant. Deviance is defined by the society or group's norms. A person who insists on being fully clothed in a nudist colony is deviant. So, too, is

Prejudice, page 190

Discrimination, page 191

a person who chooses to run naked through a town centre. In many cases the pattern is challenged by young people going through adolescence who try to establish their own values and beliefs. The rebellious young person who refuses to conform has been a constant source of complaint for adults throughout the ages!

Reference groups

One interesting aspect of socialisation is where a person aspires to membership of a different group. This reference group could be one with whom the individual may have little or no contact, but whose standards and attitudes are desired. We use reference groups to alter how we wish to be identified by others. A reference group can influence the choices and decisions made by an individual.

For example, if the reference group that you would like to be part of wears specific clothes or eats a specific diet, then you may adopt the style of dress and diet even though you are not, in reality, a member of the group. Your socialisation has been affected by your aspirations.

The reference group can be imposed on you. This is one of the bases of stereotyping. In this case a feature such as age, gender or race may be used by others to impose expectations based on their stereotypes of the group.

Such imposed membership groups include elders, people with mental or physical disability, and people who are out of work. By using stereotypes of a group to affect how an individual is treated, the individual can be socialised into the stereotype. For example, if a black teenage boy is always being stopped by the police and treated as someone who is hostile (because the stereotype is that all black teenagers hate the police) then eventually the teenager might be socialised into hating the police. The stereotype reference group used by the police has been reinforced and accepted.

Reference groups are important to a person's sense of identity. However, where they are imposed, they can have a negative effect. This is clear in the cases of the '-isms' such as racism. Access to health and care services can be affected by identifying the client as a member of a group with an 'abnormal' label. The labelling shapes attitudes toward, and expectations of, members of the group and leads to discrimination.

Influences on socialisation

In studying these influences, sociologists focus on social explanations – what is learned through interacting with others and with the environment.

Parents/teachers/carers are role models for the child's behaviour and are very influential in, for example, the learning of appropriate gender roles, that is, the patterns of behaviour which are seen to be appropriate to being male or female and linked to ideas of masculinity and femininity.

In addition to the socialising roles of the family and the school, we need to consider, although briefly, the effects of the peer group, religion and the media.

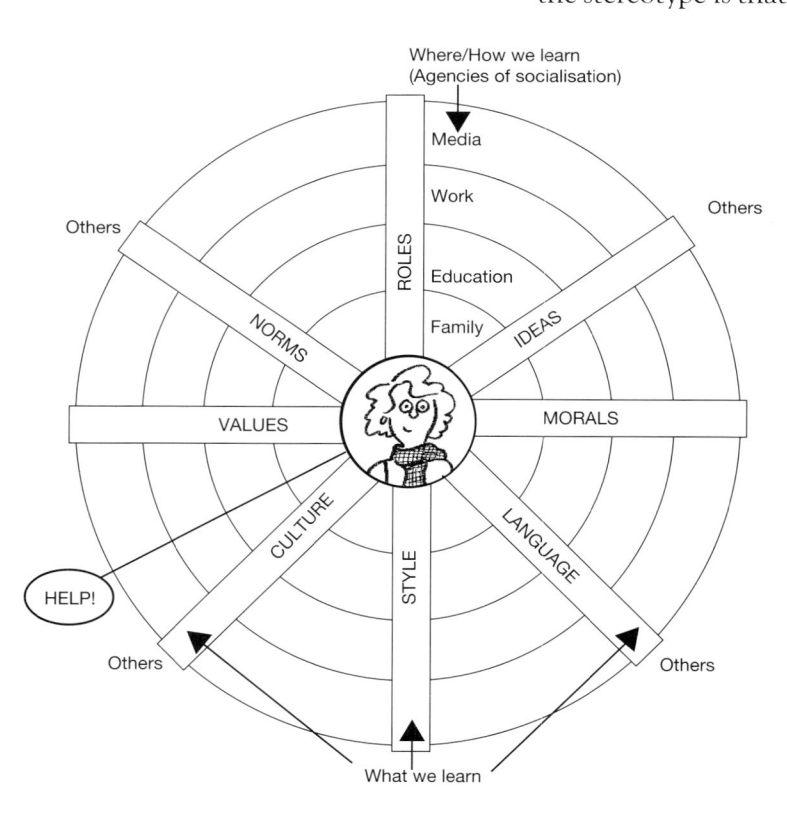

Figure 2.34 Influences on socialisation. The diagram illustrates the main influences or agencies of the socialisation process – the family, the school, the work place, the media, the peer group, and religion

The peer group, defined as a group of friends of similar age and interests, has a great influence on our behaviour. This influence becomes increasingly important in adolescence. The desire to be accepted as a group member means that individuals conform to the group norms.

Religion too, influences how we lead our lives, with many of society's norms and values relating to religious beliefs. It is also true that many of society's stated norms reflect religious beliefs, but some will argue that religion itself has become less important in broader society.

The mass media, which include television, newspapers, books, magazines, films and so on, shape our views and attitudes towards the world and direct our behaviour. For example, several studies have shown the way in which television and the media in general reinforce popular attitudes and stereotypes.

Social stratification

We have made references to the term 'social groups' and 'social class' without defining them. Social **groups** can be different, and vary in ranking to form hierarchical layers or strata in society based on power, influence, wealth and status. Thus, although there can be equality within the group, the inequality between groups can be great. This ranking of groups within society is known as social stratification: there are many forms of this.

The major ways in which groups tend to be stratified are in terms of class, ethnicity/race, gender and age.

> **FOCUS**
> Characteristics of socio-economic groups include:
> • housing
> • environment
> • education
> • employment
> • financial status.

What do we mean by social class?

A — Classes in society

Even before reading a definition of social class, you will have some ideas about different classes in society.
In three different groups imagine you are members of different classes – the upper class, the middle class and the working class.
Each group should define its class in terms of norms, beliefs, typical attitudes and lifestyles.
What would indicate the social class of a person?
Identify what makes your group's social class different from the other two groups.

It is clear that we already have some ideas about class and class differences which relate to occupation, style of dress, accent, leisure activities and so on. To have these views we must be using stereotypes, but they do provide us with a model to work from. They also provide an opportunity to demonstrate prejudice, but demonstrate, too, the influence of class on a whole range of issues.

In describing the way of life of members of different classes you have been describing different class cultures. You will have probably included factors such as accent, schooling, leisure activities, voting behaviour and so on in your descriptions. But, you have probably also listed other factors which could be described as economic and material factors, such as occupation, income, wealth (which is people's assets – houses, cars, land, etc.).

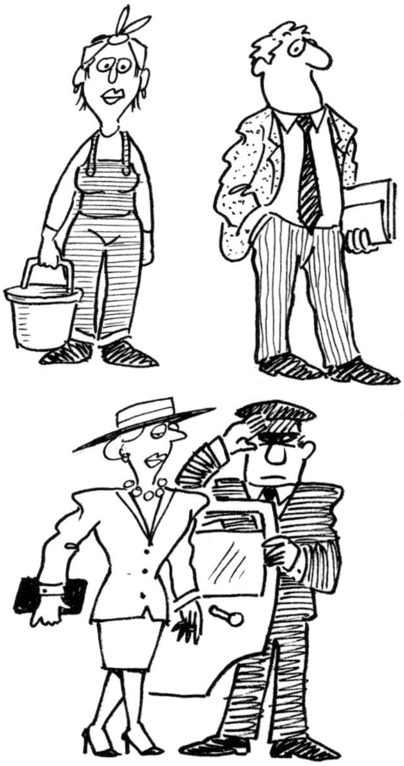

However, although income and wealth clearly influence lifestyle, these factors are not the only ones which determine which class you belong to. For example, if someone is a member of the working class (manual or 'blue collar'

Figure 2.35 Working class, middle class and upper class

jobs, either skilled, semi-skilled or unskilled) would they automatically become a member of the upper class or middle class if they won £1 000 000 on the National Lottery? Their income would change, but would their values and norms necessarily change too?

There is no one way of defining **social class**. Attempts have been made to devise a reliable method of class categorisation, but because there are so many different factors which can be taken into account, it is a daunting task.

Many researchers use occupation as the starting point for defining a person's social class, and indeed this forms the basis of The Registrar General's social class scale. Although this scale has its problems, it is the 'official' scale of social class in Britain and is widely used in official surveys.

Table 2.5 The Registrar General's scale of social class

Social class	Examples of occupations included in each social class
A Professional	accountant, doctor, dentist, lawyer, surveyor, university lecturer
B Intermediate	MP, teacher, nurse, police officer, manager
C1 Skilled non-manual	clerical worker, sales rep, secretary, waiter
C2 Skilled manual	carpenter, cook, electrician, taxi driver
D Partly skilled	agricultural worker, fisherman, postman, telephonist
E Unskilled labourer	office cleaner, messenger, lorry driver's mate

All occupations are divided into manual and non-manual and are ranked according to level of skill into five different classes.

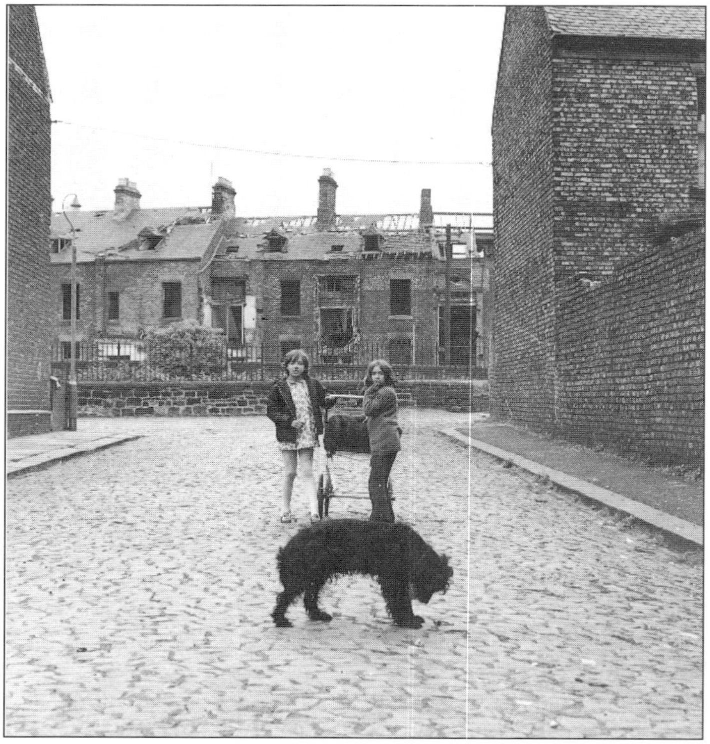

Group membership and health and social well-being

The social class an individual is born into will definitely influence their life chances and their potential for social mobility.

Life chances: opportunities within your life. These are affected by social class. The higher up the social class scale the greater the life chances.

Social mobility: movement up or down the social ladder, between social classes.

An individual's life chances are the opportunities an individual has to achieve their goals in life and reach their full potential: it also means being able to avoid those things in life one wishes to avoid.

Certainly, research has shown that the higher your social class, the greater your chances of having a long and healthy life. Class differences are reflected in the infant mortality rate, for example, Classes D and E have a higher rate of infant mortality than Classes A and B.

Figure 2.36 Housing, health risks and social class are linked. A child brought up in a poor area (financially and environmentally) has less access to health care and risks a shorter lifespan than one brought up in a middle class environment

Health and social well-being

A | Class difference in health care

Note. You will need access to the government report *Social Trends* to undertake this research.

Using tables from *Social Trends*, conduct research into factors which affect the infant mortality rate, or the factors which affect the general health of different social classes.

Infant mortality[1,2] by social class of father, 1990
England & Wales

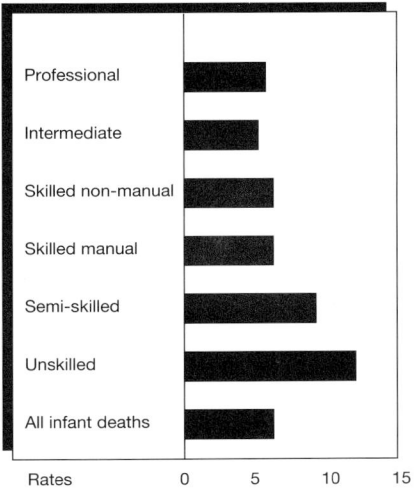

Class	Rate
Professional	~6
Intermediate	~6
Skilled non-manual	~7
Skilled manual	~7
Semi-skilled	~9
Unskilled	~12
All infant deaths	~8

Rates 0 5 10 15

1 Death of infants under 1 year of age per thousand live births
2 Data are for births within marriage only
Source: Office of Population Censuses and Surveys

Percentage of adults who went to the dentist for a regular check-up: by socio-economic groupo, 1985 and 1991

Great Britain	Percentages	
	1985	1991
Professional	66	63
Employers and managers	62	59
Intermediate and junior Non-manual	58	54
Skilled manual	41	41
Semi-skilled manual	39	37
Unskilled manual	30	36
All adults	50	48

Aged 16 and over with some natural teeth
Source: General Household Survey

Figure 2.37 Sample tables from **Social Trends**

There are several explanations for this which relate to the inequalities which exist between groups. Although geographical area, marital status, gender and ethnic status all play a part, major contributors are socio-economic factors such as occupation, income and **housing**.

A lack of material resources can mean living in a deprived, run-down area, having poor housing, eating an inadequate diet and having a generally less healthy life style.

Research has shown that class culture is important in that, for example, the middle classes are more likely to make greater use of the health services available. One of the reasons for this may be that professionals in health and social care occupations share the same social class. Communication tends to be on a more equal basis, therefore the middle class are in a better position to demand their rights.

It has been argued by many social scientists that there are social class differences in child-rearing practices and that this has an important effect on educational achievement.

In general, it is probably true to say that parents will raise their children in a manner similar to that experienced by themselves. For example, middle class parents are likely to have had a good education themselves and are likely to have a career with prospects. They value achievement for themselves and for their children. The fact that middle class parents are likely to place a high value on education and achievement means that middle class children are constantly being encouraged to do better.

> **FOCUS**
>
> **Impact on individual choice (e.g. nutrition, alcohol, smoking, and attitude to education) of:**
> - housing
> - environment
> - education
> - employment
> - financial status.

However, this one factor alone cannot account for the class inequalities in educational achievement, (see Figure 2.38).

A great deal of time and money has been spent researching the effects of poverty on educational achievement. The general findings of the research suggest that a 'cycle of deprivation' exists which transmits disadvantage from one generation to the next. The life chances of the parents are passed on to the children. Some groups in society are more at risk of being poor than others.

Figure 2.38 Factors influencing educational achievement

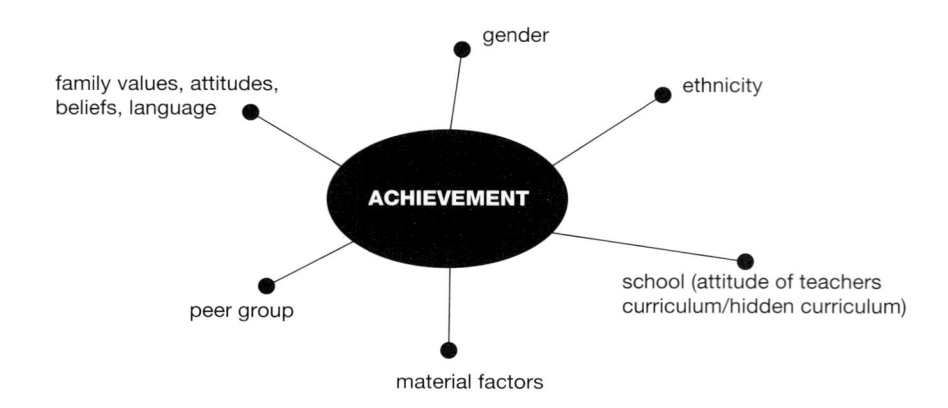

Factors linked to ACHIEVEMENT: gender, ethnicity, school (attitude of teachers curriculum/hidden curriculum), material factors, peer group, family values, attitudes, beliefs, language.

Standards of living

Case study: Project Headstart

A project, called 'Project Headstart', provided children from deprived areas with extra classes and tuition, playgroups and visits, while they were in their pre-school years. The children involved all showed noticeable improvements in their IQ scores, and in their achievements in school. But as the children outgrew the Headstart years, and went through normal schooling, the improvements seemed to vanish. They became very much more slow at school learning, and their IQ improvements disappeared.

For several years, psychologists thought that improved nursery school education without a continued improved out-of-school support system wouldn't make that much difference to the children. The scheme, which was set up in the 1960s didn't really seem to have an effect. But when the first Headstart children grew up to be teenagers, some recent research supported the scheme. I. Lazar, (1982) showed that there did seem to be improvements in the achievements of these children; at the age of 14, children from Project Headstart were scoring consistently more highly on school tests than those of the same age who hadn't had nursery education. Lazar considered that this was probably due to the way that many parents became much more interested in their child's education as a result of Project Headstart, and so they may have encouraged their child more.

Source: *Hayes, N. A First Course in Psychology*

Questions
1 Discuss how you think extra classes, playgroups and visits helped the children.
2 What problems might you come across in trying to set up a project like this in Britain?

Health and social well-being

What does Figure 2.39 tell you about which groups are more likely to experience poverty? Although the chart gives some information, it gives no insight into the standards of living that people in these groups experience. It is also possible that within one household different members might be experiencing different living standards. Recent research has shown that women often go without in order to protect other members of the family from the full impact of poverty. Although women make up a growing percentage of the labour force, this work generally tends to be part-time, low pay, low status work.

Other groups more likely to be in poverty are black and ethnic minority groups. Members of these groups are more likely to be unemployed or on low incomes, due either wholly or in part to discrimination.

A term which is sometimes used in discussions of social stratification is the idea of an 'underclass'. This term has been used by many writers in many different ways. Generally, it refers to those groups in society who are unable to participate fully in community life. These groups may well have to rely on state benefits and are likely to be the targets of widespread discrimination. Since they are living on the edge of society, they are said to be 'marginalised' or cut off from the mainstream of society.

Deprived of sufficient income, families have to adjust their lifestyle accordingly. The major expense in any family budget is food and accommodation.

It is generally agreed that where there is a lack of money in the household the diet of the family will be less healthy. Research has shown that this is not necessarily due to lack of knowledge about foods and healthy eating, but to perceptions of the cost of a healthy diet. Does a healthy diet (including fresh fruit and vegetables) actually cost more than processed foods?

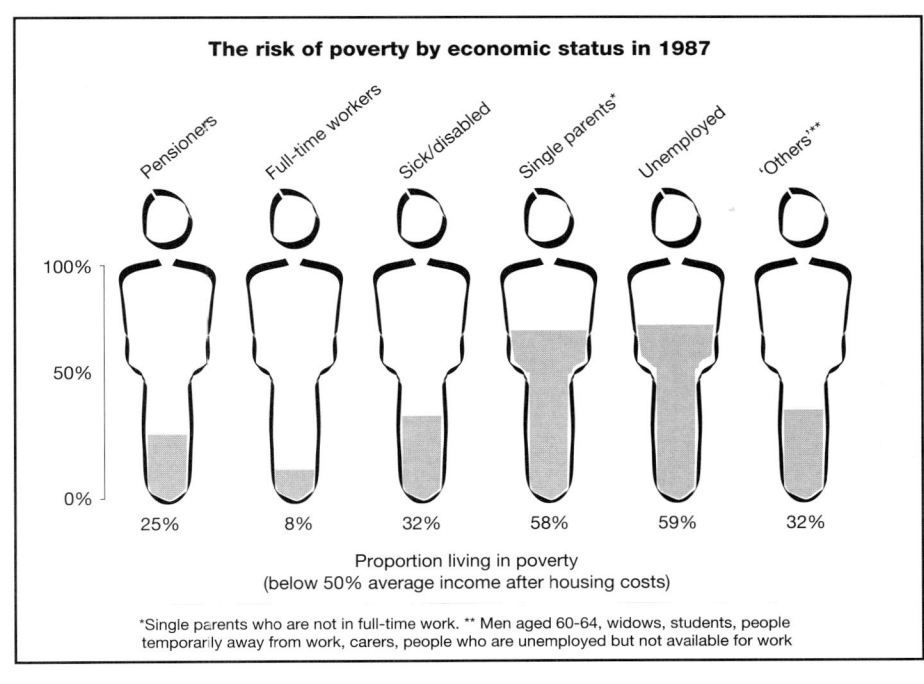

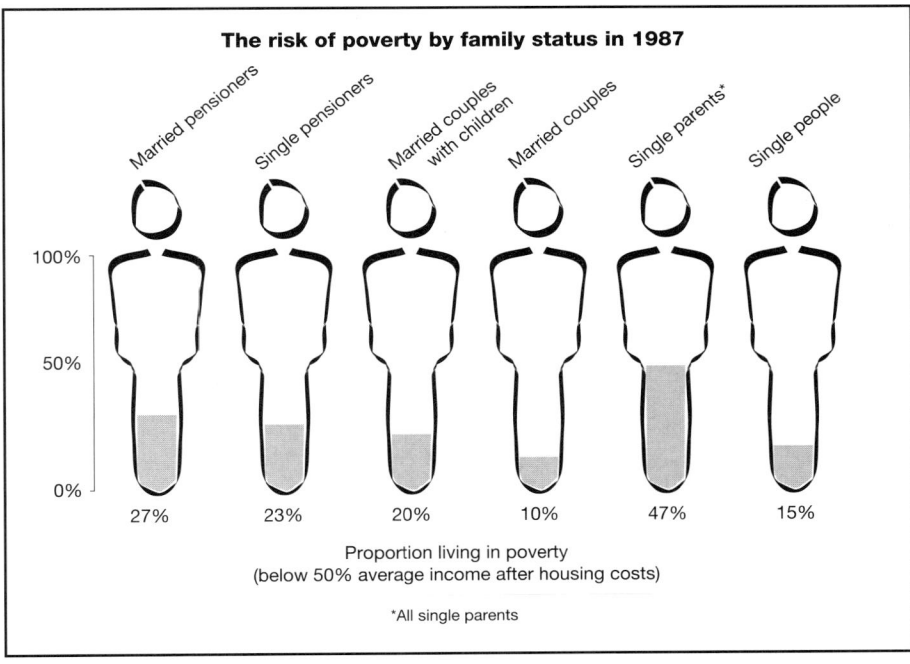

The risk of poverty by economic status in 1987

Pensioners	Full-time workers	Sick/disabled	Single parents*	Unemployed	'Others'**
25%	8%	32%	58%	59%	32%

Proportion living in poverty (below 50% average income after housing costs)

*Single parents who are not in full-time work. ** Men aged 60-64, widows, students, people temporarily away from work, carers, people who are unemployed but not available for work

The risk of poverty by family status in 1987

Married pensioners	Single pensioners	Married couples with children	Married couples	Single parents*	Single people
27%	23%	20%	10%	47%	15%

Proportion living in poverty (below 50% average income after housing costs)

*All single parents

Figure 2.39 The risk of poverty

Source: Oppenhein, C. *Poverty, the facts*

▶ Discrimination, page 191

▶ A healthy diet, page 10

105

Effects of different housing levels

A home provides us with far more than just shelter. It is a place to unwind, to relax; providing security and stability for ourselves and our children. However, for many people on low incomes housing may be overcrowded or of poor quality.

For a growing number of people a home means living in temporary accommodation, for example 'bed and breakfast' hotels, refuges, squats, night shelters and indeed living on the streets. Sometimes, such 'temporary' accommodation can last for years.

Bed and breakfast accommodation, usually one room, is totally unsuitable for family living. Young children have no space to play or do their homework and there is an increased risk of accidents. Food may be prepared on single burners in the room, or in shared kitchens. Hygiene standards may be poor. Overcrowding makes passing on illnesses much easier.

Overcrowding and lack of privacy can cause stress and frustration and strained relationships. This in turn increases the risk of family violence, family breakdown and alcoholism. There is an increased reliance on convenience foods which is more expensive and does not necessarily provide a well-balanced diet.

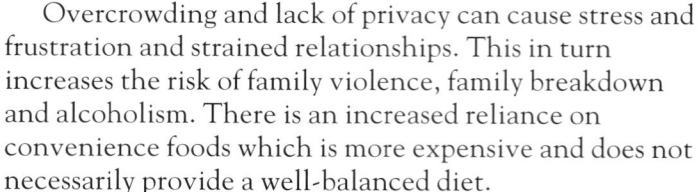

The overall effects of material disadvantage and associated stress that goes with living in such conditions has very serious implications for health and well-being.

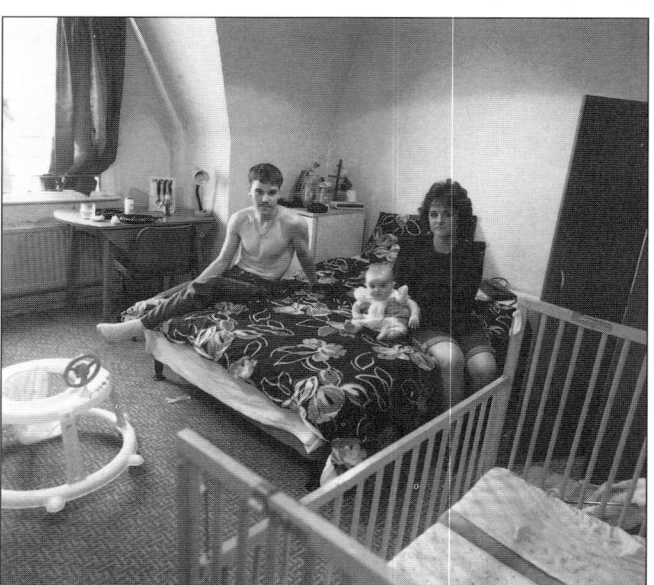

Figure 2.40 Bed and breakfast accommodation is unsuitable for family living

A Social class: is the model a good one?

1. In small groups, using the Registrar General's definitions of social class, discuss into which class you would put the following people:
   - a teacher
   - the winner of the National Lottery who gave up being a dustman
   - a former company director who was imprisoned for fraud
   - a bankrupt who used to own a supermarket chain
   - an unemployed doctor
   - an unemployed labourer
   - the ex-wife of a doctor.

2. Consider now the position if in each case the person were from an ethnic minority group. Does the Registrar General's definition reflect society's generally racist views?

When you have discussed the different people, come together as a large group and share any conclusions.

How accurate is the Registrar General's classification?

Are there any groups of people who do not fit into the classification?

How does the social classification reflect the UK's multi-cultural society?

▶ Registrar General's scale of social class, page 102

Assignment

DEVELOPMENT AND CHANGE

Setting the scene
You have been asked to write an article on development and change for a magazine.

Note. You need to preserve confidentiality if personal interviews are used in this assignment.

Task 1
In the form of a fictional biography, produce an illustrated report on how people pass through the different life stages. You could use appropriate photographs and/or pictures from newspapers and magazines. Physical, intellectual, emotional and social development during childhood, adolescence, adulthood, mid-life and old age will be covered in the report. You should describe how an individual develops self-concept and the factors that can affect self-concept.

Task 2
Using the person that you used for Task 1, produce a case study related to the (auto)biography. Using two other people in their life, produce two more case studies: one person should be of a different gender, and the other of a different ethnic origin from the original person.

Use the case studies to explain some of the major events that can take place in our lives. Show how the people in your case studies faced and coped with change. Your research for the case studies could include personal interviews, and/or using materials from television programmes or films, etc.

In each case, the examples you produce should describe:
- one major predictable event which affects the person's life
- one major unpredictable event which affects the person's life
- the ways in which that person may manage the change caused by the predictable and unpredictable event.

Example of what you might do
Use a magazine or newspaper story of, for example, a wedding to illustrate a predictable event and describe the change that one of the people involved in the wedding will face and the ways that they might use to cope with the change. You could also refer to caring organisations and people that might support the individual through this change in their life.

Opportunities to collect evidence
On completing these tasks you will have the opportunity to meet the following requirements for Intermediate GNVQ Health and Social Care.
Unit 2
Element 2.1 PCs 1, 2, 3, 4

Core skills

The major core skill developed is communication.

You may have opportunities to develop information technology if you use computers to produce your report or seek articles from newspapers on CD-ROM. Application of number may also be used, for example, in assessing and calculating the costs involved in moving house or retiring.

Grading

The grading themes addressed most easily are planning (to meet the requirements of the different case studies), information seeking (to provide credible examples of case studies) and quality of outcomes.

Assignment

RELATIONSHIPS

Setting the scene
The person whose (auto)biography you wrote for the assignment 'Development and Change' page 107 formed many relationships in a long life.

Task 1
Illustrating your points from the relationships in their life, write a short report to outline the different types of relationship that occurred in:
- the family
- social settings
- at work.

Note. You need to preserve confidentiality if personal interviews are used in this assignment.

▶ Confidentiality, page xxi

Task 2
Show how and why as an adolescent, as a middle-aged person and as an elderly person:
- relationships formed
- relationships changed (particularly as the family or the person developed)
- relationships broke down.

You will find plenty of information to help you in magazine articles or short stories aimed at the particular target market (for example, teenage magazines for adolescents). There are a variety of other ways to collect information, including personal interviews or questionnaires.

Opportunities to collect evidence
On completing these tasks you will have the opportunity to meet the following requirements for Intermediate GNVQ Health and Social Care.
Unit 2
Element 2.2 PCs 1, 2, 3, 4, 5

Core skills
The major core skill developed is communication. You may have opportunities to develop information technology if you use computers to produce your report or if you seek articles from newspapers on CD-ROM.

Grading
The grading themes addressed most easily are action planning (to meet the requirements of the different case studies), information seeking (to provide credible examples of case studies) and quality of outcomes.

Assignment

ROLE IN SOCIETY

Setting the scene
If you think of yourself and your relationships with different people then you start to see that people are members of many groups. You are going to compare two individuals within four different group settings. (Many of us feel uncomfortable using our own lives and relationships for assignments – so you don't have to do that.)

Part 1

Task 1
Choose two individuals: they could both be members of the same family, if you prefer. One may be someone you know well and who is comfortable about being the (anonymous) subject of this assignment. Write down the different roles the first person has in society. These may include:
- being a student
- their place in the family
- their work (if they have any paid or voluntary work)
- their recreation activities
- their position in the community.

One way of presenting this may be to use a sheet of paper with their name in the middle, and then identify the groups in boxes around the name.

Do the same thing for the other individual, it may be their parent or close relative. You may already know most of the information, but check by asking questions.

Task 2
For each of the roles identified in Task 1 for the first individual/s identify the laws, rules and conventions that govern their role. Remember that many of these are unwritten and come from their own or society's expectations. Some of the rules may be those of a club.

On your diagram from Task 1, write in the main rules, laws and conventions that are part of being a member of the group.

You do not need to identify the laws that generally cover all members of society unless you know they have an effect on the way a role is defined. (You do not need to know the law that makes them a taxpayer. It would be useful to identify the law(s) that control the role of the second individual if they were a health and safety representative in work.)

Task 3
Having identified the different roles that other individuals have within different groups, identify the roles that they take in four of the different groups of which they are a member. (For example, within the family group others will have roles as parents: in work they may be an employee and the other person may be their manager or employer. In these cases the roles differ amongst members of the groups.)

Part 2

Task 1
You will have seen from the Registrar General's classification that people can be categorised into different social classes.

Search through newspapers and magazines for reports that identify the income, health, housing and education of individuals. Using this classification system or any other that you may have found, try to identify the social class of the people described in the newspaper.

Task 2
As a group, bring together the articles that you have found. Display the articles around the room. Individually, read each article and try to identify the social class and wealth, state of health, education and housing of the people involved. You will not be able to do this for all people for all categories but each article should have been selected to identify at least one of these.

Task 3
The Registrar General's classification is based on the work role of the main wage earner in the family. As a group discuss how housing income, education and health vary for the different classes. Produce an individual summary of the features of the different classes and the evidence that you have used to support your conclusions. If there are any people who do not easily fit into the model, then identify them as special cases (for example, people who are rich but social class E, people who are social class A in a school with a poor record of achievement, unemployed people).

Task 4
Use text books and journals (for example, copies of *Social Trends* and the *Black Report*) to see if any of your conclusions fit in with nationally identified trends in the population. (For example, does your evidence from the newspaper articles show that people from social classes D and E have poorer health?)

Task 5
From all the information that you have gathered, produce a short piece of written work that identifies the effects that the social class of an individual has on their choices in terms of health (including diet) and education. Use your list of special cases identified in Task 3 to produce a critical assessment of the use of social class to predict individual choices.

Opportunities to collect evidence
On completing these tasks you will have the opportunity to meet the following requirements for Intermediate GNVQ Health and Social Care.
Unit 2
Element 2.3 PCs 1, 2, 3, 4, 5

Core skills
All core skill areas may be addressed. The application of number will be covered if you use statistical or graphical techniques to help you look at the classification information from the magazines and newspapers.

▶ The Registrar General's scale of social class, page 102

Grading

All grading themes are addressed.

Action planning is important in organising the sequence of your activities and making good use of resources. As the assignment is a long one you will need to monitor and adjust the time-scale of your plans.

Information seeking is an essential theme in gathering together the newspaper and magazine articles.

Evaluation will need to be used both in selecting the material to be used and identifying alternatives that may be used. Because of the complexity of the assignment you will have a clear opportunity at the end to evaluate the success of your efforts and identify how you might have changed the way you worked.

Quality of outcomes will be demonstrated in the reports and conclusions that you make.

Health and social well-being

Questions

Each question shows more than one possible answer, **a, b, c** and **d**; only **one** is correct.

1. The period in a person's lifetime roughly between the ages of 45–65 years is a stage in life referred to as:
   a old age
   b mid-life
   c adulthood
   d adolescence.

2. Chemicals produced by the body during puberty, for example testosterone, oestrogen and progesterone, are called:
   a menstruation
   b menopause
   c cartilage
   d hormones.

3. The ways in which people react to us has an important effect on our:
   a self-concept
   b conception
   c concept
   d culture.

4. A person's self-concept can best be strengthened by:
   a criticism
   b a joke
   c an insult
   d a compliment.

5. A group of people who live in a particular area or neighbourhood and who share a sense of belonging are said to form a:
   a community
   b town
   c family
   d relationship.

6. Factors, such as employment status, wealth, housing, are referred to as:
   a economic factors
   b cultural factors
   c socio-economic factors
   d social factors.

7. The process of thinking, reasoning and understanding is known as:
   a self-awareness
   b self-esteem
   c cognition
   d culture.

8. The beginning of sexual maturity leading to changes from girl to woman and boy to man is known as:
   a childhood
   b adulthood
   c independence
   d puberty.

9. Wrinkles, declining eyesight and hearing are some of the changes associated with ageing. Such changes are referred to as:
   a physical changes
   b psychological changes
   c social changes
   d economic changes.

10. Bonding with a parent is a characteristic of:
    a physical development
    b intellectual development
    c emotional development
    d social development.

11. The biological term for the time of rapid growth in both sexes in early teens is:
    a adolescence
    b childhood
    c menarche
    d puberty.

12. The patterns of behaviour which are linked to masculinity and femininity are known as:
    a role models
    b family roles
    c gender roles
    d role conflict.

13. Stages between life and death, for example childhood, youth, adulthood and old age, make up:
    a the life cycle
    b a generation
    c the reproductive cycle
    d old age.

14. The way of life of a given society is known as:
    a economy
    b sociology
    c culture
    d politics.

15. The expected behaviour which accompanies a particular employment status is known as:
    a image
    b status
    c a norm
    d a role.

16. Which one of the following factors is **not** indicative of a person's social class?
    a educational background
    b occupation
    c age
    d accent.

17 One consequence of marital breakdown is:
   a an increase in the number of one parent families
   b an increase in the number of nuclear families
   c a decrease in the number of step families
   d a decrease in the number of one parent families.

18 Individuals with a poor self-image are more likely to:
   a find it easy to establish a loving relationship
   b be psychologically stable and settled
   c be able to settle in quickly to new surroundings
   d find it difficult to establish a loving relationship.

19 A family group which includes other relatives in addition to parents and children is often referred to as:
   a a wider family
   b a step family
   c a new family
   d a modern family.

20 The growth of love and attachment between parent and child, which is encouraged by interaction, is known as:
   a non-verbal communication
   b bonding
   c socialisation
   d maternal deprivation.

21 Individuals have ideas and beliefs about themselves as people. This is their:
   a stereotype
   b role play
   c self-concept
   d sex role.

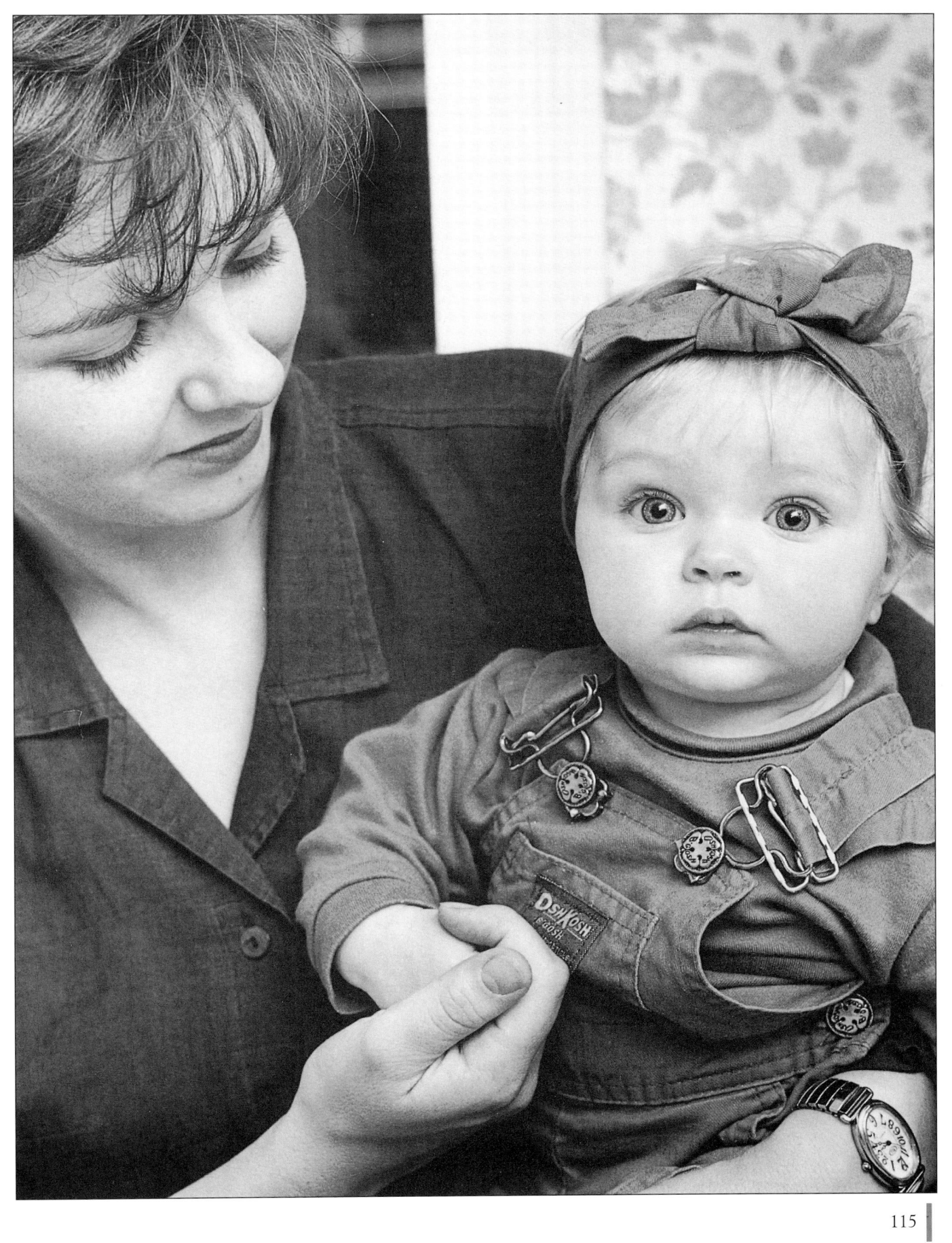

Health and social well-being

3 | Health and social care services

Most of us will, at some time in our lives, need help from the caring services. We have come to expect that whenever we need a doctor there will be one available; if we need social care then Social Services can be approached. There are other organisations we can get help from, for example the NSPCC can help children in need of support.

In this unit we will investigate the provision of services, the people who might need to use them and the people who work to provide the services. This unit cannot list all the services, but identifies the main areas and helps you to find out more about provision in your local area.

Public sector social care

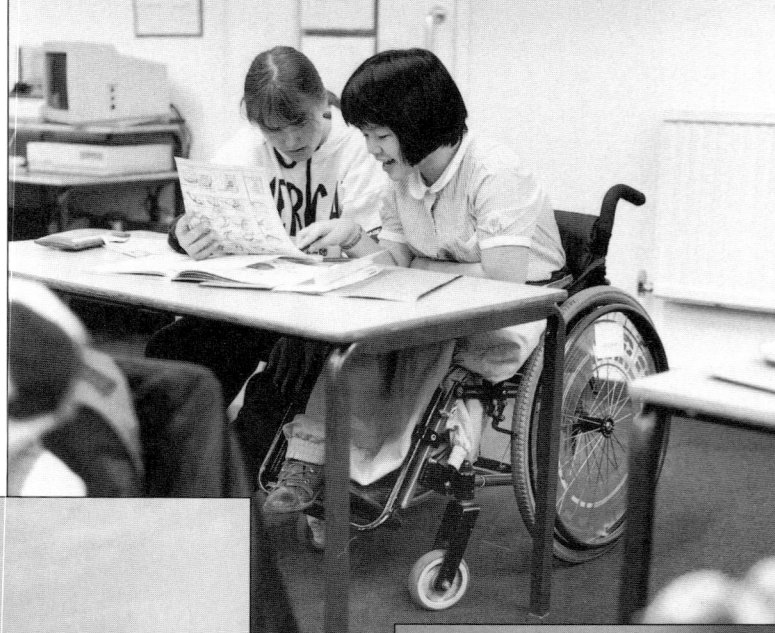

Health Care

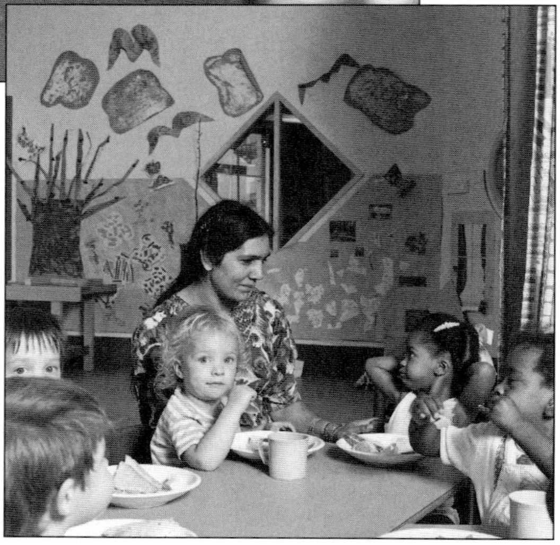

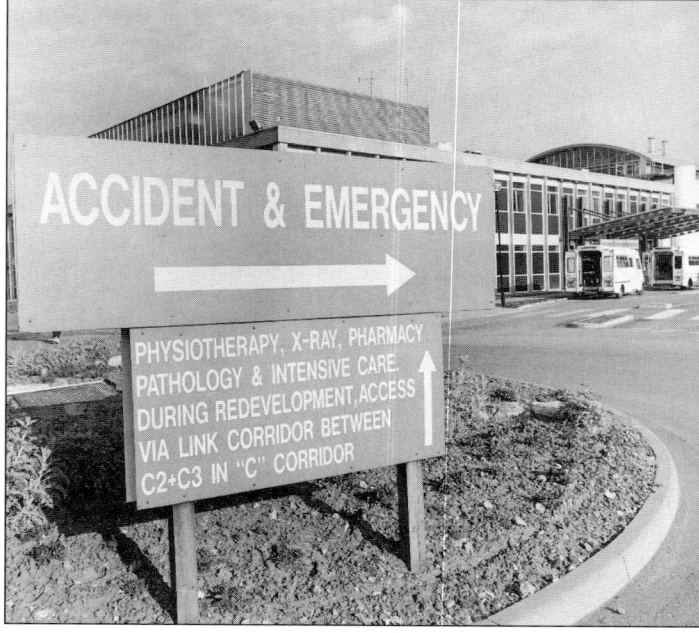

Figure 3.1 *We all need caring services*

Private sector social care

The Elements

Investigate the provision of health and social care services

- explain the organisation of statutory health and social care services
- describe the health and social care services provided by non-statutory and independent sectors
- describe the forms of health and social care which are provided by informal carers
- explain the methods of funding non-statutory sectors.

In this you will investigate the scope, coverage and funding of services and facilities which are provided locally by the statutory services. You will also investigate the important roles of the non-statutory and independent services, and informal carers.

▶ Health and social care services, page 118

Describe how the needs of different client groups are met by health and social care services

- describe the needs of client groups using health and social care services
- describe the services provided to meet the needs of client groups
- explain methods of referral to services for different client groups
- describe support for client groups to make use of services.

This section focuses on the needs of different client groups in terms of the use they might make of health and social care services and facilities. You will consider methods by which clients are referred to health and social care services and facilities, and how they can best gain access to the service.

▶ Who needs care?, page 136

Investigate jobs in health and social care

- identify the main jobs in health and social care services
- describe the day-to-day work of people with jobs in health and social care
- describe the career routes of people with jobs in health and social care
- compare the actual role of people who work in health and social care with stereotypes of these roles.

Here you will investigate the roles of people who work in health and social care, and consider the broad tasks which they perform. The section describes the broad functions of the practitioners, from which you can conduct your own investigation into local workers and their roles. Examples are given of career paths into the caring services. You will be expected to investigate these further for yourselves.

▶ Who delivers care? –2, page 147

Health and social care services

HELP....!
- My brother has broken his leg.
- I've just been diagnosed as HIV positive.
- I need to go into hospital soon. Who will look after my children?
- My wife has Alzheimer's disease and I need a break.
- The two young children next door are left alone most nights.
- I'm pregnant. What happens next?
- I've got this terrible toothache.

In all of these situations one or more of the health and social care services need to be involved. Sometimes the need is an emergency; at other times the need can be planned for. The care need may be for nursing care, companionship or help in the home. In each case we need to find a way of reaching the right service.

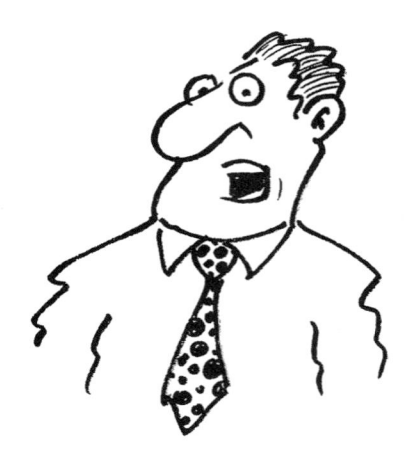

A Who delivers care? – 1

Spend five minutes writing down as many people, or organisations, associated with care as you can. Share your list with others in your group, then divide the group list into different categories (see below). The people or organisations may be in more than one category. Keep the list of 'don't knows' – by the end of the unit you should be able to allocate some of them to the right groups.

Categories should include:
- those delivering health care
- those delivering social care
- those funded by Government both Central and Local
- those that make money from caring
- those that are charities
- don't know.

Your lists will have started to help you classify organisations involved in care. There are two groups or sectors normally identified with health and care services:
- statutory sector
- non-statutory and independent services (private sector, voluntary sector).

It is possible to identify a third group sector that provides a great deal of care: those people who care informally for others.

We will look at all three of these sectors in more detail.

The statutory sector

The statutory sector: organisations that have been set up by law. It includes the Health (under the NHS), Social, Probation and Education Services.

We will look at the Health Service and the Social Services. Before looking at them in detail, it is important to understand something about government control and why there are two parts to the statutory sector in health and social care.

> **FOCUS**
>
> Organisation of statutory services:
> - overall structure (goverment department level, regional level, area level)
> - purchaser and provider
> - function of services
> - inter-relationships of services
> - funding of services.

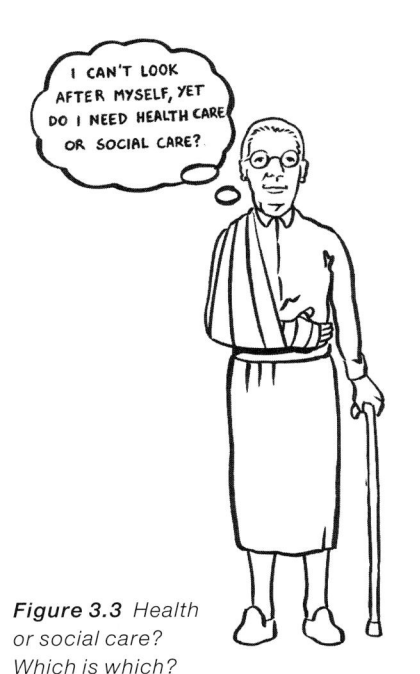

Control at government level

The Health Service and Social Services are both under the control of central government. The overall policy-making and funding comes from the government department that controls them. For the Health Services, only one department is involved – the Department of Health. Several different Government Departments are involved in the overall provision of Social Services as can be seen in Figure 3.2.

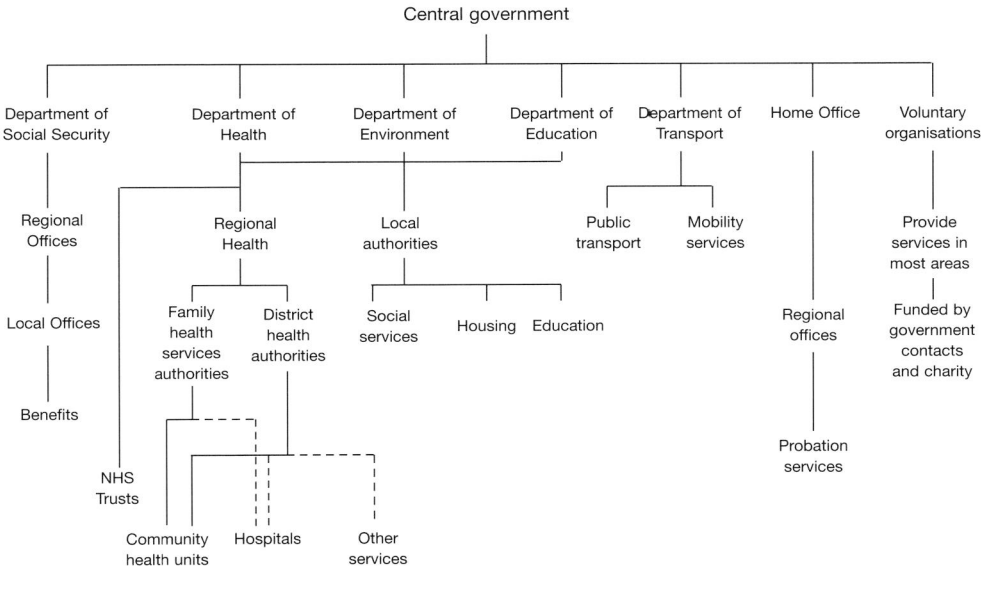

Organisations involved in health and social care

```
                              Central government
   ┌────────┬──────────┬──────────┬──────────┬──────────┬──────────┬──────────┐
Department  Department  Department  Department  Department  Home Office  Voluntary
of Social   of Health   of          of          of                       organisations
Security                Environment Education   Transport
   │           │           │           │           │           │            │
Regional    Regional    Local                   Public    Mobility      Regional    Provide
Offices     Health      authorities             transport services      offices     services in
                                                                                    most areas
   │       ┌───┴────┐   ┌───┬────┐                          │              │
Local    Family   District Social Housing Education                    Regional   Funded by
Offices  health   health   services                                    offices    government
         services authorities                                                     contacts
         authorities                                                              and charity
   │
Benefits                                                              Probation
                                                                      services
         NHS
         Trusts

         Community  Hospitals  Other
         health units          services
```

Figure 3.2 Organisations involved in health and social care

Source: Based on *GNVQ Advanced Health and Social Care* by Clarke, Sachs and Waltham, published by Stanley Thornes Publishers.

Health and social services

Why do we have separate health and social care services? Where are the boundaries between health and social care? More importantly – What does the division between health and social care mean to you and me, the users of the services?

The divisions can be explained by looking at how the two sides of the caring services developed.

Figure 3.3 Health or social care? Which is which?

Health and social care services

The formation of the health services

The National Health Service (NHS) came into existence on 5 July 1948. It was set up as a result of the National Health Services Act in 1946. The function of the NHS was to provide health care to all. It was to be paid for with national insurance contributions from all working people. It was initially thought that the health of the nation would improve and so the cost of the NHS would fall, with fewer people needing treatment.

Before the NHS was formed there had been a variety of insurance systems that paid for health care in privately owned and run facilities. After the formation of the NHS the bulk of health care was controlled by the NHS with some care remaining in the private sector.

The structure set up under the Act had a major effect on the NHS as it set up a bureaucratic (rigid) system that many people felt created both problems in management and increased costs. In fact, the organisation has changed over the years until the current structure shown below was established. This structure has developed since the NHS and Community Care Act, 1990 started to be implemented and is likely to develop further in the future.

Key legislation, Appendix III page 224.

Before April 1994
1 Northern
2 Yorkshire
3 Trent
4 East Anglia
5 NW Thames
6 NE Thames
7 SE Thames
8 SW Thames
9 Wessex
10 Oxford
11 South Western
12 West Midlands
13 Mersey
14 North Western

After April 1994
1 East Anglian & Ox.
2 North Thames
3 South Thames
4 South West
5 West Midlands
6 North West
7 North East & Yorks.
8 Trent

Source: Guardian, 22 October 1992

Figure 3.5 Regional Health Authorities in England before and after 1994

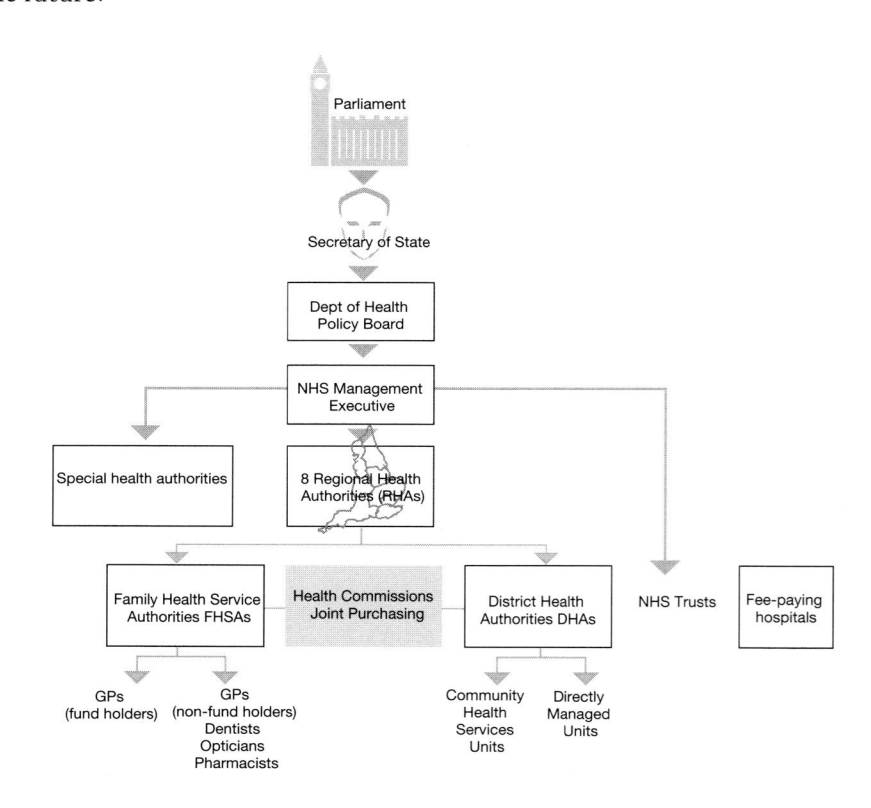

Figure 3.4 The structure of the NHS in England. The structures in all four countries of the United Kingdom vary: you need to identify the current structure in your country

Note. These structures are currently under review and you will need to gain access to the most recent information for further developments.

Regional Health Authorities (RHAs)
England has eight Regional Health Authorities. Each RHA is divided into smaller District Health Authorities and Family Health Service Authorities.

Wales is similar to England except that the whole of the country can be considered as one regional health authority run by the Welsh Office. Within Wales there are nine District Health Authorities.

Scotland can be considered to be like Wales. The whole of Scotland is organised like a Regional Health Authority run through the Scottish Office. Within Scotland there are 15 Health Boards that combine the roles of District Health Authorities and Family Health Service Authorities.

Northern Ireland is organised quite differently. It has four Health and Social Services Boards that provide both health and personal social services.

RHA responsibilities
RHAs make regional plans and share out resources. They:
- identify the needs in the region
- determine priorities, such as how much specialist surgery will be provided compared with care for elderly people
- plan where any new facilities should be set up or built within the region
- identify hospitals that are regional centres for specialist treatments (for example, heart transplant surgery is normally located in a few regional centres)
- share out the available money to the District Health Authorities, Family Health Service Authorities and fund-holding General Practitioners
- monitor the activities of the organisations that they fund, and work to help co-operation.
- employ senior medical and dental staff.

District Health Authorities (DHAs)
DHAs are responsible for:
- assessing the health needs of the local population
- purchasing health care services for people living in their district
- managing the hospitals and other services which are directly under their control (for example, Directly Managed Units, DMUs) including employing medical and other health-related staff.

Their role is becoming one of predicting local health care needs and contracting with health care providers to meet the needs. As such they are becoming purchasers of health care. The contacts are with the NHS, private or voluntary sector organisations.

▶ NHS purchasers, page 127

Family Health Service Authorities (FHSAs)
These are responsible for the provision of primary care services in the community. The services are provided by:
- General Practitioners (GPs) – the doctor with whom you will be most familiar
- dentists – many now work only in the private sector and are not funded by the FHSAs

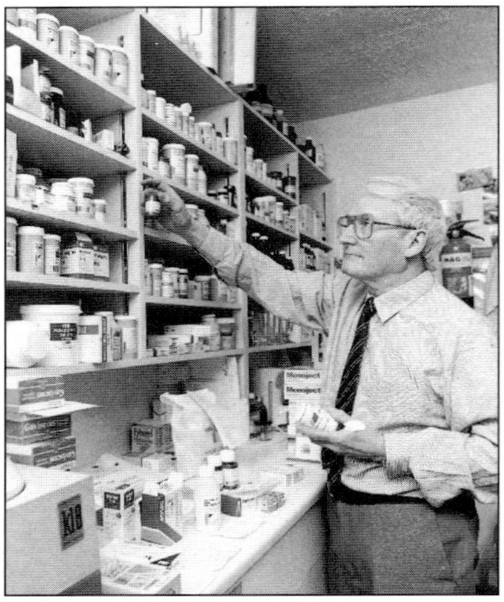

Health and social care services

Figure 3.6 Pharmacists provide medicines prescribed by doctors

- opticians – who test eyesight and prescribe lenses to correct vision defects
- pharmacists – who are responsible for providing medicines prescribed by doctors.

In recent years the role of the various bodies has been changing and it is likely that these trends will continue:

- the number of RHAs has recently been reduced considerably (from 14 to 8) and in the future their role is likely to change further – for example, by effectively becoming regional offices of the National Health Service Management Executive
- although both FHSAs and DHAs continue to be providers of services themselves (for example, by employing doctors and running directly Managed Hospitals), their role is increasingly becoming one of assessing the local health-care needs and drawing up contracts with providers to purchase these services
- in many areas the trend is for DHAs and FHSAs to work together in Health Commissions, with major responsibility for purchasing all the health care for the local population.

NHS Trusts

NHS Trusts are a further division in the structure of the NHS. The NHS and Community Care Act made it possible for organisations (units) within a district to opt to become self-governing trusts. These units could be individual hospitals, Community Health Services or services like the ambulance service.

The NHS trusts have a responsibility for managing their own money. They employ their own staff. The NHS trusts compete for the contracts alongside private and voluntary sector providers. The original expectation was that this competition for money would increase the value for money of the health care provided.

The trusts provide the health-care services identified as necessary by the RHAs, DHAs, FSHAs and fund-holding GPs.

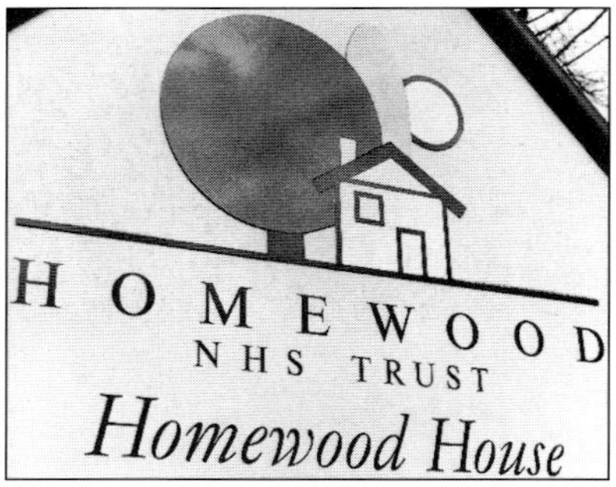

Figure 3.7 A trust hospital is entirely self-governing

Special Health Authorites (SHAs)

These report directly either to the Department of Health in London or the NHS Management Executive. There are at present three kinds of SHA although this is changing as the NHS itself changes under the current reforms.

1 Non-Hospital SHAs provide a service for the NHS as a whole, for example, The NHS Supplies Authority based in Reading buying hospital supplies for the NHS and accountable to the NHS Management Executive. Another example is the Health Education Authority.

2 Special Hospitals which deal with the care of seriously disturbed offenders. There are three: Broadmoor, Rampton and Ashworth. There are no plans at present for these to become NHS Trusts.

3 Until April 1994 there were a number of specialist postgraduate teaching and research hospitals in London. By April 1994, six of the eight hospitals had become NHS Trusts and were no longer SHAs leaving only two that were SHAs. These are likely also to become NHS Trusts.

NHS purchasers and providers, page 127

Health and social care services

Subdivisions of the health services

Health care is divided into four classes that reflect the differing needs. They are:

- **primary care** – describes care delivered in the community and is usually the first to be used, for example GP, practice nurse, health visitor. The care is often of a preventative nature

- **secondary care** – provided in hospital situations. The care is often aimed to bring about a cure

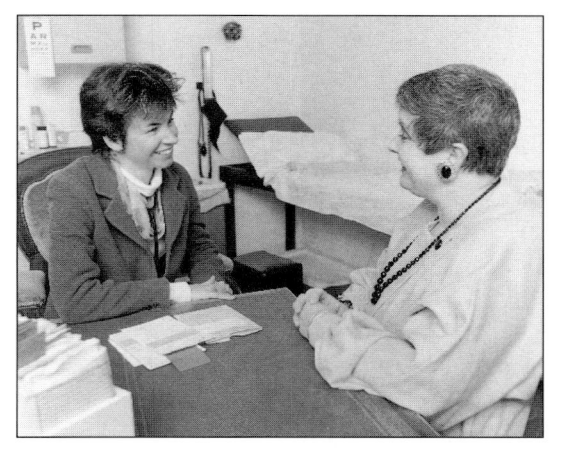

Figure 3.8 *Primary Care*

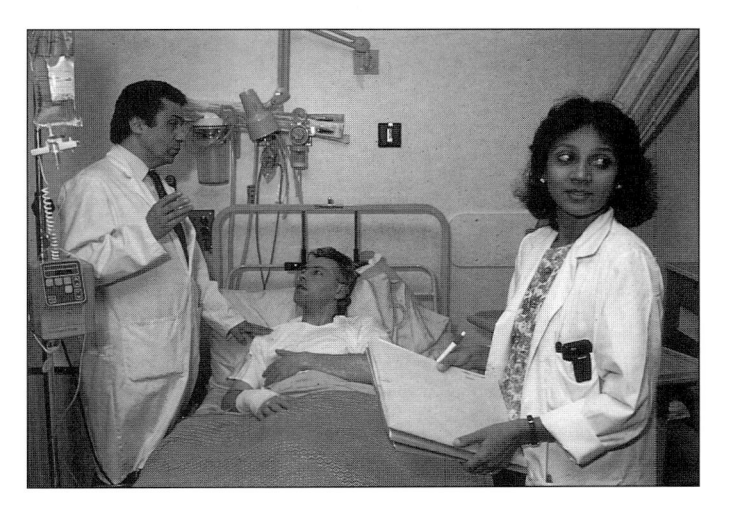

Figure 3.9 *Secondary Care*

- **tertiary care** – provided through long-term rehabilitation. This may be in a long-stay hospital but more and more it forms part of community care.
  Rehabilitation: *returning a person to as near normal a state of health as possible.*

- **community care** – these services are based on the delivery of care as much as possible within the community and, in many cases, within the client's own home. For this to happen there has to be close co-operation with the Social Services.

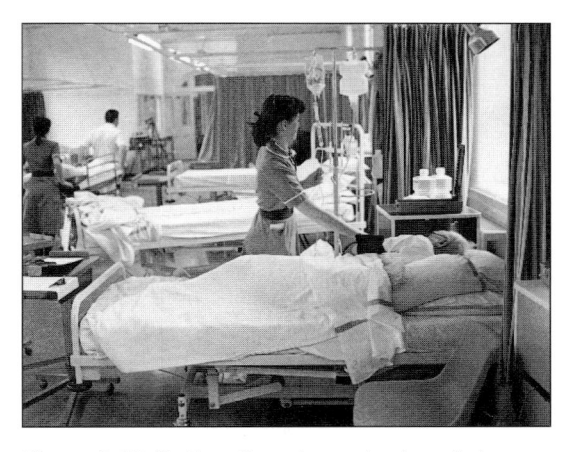

Figure 3.10 *Tertiary Care, long-stay hospital*

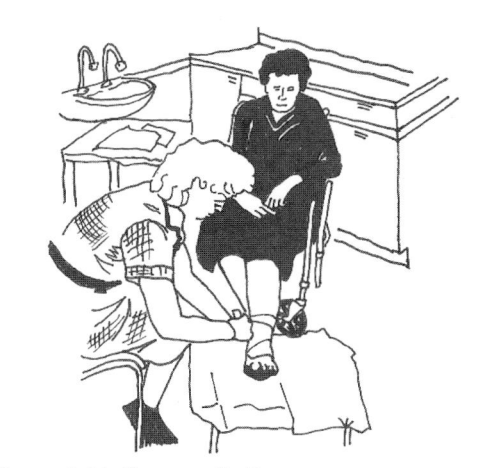

Figure 3.11 *Community Care*

FOCUS

Statutory health and social care sectors:
- NHS (primary, secondary, tertiary care, community care)
- personal social services.

123

Health and social care services

Except in the case of emergencies, it is normal for a person to receive care from the primary care team, for example GPs, before being referred to hospital. Following hospital treatment there may be a need for further rehabilitation. This may take place in the hospital itself or more often in the person's own home as part of Care in the Community. For this to work there must be close links amongst the care providers (and purchasers) to ensure that a person is not discharged from secondary care without the tertiary or community care being available.

There are times when a service may provide both primary and secondary care. For example, a paramedic treating someone at the scene of an accident is providing primary care, whereas the same paramedic working in an ambulance service collecting a client for treatment at a hospital is an example of secondary care.

▶ Purchasers and providers, page 127

The formation of the social services

The personal social services are those which look after the needs of a wide range of client groups including families, children and young people, people with disabilities and/or learning difficulties, and elderly people. These services are the responsibility of the local authority, although as we shall see later in this unit, many services are also provided by voluntary organisations of various kinds.

Going back in history, many of these services were set up in response to social conditions associated with poverty, and they provided a safety net for vulnerable groups in our society. Today's services have a wide variety of origins, including those provided by law by local authorities and those provided by charitable organisations. Those charities include Barnados (formerly Dr Barnardo's) and the Children's Society (formerly Church of England Children's Society).

Local authority social services really began to develop as we know them today after the Second World War: for example, in 1948 Local Authority Children's Departments were set up.

In 1970, following a major report, Social Services Committees were formed in each local authority. These had responsibility for:
- child-care (including fostering and adoption)
- provision and regulation of residential accommodation for older people and people with disabilities
- welfare services for older people, people with disabilities and the chronically ill. Also statutory powers under the Mental Health Act
- delegation to other appropriate organisations of some of the social care provision.

The 1970 Act largely brought social care within the control of local authorities, and their Social Services Committees.

The diverse origins of the Social Services and the structures of local authorities mean that it is not easy to define the national management of statutory social services. Even the formation of the Social Services in 1970 did not provide an overarching structure like the NHS. You will need to investigate your own local organisation. A large public library will usually have most of the information that you need.

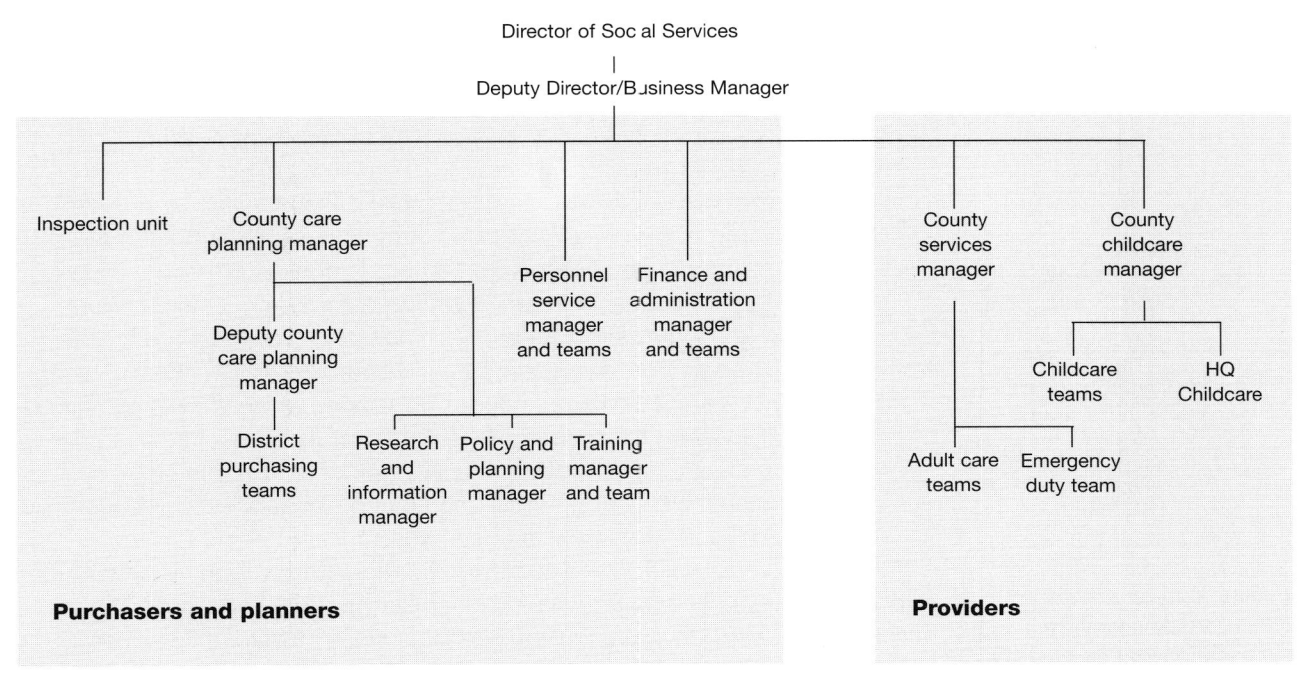

```
                        Director of Social Services
                                 |
                   Deputy Director/Business Manager
```

Figure 3.12 The structure of a typical local authority Social Services Department. The Probation Service, Housing and the social care aspects of Education are not mentioned: these areas come under different control. This reflects the control from central government

Purchasers and planners (left side): Inspection unit; County care planning manager → Deputy county care planning manager → District purchasing teams; Research and information manager; Policy and planning manager; Training manager and team; Personnel service manager and teams; Finance and administration manager and teams.

Providers (right side): County services manager → Adult care teams, Emergency duty team; County childcare manager → Childcare teams, HQ Childcare.

Source: Based on *GNVQ Advanced Health and Social Care* by Clarke, Sachs and Waltham, published by Stanley Thornes Publishers.

The National Health Service and Community Care Act 1990

The divide between health care and social care was always an artificial one which affected local authorities' ability to plan care for people in the community. The NHS Community Care Act 1990 was a wide-reaching piece of legislation covering the following principal areas:
- community care plans
- assessment and care management
- purchasing and contracting
- inspection units
- specific grants for mental illness.

Care planning

The NHS and Community Care Act 1990 focused on care planning. Local authorities are now required to publish an annual community care plan. (Your local library will probably have a copy.) Another drive towards planning was the change in funding. The Act defined two roles; those of purchaser of care and provider of care. Those people with control of funds (Local Authorities and District Health Authorities) purchased the care required from providers in any sector.

Predicting care needs

In order to purchase care it is necessary first to predict what care is going to be needed.

▶ Key legislation, Appendix III, page 224

Health and social care services

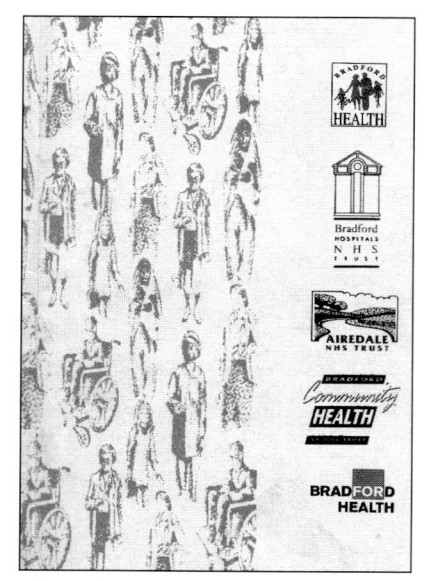

Figure 3.13 *Health care organisations in Bradford work together to produce local patient's charter information for the community*

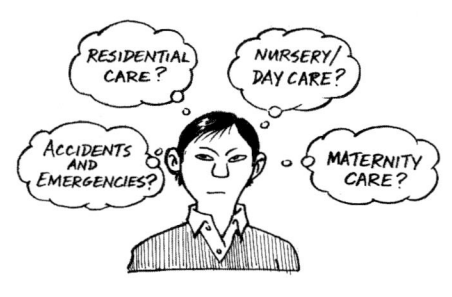

Figure 3.14 *Many things need to be considered when planning care*

A. Care needs in your community

How would you predict care needs in your local community? What information would you need to have?

1a Working in twos or threes, design a questionnaire or survey sheet to collect information on current care needs. Ask each member of the group to collect information from about 30 people drawn from family, friends and neighbours. The information you collect should include relevant background information, for example age (age group) and gender. Try to include people from all age groups and both genders, to enable you to find out if there are different needs for male/females/different age groups.

b Without invading their privacy, try to find out what sort of care needs different people have had over the last year or so. Explain that the information they provide will be treated confidentially – the questionnaire should not ask for names, or addresses.

As a group you should aim to obtain information from a cross-section of the population – old and young, male and female. Try to get between 100 and 200 results. Why do you think you need this many? Could you use only 20 results to predict the needs of the local population? Share the list of needs with the full group to compile an overall list of the care needs you have identified.

Can you think of a way to quantify this type of information? Get a rough idea of how many hours/days people have used the services. For example, you could estimate that a visit to the doctor/GP requires an average of, say, ten minutes of the doctor's time. What else does it require? What does a visit to casualty/the accident and emergency department in a hospital require? Can you estimate this for each area of care? This will help you to find which kind is needed most.

To help analyse your results set up a database or spreadsheet.

If you can quantify the information, you can use your results to estimate the total number of hours required of each type of carer.

2 Find out the population of your local health authority. Use your result to predict care needs in your area.

Possible methods:

- work out what fraction of the population you have asked. Use this information to work out what would be required by the whole population. For example, if you had asked one half of the population, you would need to double your results. If you had asked one tenth of the population, you would need to multiply your results by 10

- work out what percentage of the population you asked. For each of your results, divide by this percentage (to find 1%) and multiply by 100 (to find 100%)

- use pie charts. All pie charts use 360° regardless of the number of people questioned. Any pie chart you produce from your sample could be thought of as being produced by the whole population. Work back to find what results this would imply. Do television 'soaps' suggest any gaps, for instance?

3 Have you included all possible areas of care in your survey? Are there care needs which have not appeared on your list, but which could arise? Are there others you could not include? Are there areas you could not quantify? If so, how would you be able to predict care needs in the areas? How reliable is your information likely to be? What are the drawbacks to the methods used here?

4 Produce a report using your statistics, explaining how you reached the main predicted care needs in an area, and stating the limitations of your predictions. This kind of information could help you to plan care in your community.

Having identified the care needs, the purchaser then asks the care-providing organisations to identify what they can provide and the cost of the provision. Contracts for delivery of care can be signed and the care delivered. The contract is not necessarily with the cheapest provider, as other issues such as quality of care and waiting times may be taken into consideration.

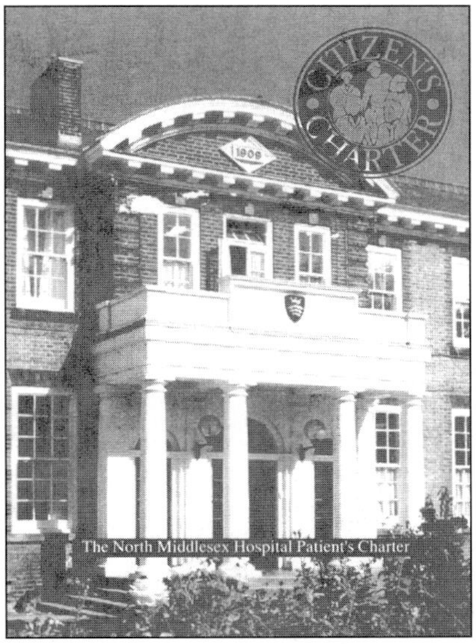

Competition

The ideas behind the purchaser/provider split are based on increased competition. No organisation can assume that it will get a specific contract and so the costs of the services have to be kept to a minimum. At the same time, organisations are aware of the need to maintain or improve the quality of care and 'customer service'. Improvements in efficiency (doing more for the same money or work) can mean that money is saved and used to improve the quality of care.

Improvements in efficiency can come from increased medical knowledge. Improved techniques may mean that recovery times from operations can be reduced. A patient may occupy a bed for less time and so free it for another patient, reducing waiting times.

In residential care efficiency cannot sensibly be measured in throughput of clients. If the service were so bad that clients died after ten days, then the throughput would be high! Client satisfaction and improved customer care may be better indicators for purchasers to use when considering bids from different organisations.

Figure 3.15 *National and local charters are designed to improve quality of service*

NHS purchasers and providers

Purchasers

In the health services the main groups of purchasers are:
- Regional Health Authorities
- District Health Authorities
- Family Health Services Authorities
- fund-holding GPs.

Purchasers: *the organisations or parts of organisations that fund the care. They buy (purchase) the caring services from an organisation that undertakes caring. To do this they need to have systems (plans) to predict the needs for care in the areas for which they are responsible.*

Fund-holding GPs: *have money allocated by Regional Health Authorities to provide for a variety of health requirements. The GP must identify the priorities for the health care of his/her patients. Fund-holding GPs are becoming more common. A non fund-holding GP relies on the services for patients that are purchased by the other authorities.*

Health and social care services

Each of these groups has money allocated to purchase the care needed by their clients. They predict and plan the health-care requirements of the population in their area and then ask health-care providers to bid for the work.

Providers

The providers may be:
- under the control of the purchaser (for example, a non-NHS trust hospital – there are fewer and fewer of these Directly Managed Units – DMUs)
- an NHS trust
- from the private sector
- from the voluntary sector.

Providers: *the organisations and people who deliver the care that is bought by the purchasers. In some cases a purchaser may also be a provider. A fund-holding GP may provide care through a contract with the Family Health Services Authority (a purchaser). The GP may also purchase care (for example, an operation) from a hospital trust (a provider of care).*

In social care similar systems exist but often the local authority may be a purchaser of care as well as a provider (for example, the authority may purchase nursery day care for a child as well as provide the care in a Social Services-run day nursery).

Figure 3.16 Fund-holding GPs are purchasers and providers. They are purchasers when they buy services for patients (e.g. some operations) and providers when they diagnose and prescribe.

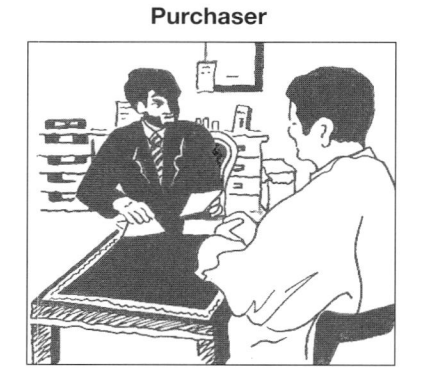

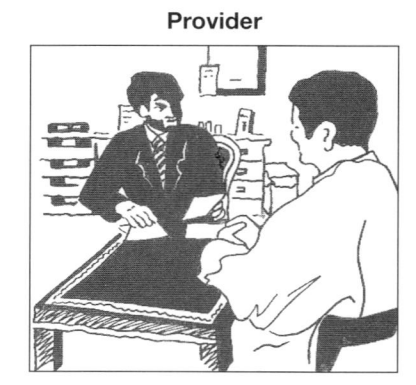

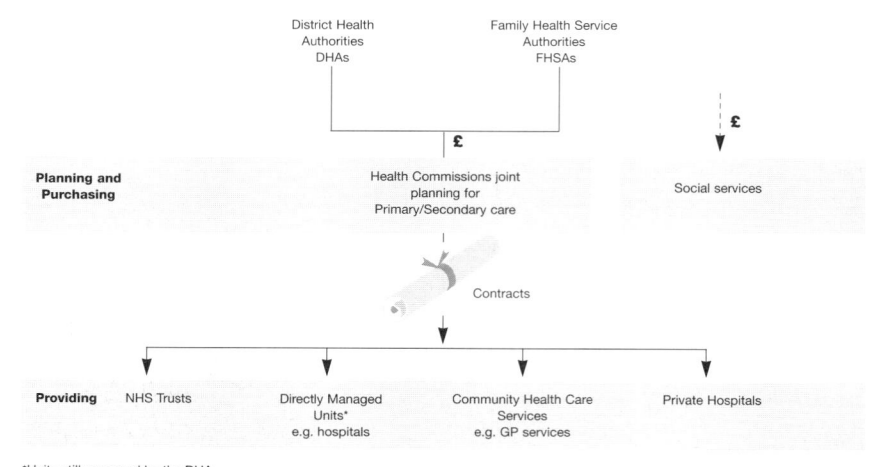

Figure 3.17 Purchasers and providers in Hampshire

Planning and Purchasing

District Health Authorities DHAs → Family Health Service Authorities FHSAs → £ → Health Commissions joint planning for Primary/Secondary care

£ → Social services

Contracts

Providing: NHS Trusts | Directly Managed Units* e.g. hospitals | Community Health Care Services e.g. GP services | Private Hospitals

*Units still managed by the DHA
Note: Under the NHS and Community Care Act these bodies must publish an annual plan for the distrct they covered – they must work together!

Health and social care services

The emergence of Health Commissions

Example: Hampshire
The North and mid-Hampshire Health Commission was set up in September 1992 as a partnership between:
- North Hampshire (District) Health Authority
- Winchester (District) Health Authority
- Hampshire Family Health Service Authority.

The aim of the Health Commission is to combine the purchasing power of each of the three constituent bodies. It is responsible for assessing the health needs of local people and setting contracts with hospitals and community units to secure health services to meet these needs. It also works closely with Social Services in the joint planning and commissioning of services for the population.

In Hampshire, and elsewhere, the following structure is developing.

Social services purchasers and providers
In the past Local Authority Social Services Departments were major providers of services to elderly people, children, families and so on.

The NHS and Community Care Act has, however, changed the emphasis in their role from being chiefly a 'provider' of services to that of a 'planner' and 'purchaser'.

Using money provided by Central Government, Social Services Departments are responsible in law for making sure that sufficient services exist for the groups mentioned.

Although it does provide some of these services itself (for example, Local Authority elderly care homes), increasingly it has to act as a purchaser of services. This means that following an assessment by a social worker, the department will purchase the 'package of care' needed from private organisations (for example, elderly care homes, home help services), voluntary bodies (for example, day care) or even from private individuals (for example, foster care).

▶ The structure of a Social Services Department, page 125

Individual care planning
Alongside the broad care plans written by the various authorities, each person receiving care has to have an agreed individualised care plan. The degree to which this is implemented depends upon the resources available. Planning creates some concerns because there are frequent conflicts between client needs or wants and the funding available.

Care in the community
The act has led to the closure of many mental hospitals and other long-stay institutions. Care plans for many of the 'patients' in these hospitals have identified that community-based care is more appropriate. Many of the patients are able to take on an independent or supported role in the community.

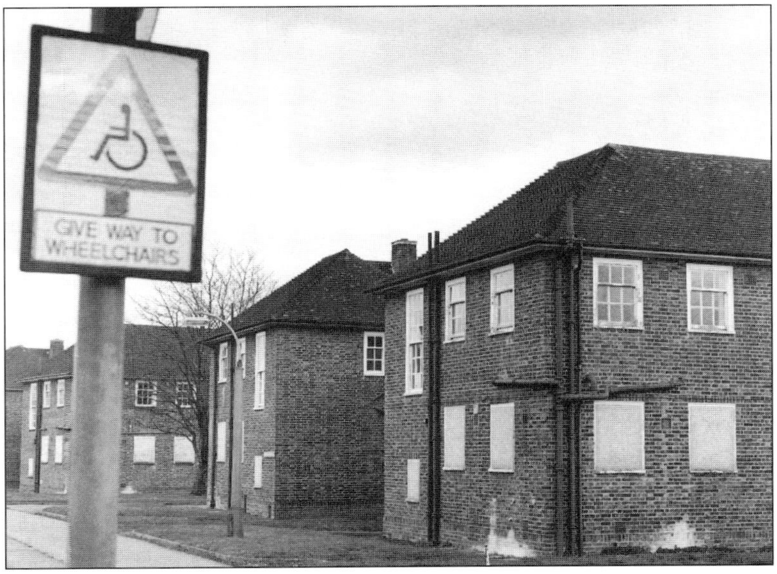

Figure 3.18 *Institutions such as these are being replaced by care in the community*

129

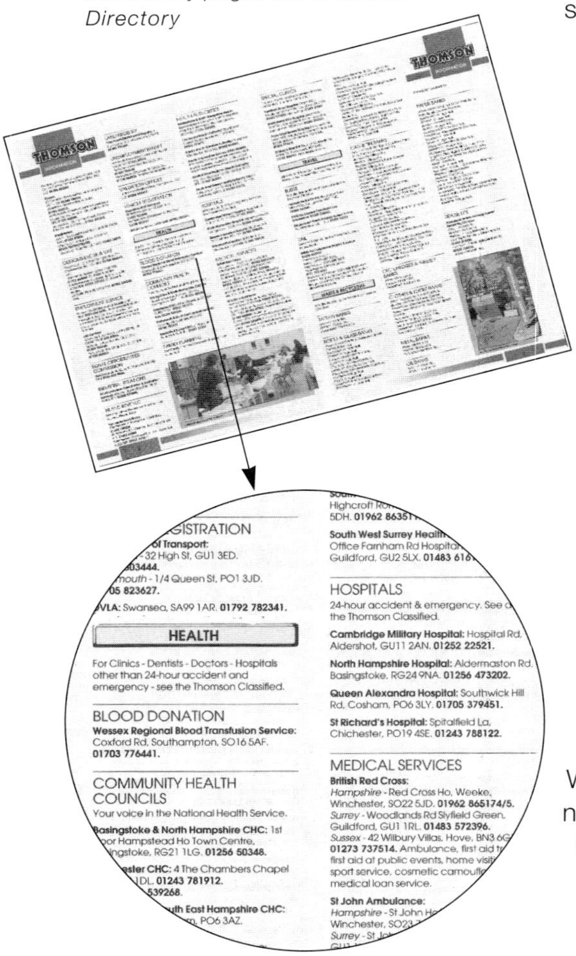

Health and social care services

Figure 3.19 *An extract from the community pages in a Thomson Directory*

▶ Bibliography/useful addresses, page 214

A Provision in your local area

All areas of the country have slightly different ways of organising caring services. For this activity you should look at caring services in your area.

1. What information is available in the various directories – *The phone book, Thomsons, Yellow Pages*?

   Look up:
   - Social Services
     - how the organisation is split up
     - what services are offered (for example, *The phone book* for Bradford has over 100 listings including Day Centres, Family Centres, Give Mum A Break)
   - Health Services
     - what types of service there are
     - where the private services are listed
   - which directories give most information about
     - Citizens Advice Bureau(x)
     - the local hospitals
     - the Family Health Services Authority
     - health centres
     - how many GPs there are
     - where a person with mobility difficulties might be able to seek advice about benefits
     - where you could get advice about contraception and abortion
     - your nearest blood-donating centre
     - provision available for under fives – playgroups, nurseries, etc.

   Write a summary of the types of information in the different directories. Do not try to list all the organisations.

2. Individually or in groups investigate what some of the services provide. Cover a broad range. Try to find out as much as you can, without causing extra work for organisations. Many produce leaflets and information sheets that are available in your local library.

The range of social services

A broad range of care is provided by the statutory social services. The internal structure of the social services departments often reflects the areas in which they provide support. You may have found sections dealing with the main areas of social care:

- families – providing support to families during times of stress
- children – services may include fostering and adoption and children's homes. There may also be an inspection service for child-care provision (e.g. private day nurseries and childminders)
- young people – often there are specfic sections for helping adolescent children, in particular in a family setting
- adults – many adults need support. This area of work has increased, with more care in the community for people with mental health problems. This section also includes working with elders. As with children, there may be inspection services for care provision for elders (for example, private residential care homes).

The voluntary sector

The voluntary sector refers to **non-statutory**, non-profit making organisations whose management committees are unpaid. The term 'voluntary' in the title does not mean that the people involved are necessarily unpaid volunteers. Almost all of the larger voluntary organisations pay their staff. These staff are normally qualified in the same way as those working in the statutory sector. It might be better to describe the sector as a non-statutory sector.

Many of the voluntary sector organisations are charities: some of these were the earliest organisations, formed in the nineteenth century, to provide care. Examples are the NSPCC (National Society for the Prevention of Cruelty to Children), the Children's Society and Barnardo's. Other examples of services in the voluntary sector are the WRVS (Women's Royal Voluntary Service) and Age Concern.

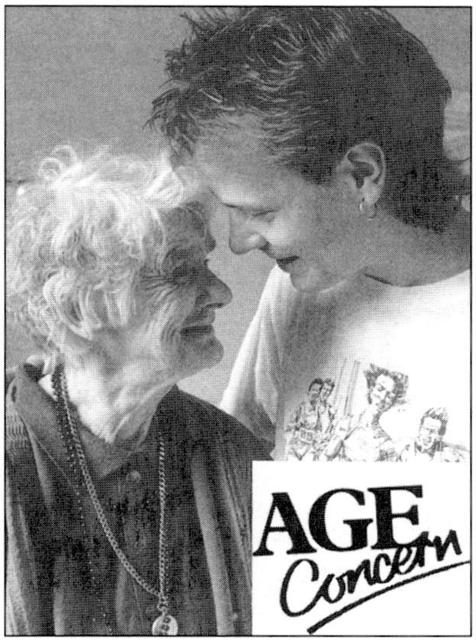

Co-ordinating the voluntary sector

The National Council for Voluntary Organisations (NCVO) is an umbrella organisation that co-ordinates the work of the 200 or so Councils for Voluntary Service (CVS). These co-ordinate, support and advise organisations within their local voluntary sector. Both the NCVO and the individual CVS advise government (both local and national) about issues concerning the voluntary sector and voluntary sector organisations. In many cases they are responsible for the administration of funds directed towards the voluntary sector from central and local government and, more recently, the European Union.

Why have a voluntary sector?

The organisations work in co-operation with the statutory sector, often identifying areas of need that are not well covered by statutory organisations. The original charities were formed because the very limited legislation at the time left many in need of care.

In spite of the development of a welfare state, there are people who need assistance in some other form. The voluntary sector provides support in areas that complement those covered by the statutory sector. The co-operation between the sectors means that the spread of care is greater, and wider sources of funds can be used to provide care. Links have been firmly established with Care in the Community, as Social Services departments purchase services from voluntary sector providers.

Figure 3.20 Age Concern is a voluntary organisation

A — Voluntary services

Use local directories, your local library and the Council for Voluntary Services to identify a range of sector organisations active in your area. If possible, obtain copies of leaflets about the local activities.
Try to discover the following kinds of information:
- target groups of clients
- nature of assistance/service offered
- address and telephone numbers of local office
- times when office open/telephone staffed.

Record the information you find under these headings or others which you find more suitable.

FOCUS

Funding for non-statutory services:
- donations
- government grants
- contracts
- direct payment
- insurance.

Health and social care services

Devise a suitable way of presenting the information to other members of the group, and try to find a way of highlighting any links between the organisations. (If three groups aim to support the same client group, one with counselling, one with emergency accommodation and one with financial help, how can you indicate that?)

Note. If you are doing this as a member of a group please organise yourselves so that you each tackle different areas. Please co-ordinate your work, telephone to make appointments and do some research before you start asking questions, to reduce the time the organisation has to spend on your enquiries.

▶ The National Society for the Prevention of Cruelty to Children; Barnardo's, Page 139

Example organisations:
NSPCC
Barnardo's
Women's Royal Voluntary Service
Help the Aged
St. John Ambulance

Funding the voluntary sector

Donations from the public are one source of funding, other sources include:

- grants from government, the European Union, etc.
- direct payments by clients for services (often these are based on ability to pay and do not cover the full cost of the service)
- payments from others for services purchased on behalf of clients (local authorities buying services for Community Care)
- grants from the National Lottery.

Some voluntary sector organisations have annual budgets of millions of pounds, whilst others survive on figures in the hundreds of pounds.

Private sector

The private sector was involved in care before the statutory sector was formed. In this sector the organisations charge for the care provided and normally seek to make a profit. Organisations include:

- hospitals (both private hospitals and private-sector work in NHS hospitals)
- residential homes
- nursing homes
- some pre-five nursery provision (there are several companies running a number of nurseries).

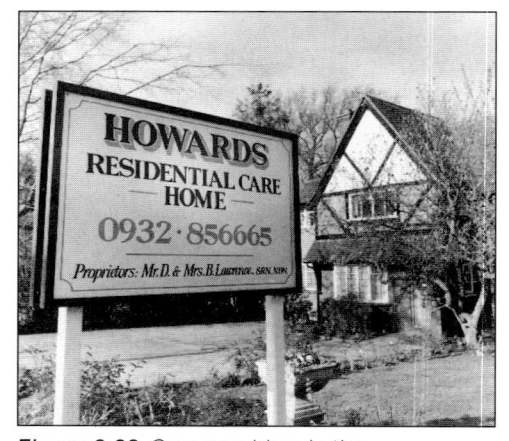

Figure 3.22 Care providers in the private sector

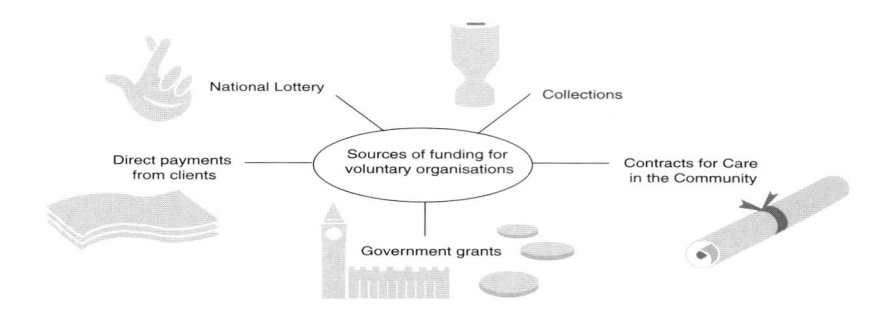

Figure 3.21 Sources of funding for voluntary organisations

There are many people who run an individual residential home or nursery and are self-employed. One of the largest groups of self-employed carers is childminders, who work in their own homes looking after children, and must be registered with their local Social Services Department. Foster carers often fit into the category of the self-employed. They are normally given an allowance to cover the costs of the person being fostered. In some cases they are paid a further amount for the care they provide.

For many care organisations in the private sector much of the income comes directly from the people requiring the care. Others, in particular private residential homes, have relied on fees being paid by the Department of Social Security. Since the NHS and Community Care Act there have been changes in the funding strategies, with the effect that the fees paid by the local authority need to be 'topped up' by the individuals in care or their families.

In health care the development of the purchaser/provider divide means that the distinction between private hospitals and NHS hospitals is less clear. A District Health Authority can purchase services from either NHS hospitals or the private sector. The distinction between the two types is that the private sector is profit-making.

Private health care is available. The individual is expected to make arrangements for the health-care provider to receive payment. In many cases the costs are met by an insurance company. The individual pays for the care through insurance premiums, for example through subscriptions to organisations such as BUPA.

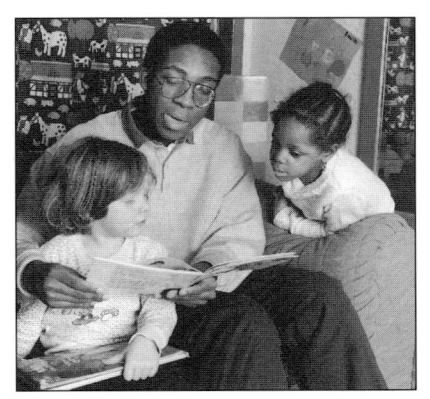

Figure 3.23 Childminders are registered carers

Complementary medicine

When we consider health we normally think of doctors, nurses and hospitals. Within this structure are people working in professions allied to medicines, such as physiotherapists, chiropodists and, increasingly, osetopaths. These services can be offered as part of private health care.

The inclusion of osteopaths in this list is a new one. Osteopaths have hitherto been viewed as part of a complementary health service.

Complementary health service: *people who practice forms of health care that are often related to ideas that have little scientific support. This does not mean that they do not work, it just means that they are not part of mainstream medical provision.*

Included in a list of complementary practitioners would be:
- osteopaths – people who use massage and manipulation to correct imbalances in the musculo-skeletal system
- chiropractors – people who manipulate bone and joints, particularly the spine
- acupuncturists – people who use needles to stimulate specific points of the body, using Chinese models that represent energy flow. Acupuncture is a total medical system, involving the whole body, rather than concentrating on just one small area
- homeopaths – people who use infinitesimally small amounts of a material to promote a cure. The principle involves giving a substance that causes similar symptoms to the problem that is being treated
- masseurs – people who use massage. There are many forms of massage that can be used.

The list could be extended, but this gives an idea of some of the forms

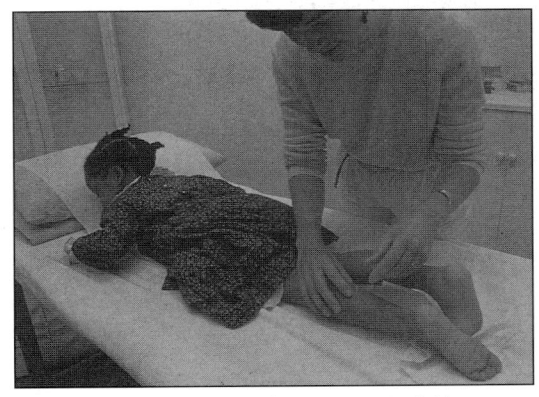

Figure 3.24 An acupuncturist is viewed as a complementary practitioner

Health and social care services

of complementary medicine. The ones listed often have supporters in traditional medicine and in the case of osteopaths and chiropractors are now becoming part of mainstream health care. Generally, people refer themselves to complementary medicine and pay for the services.

Not-for-profit services

Within the private sector there are organisations that charge for the care they provide but do not expect to make a profit. Such organisations tend to use any excess of income over expenditure to fund further developments in the care sector that will benefit their clients.

Informal carers

For many people informal care is provided by members of the family, close friends and neighbours or local support groups. This care is expected of parents when they have children and so child care by parents is not unusual. As parents live longer, an increasing number are cared for by their children.

Help in the home enables a person to cope with everyday life. The help could involve going to the shops, cooking a meal, cleaning the house or any other 'activity of daily living'. It could also involve tending somebody's garden so that they are still able to get pleasure from having a garden, even though they are no longer able to do the work themselves.

By helping undertake such tasks, the informal carer can help reduce worry and stress for the person they are caring for.

Care provided by informal carers may be recognised within the care plan for the individual. It normally requires a sacrifice of time, and often income, to undertake the care. Peter's story provides one example of informal care.

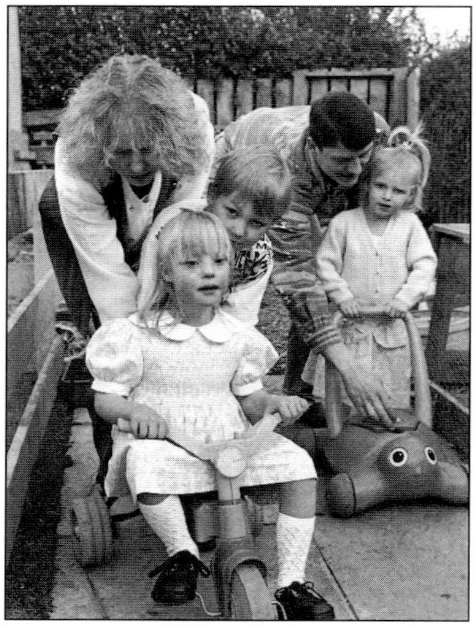

Case study: Peter's story

Peter was born with Down's syndrome. He was the fifth of five children and was born when his mother was in her early forties. As a child Peter played with his brothers and sisters and, for a while, went to school.

Eventually the school was unable to provide for Peter's needs and so he transferred to a special school for children with learning difficulties. During this time his brothers and sisters left home and started their own families.

Peter left school and started attending a training centre and sheltered workshop run by the local Social Services department. As a teenager and young adult he demonstrated an affection for his family and also an ability to learn and work in the training centre. However, in order to make progress he needed one-to-one attention almost all the time. The training centre could not provide this and so slowly Peter stopped doing things for himself.

When Peter was twenty-nine his father died. His mother was left on her own, with Peter to look after the whole time he was not at the training centre. She was not able to provide the one-to-one attention that he needed, as she had to carry on all the tasks of running the house. By this time she was in her seventies.

Peter gradually became less and less able to do things for himself. At home he spent most of his time watching television or flicking through the pages of magazines. At the training centre he sat on a chair doing very little.

FOCUS

Informal carers:
- children
- parents
- friends
- neighbours
- local support groups.

Figure 3.25 Family members have a role as a informal carers

FOCUS

Forms of health and social care provided by informal carers:
- nursing
- companionship
- help in the home.

He contributed nothing to the work of the centre. He was able to feed himself but as he got older he was having more and more toilet accidents. This of course meant more work for his mother.

Eventually, when she was in her mid-eighties, Peter's mother decided that she was unable to cope with him any more. He needed lifting and was becoming too heavy for her to move around. His incontinence (toilet accidents) meant that she was having to wash him, his clothes and bedding several times a day. Peter moved into residential care. The only place that would take him was too far from his home for his mother to visit him regularly.

Within two years of Peter moving into residential care his mother also had to enter residential care herself.

When he was forty nine Peter died in care. His mother died ten days later.

Peter's family, particularly his mother, looked after him for over forty years. His mother spent her 'retirement' looking after him. She had no time from having her first child, to Peter's entry into residential care, when she was not looking after her children.

Peter's story is an example of care in the community where much of the care is provided by relatives. The increasing number of people requiring care in the community will mean that more care will be given by the community itself. Often it will be by members of the family. Occasionally neighbours take an important role befriending and keeping an eye on the health of a person in need. More self-help groups are being set up to provide time off for the full-time carers of people like Peter. These groups are part of the voluntary sector and provide a considerable amount of care.

They are increasingly being supported by the statutory services as their role in providing care is recognised.

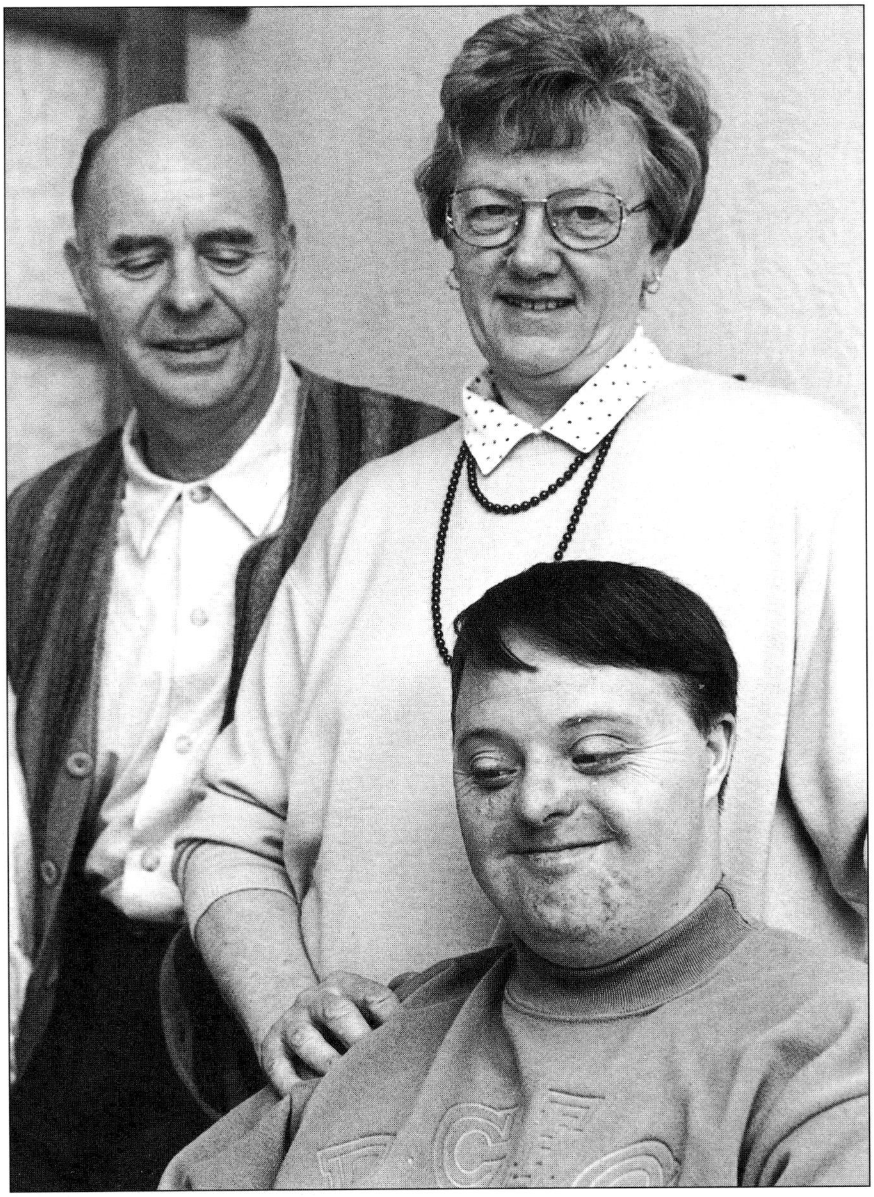

Figure 3.26 Care for many people extends beyond childhood.

Health and social care services

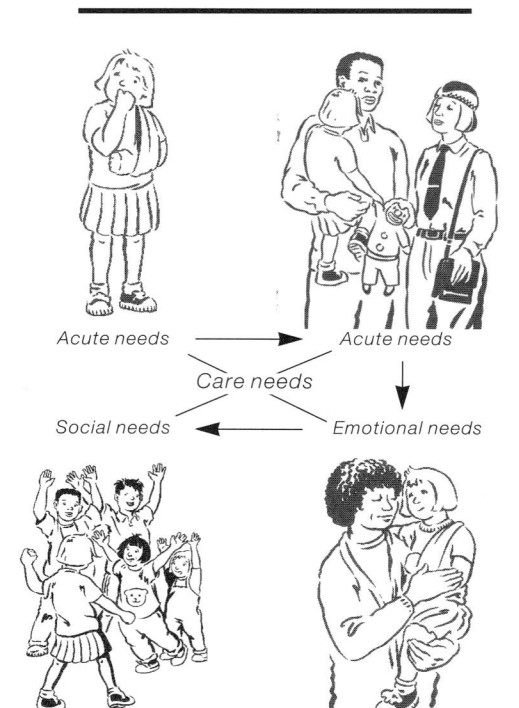

Figure 3.27 Acute social care is occasionally required

FOCUS

Needs can be:
- physical (acute and chronic)
- emotional
- mental
- social.

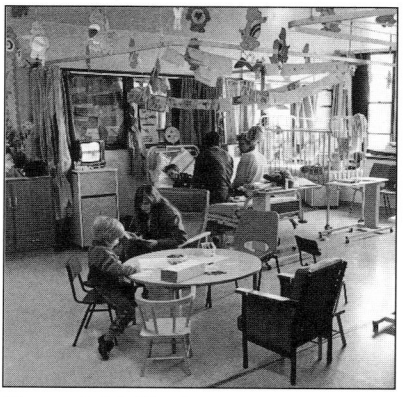

Figure 3.28 The importance of parental involvement in hospital is now recognised

Who needs care?

Everyone needs care at some time in their life. The needs can be for physical, emotional or social care. Sometimes the need is acute (urgent) in which case the services need to be available at all times.

Physical care needs

It can be easy to identify somebody requiring acute physical care. The person may have been injured in an accident or require urgent treatment for an illness. The acute need may be for support in giving birth. Health services are set up through the primary and secondary health-care services to meet acute health-care needs.

Often the need is for long-term health care. A diabetic person needs regular planned checks on his/her health and also needs regular medication. A need for ongoing care is described as a chronic need: tertiary health-care services often provide for these needs.

Occasionally in social care the need is acute. A child who is being abused may need to be provided with care the same day the need is discovered. In these cases the acute care may be provided by social workers with the assistance of trained foster or community parents.

Emotional needs

Everyone has emotional needs. It is important for caring services to provide specifically for these, not only for the **client**, but also for family members. Any person in need of care is likely to be suffering from some form of stress or anxiety.

A Recognition of the emotional needs of children

Many years ago children would enter hospital and be taken away from their parents. The hospital services thought that the parents of a young child would be in the way and make the child upset. They thought that parents had a disturbing effect, because the children seemed upset after visiting time. Visiting times were therefore restricted and the number of visitors limited. The brothers and sisters of the child in hospital were often not allowed to visit at all.

Hospitals failed to recognise the emotional needs of the children. They saw the child as a patient who needed treatment. The hospital would provide the treatment and the patient would get better: any physical needs would be provided for by the hospital, emotional needs were not considered.

1. Why do you think that the children were upset?
   How do hospitals now deal with children and their carers?
   Find out the visiting times for parents/carers in your local hospital.
2. What extra burdens are put on hospital staff, accommodation, and other resources by allowing parents to visit freely? Are there any security issues? What burdens on hospital staff can parents remove? What evidence is there that happier, more relaxed children recover more quickly?

Research the topic of children in hospital. There are many books on the subject, including those for children which provide emotional support to those about to enter hospital.

Do a presentation on the subject, for example diagramatically showing the pressures on a child that come from being in the hospital environment, and the deprivation (what the child is feeling through being out of the home environment).

Social needs

As social animals, people enjoy and need contact with other people. There is a risk of people in need of care becoming isolated. This may be because they are unable go out and meet people. It may also be that people are unwilling to visit them because of fear of infection, or embarrassment about the need for care. The carer, too, may become isolated: in the case of Peter, his mother was isolated because people did not visit when he was at home. They did not know how to react to Peter, an adult who spoke little and had no social skills.

In the next part of this unit we will identify different care provision for different client groups. When you read about the provision, think about how the physical, emotional and social needs are being met.

Case study, Peter's story, page 134

Children and families

All children should be entitled to a family life which safeguards all aspects of their health and social well-being. This means that all agencies try to work together to provide for the health and social care needs of families, children and young people.

There are some services that all children need, for example health-care services and education. General services, for example leisure facilities, play schemes and out-of-school activities are provided by District Councils.

Many families in a community will need a little extra help in order to cope with life's ups and downs. For many families, the support provided by the extended family, friends and neighbours is invaluable and will see them through even the toughest times. However, there will be times when the help and support of professional services are needed. Such services are provided by national and local government and the voluntary organisations.

FOCUS
The range of social care services can be listed by client groups:
- babies
- children (and families)
- young people
- people with disabilities
- elderly people
- low income families.

Informal carers, page 134

Care provision for babies, children, young people, families, adults and elderly people

What help is available to children and families?

Jointly, Health and Social Services work together as care services with the aim of providing help and support to promote good health even before birth and continuing to provide support throughout childhood and adolescence if it is necessary.

In order to promote good health and ensure that potential problems are identified, early screening checks are carried out at regular intervals, for example at birth, 6 – 10 weeks, 7 – 9 months, 2 years, 3 – 4 years and throughout the child's school career. These checks are carried out by health professionals in the field of child health. These specialists include children's doctors, school nurses, health visitors and GPs. As part of this process, immunisation is available against diseases which include polio, mumps, diphtheria, measles, whooping cough and typhoid. Importantly, the screening process also looks at the physical and developmental progress of a child and if necessary they will be referred to a specialist paediatric or child-development clinic for further action. In addition to this, the GP provides a regular source of help and treatment if a child exhibits symptoms of an illness.

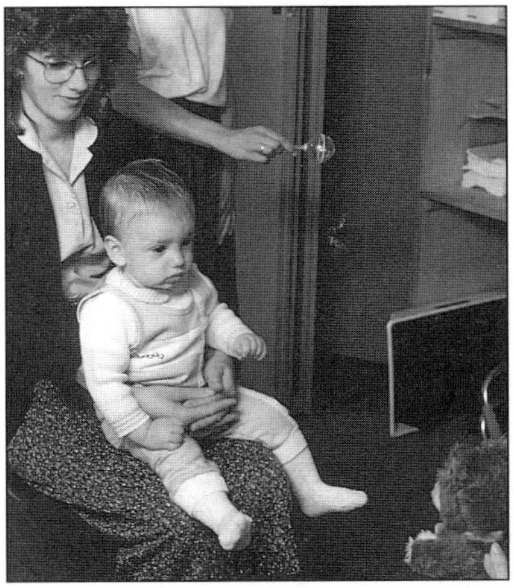

Figure 3.29 These health professionals are carrying out screening for hearing problems

Community-based health services, page 151

Health and social care services

Access to Health and Social Care, page 143

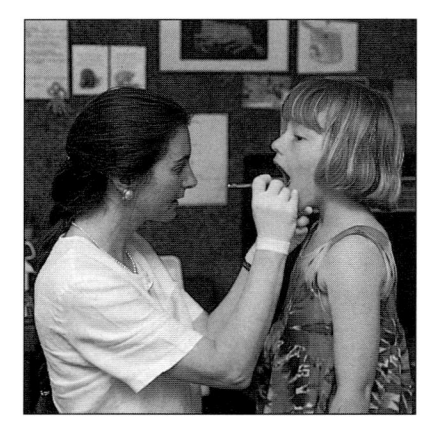

Figure 3.30 Dental checks in school are used to identify problems and potential problems. Children would be referred on for a more thorough check and treatment

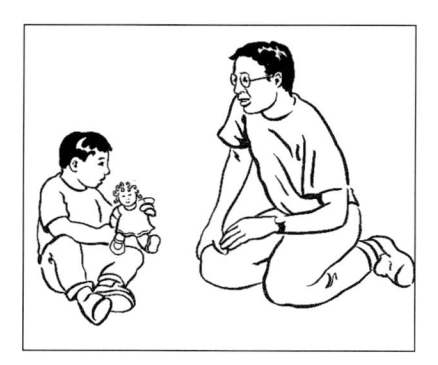

Figure 3.31 Social workers have to be able to work with children to identify their needs and provide the support required. Many children may well need to talk using dolls and toys to explain what happened to them

Methods of referral

Child welfare services also identify and respond to any problems which may emerge, and provide support for families and protection to children. These problems may be behavioural or emotional, such as the breakdown of relationships within a family unit as a result of a poor physical environment. The help required might be practical support of a child with a disability or responses to drug or sex abuse. Where the Health or Social Services may be inappropriate they may be able to refer families to other agencies who can help them with housing or benefits problems. Social Services also provide day care or residential care where needed. In some areas, such as physical or sexual abuse, a multi-agency approach is required, and in the case of abuse both the police and social services would be involved.

A multi-agency approach is also common in the provision of treatment or therapy. Both health and social services work together to provide help and assistance to children with disabilities, for those who have chronic health problems or those who are victims of abuse. The type of support given will depend upon an assessment of an individual's needs.

Getting the help which is available is made as easy as possible: there are a number of starting points, and local doctors, voluntary organisations, as well as social services, can act as the initial point of contact. Initial contact will be followed by advice which may include referral for assessment by a health or social worker. Part of the assessment will involve deciding whether help is needed and what sort of help is most appropriate. This help will be reviewed over time, and changes made if needed.

The Health Service professionals working in child-care include:
- paediatricians
- GPs
- health visitors
- school nurses
- child development clinics
- dentists.

Other more specialist services are provided by community child health doctors, physiotherapists, mental health specialists, speech therapists and occupational therapists.

Social Services professionals in child-care include:
- social workers
- residential social workers
- nursery workers
- family home carers
- child disability social workers
- day care workers.

Trained foster parents are available to take children into their homes for short- or long-term care. The need can arise as a result of many different circumstances: from a parent being taken into hospital through to family abuse.

Social Services Child-care teams also provide support and guidance for:
- children and their families involved with the police
- young people living away from home
- personal and family problems
- nursery placements
- families experiencing practical difficulties in the home

Health and social care services

- young children who may need day care
- children with disabilities and their carers.

Social services may also be able to provide residential home accommodation and will also have specialists in all these fields.

The Children Act, 1989, made it the responsibility of councils, and hence social services, to monitor and register child-care provision (other than education) in their area. This means that all voluntary and private organisations working with children are registered, and social services departments can provide lists for people seeking different types of child-care. These include:
- childminders
- playgroups and nurseries
- self-help groups
- counselling services for those with particular needs.

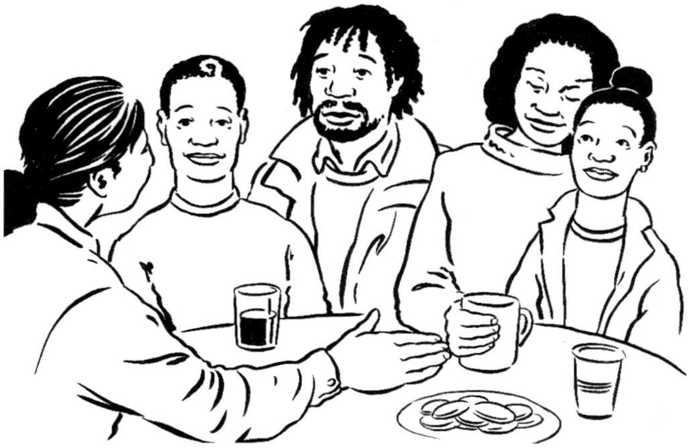

Figure 3.32 Counselling for families is important in resolving conflicts. Parents and teenage children often find it difficult to communicate. Counselling can help

The National Society for the Prevention of Cruelty to Children (NSPCC)

This organisation in the voluntary sector works very closely with social services in looking after children's needs. In particular, the NSPCC may receive reports of abuse which their social workers investigate. They aim to provide support to maintain the family structure, and only as a last resort seek to take children into care. They do this with the knowledge and co-operation of the statutory services.

Barnardo's

A second voluntary organisation that works closely with children is Barnardo's. This organisation, formed in 1866, was one of the first charities, working with young children. Barnardo's now works with more than 20 000 children, young people and their families who face disadvantage or disability. They work in partnership with parents, local authorities and other agencies.

Barnardo's:
- runs over 160 community based projects
- runs day-care centres for children at risk
- supports families under stress and young people leaving care
- finds new families for older children and those with special needs
- helps young people with learning difficulties to live and work in the community
- runs intermediate treatment programmes for young offenders helping them to stay out of trouble
- offers residential provision for children with severe learning difficulties and/or behavioural problems.

If help is needed, how can it be arranged?

The ways in which help can be obtained varies from case to case and the nature of the problem.

If a child's development gives cause for worry or if a child with disabilities is proving difficult to cope with, a potential client would probably turn initially to the GP. The GP would arrange for specialist help and treatment, for example by arranging for speech therapy. Specialist children's doctors could also refer children for further specialist support. The Health and Social Services would liaise with each other to make sure that specialist equipment was made available.

If a child was having behavioural problems, for example, the GP would be likely to refer the child to a child psychologist or a child psychiatrist. If, in addition, the child was at risk, a social worker would also be brought in and assigned to the case.

Based upon the assessment of the professionals involved, the required services would then be identified and provided. The work of the Health and Social Services does not apply simply to young children; teenagers, too, can be helped, together with their families, if problems emerge. For example, drug abuse or drink problems might involve both health and social services input.

Social services do not only deal with problems and crises to do with children. For example, the social service department is responsible for registering all childminders, nurseries and playgroups and makes sure that these facilities are safe, well-regulated and staffed by properly trained workers. The main purpose of this is to ensure that children will come to no harm in using them.

Services for people with physical and sensory disabilities

Anyone can become disabled: some people have disabilities from birth, others become disabled suddenly through accidents, yet others gradually through illness. Health and social services aim to provide help and support to those with disabilities of varying sorts and severity. The nature of the help needed varies enormously and can be connected with day-to-day living, work or leisure. The help may be therapeutic or it may be practical aid to ensure that the problems associated with the disability can be overcome or reduced.

How can help be obtained?

The starting point can be with a number of service providers. The GP, the Social Services office or a voluntary organisation can all be access points to a range of services for people with disabilities. The process invariably includes assessment to determine an individual's full range of need and their eligibility for help. It may be followed by referral to specialist agencies, in the form of local support groups or national bodies, for example RNID.

The help available is very wide ranging and includes home help, equipment loans, housing adaptations, guidance, and access to specialist therapists (occupational, speech, etc.). For example, if a person is due to be discharged from hospital, social workers will help to co-ordinate plans for transport, home-care and other support such as day-care or a home help. Each person with a disability has his or her own particular needs and the duty of the social and health care services is to match needs with appropriate levels of support.

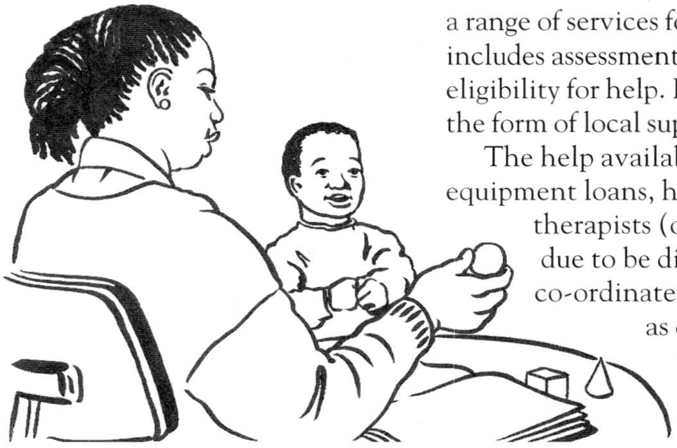

Figure 3.33 Speech therapists work with children and adults to help them to communicate.

Services for people with learning difficulties

There are large numbers of young people and adults who have learning difficulties (the expression 'learning disabilities' is also used). Having a learning difficulty is not an illness which can be treated; it is a condition which makes learning difficult. The severity of learning difficulties varies from person to person. Learning difficulties may have a number of different causes. A person may have damage to their brain which is due to injury at birth, it could be inherited, it may be due to illness or to an accident. Whatever the cause, extent or type of learning difficulty, support and opportunities are available.

How may help be obtained?

There is a range of people and/or agencies where initial help and guidance can be obtained. Doctors, social services or voluntary organisations will all refer a person with learning difficulties and their carers for assessment of need and the services required. These may include health and or social services.

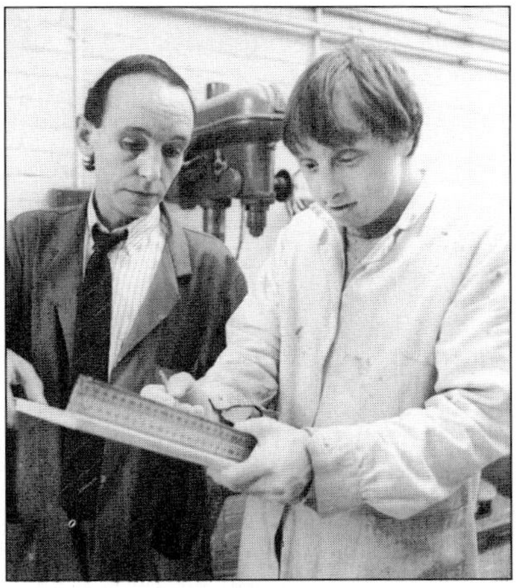

What help is available?

Children with a learning difficulty and their parents may need a wide range of services. These services include playgroups and nurseries with appropriately trained staff, residential homes for long- or short-stay care, schools and units with specialist services for those of school age. The education of children with special needs is moving more and more into mainstream schools, with additional support being provided. Services which focus on specialist equipment needs also exist: a child with learning difficulties may need equipment to make such activities as walking, dressing, eating and washing easier.

Adults with learning difficulties will also need appropriate levels of help and support and, depending upon the assessment of need, these may include:
- work-skills development
- life-skills development
- help in obtaining work
- advocacy services to help in expressing views and making decisions
- help to enable independent living
- information on the range of services available
- advice on access to educational opportunities.

In all cases the emphasis is upon individual need and the needs of the carers (if any).

Figure 3.34 Training centres and workshops provide opportunities for people with special needs to develop skills for work and daily living

Services for older people and their carers

As with other groups, an individual assessment of need and the eligibility of an older person or their carers to the range of services available is the starting point in the process. The needs and wishes of an older person will have an important bearing on the range of services required.

If an older person wishes to stay in their own home, the health and social services would be able to work together to enable this to happen. The help available is wide ranging and the assessment process would identify which services were appropriate. Examples of such services are:

Health and social care services

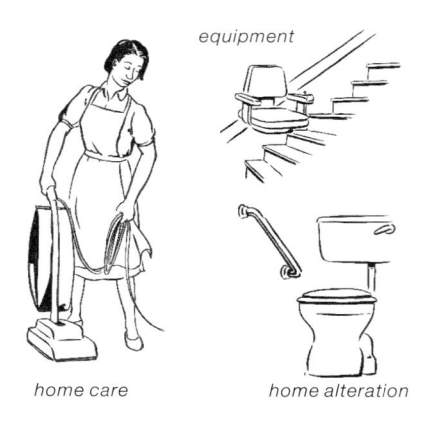

Figure 3.35 Services and equipment can be provided to help elderly people maintain independence in their own home

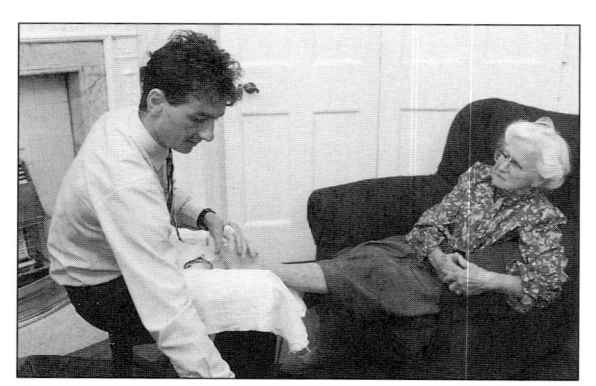

Figure 3.36 Chiropody is one of the many services which can be provided

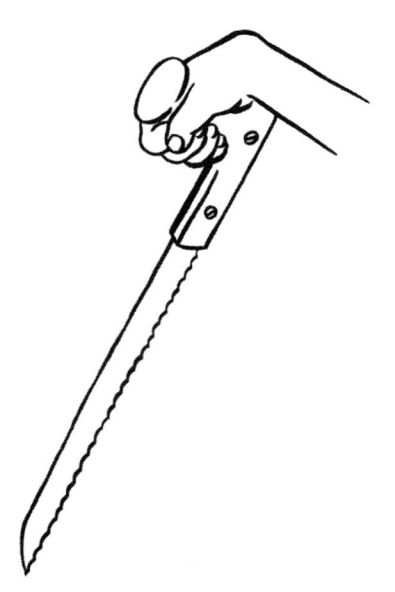

Figure 3.37 Tools can be adapted to make them easier to use by people with arthritis

- home care
- meals on wheels
- home alterations
- equipment
- telephones
- help with holidays
- day centres
- benefits information
- chiropody
- ophthalmic services
- physiotherapy
- advice on incontinence
- specialist nursing services
- annual health checks (over 75 years of age)
- transport for hospital appointments.

In some cases older people may need to be cared for in a residential home. This may be because the person can no longer cope with living in their own home. Social services staff will help an older person in the decision-making process and can, if necessary, make financial help available towards the cost of residential care.

Homes are provided by statutory, private and voluntary organisations. The homes are geared to the particular personal care needs of an older person. Social services also have a responsibility for registering and inspecting residential homes in their local area to ensure that standards are maintained. Nursing homes are also available for those older people who can no longer manage at home and who are ill and in need of nursing care. All nursing homes must be registered and regularly inspected by the Health Authority. Some homes have dual registration offering both types of care.

For carers, too, the social services department also has an important role. They can offer care for a dependant older person whilst carers have a break (respite care), they can provide equipment and gadgets to help in caring for an older person and will also act to put carers in touch with a range of voluntary organisations which can offer them help and support.

Services for people with mental health needs

Health and social services, voluntary organisations and private health services are available to support people with mental health needs. Referral for assessment may come from a GP and can be obtained on an emergency basis if that is what is needed. Most areas have community mental health teams which comprise a group of specialists who can provide help in the home or in community mental health centres. Observation, assessment and treatment can be offered in day hospitals or through in-patient care, on a 24-hour intensive basis.

Where long term help is needed, the agencies prefer to provide help at home based on a specific programme tailored to the needs of an individual with mental health needs. This programme should be reviewed on a regular basis and changes are implemented as needed.

Services are also available in this field to provide support for carers. The help may include counselling, respite help or practical advice.

Access to health and social care

How are individuals referred to caring services?

There are three ways in which a person can be **referred** to care. These are:
- self-referral – where the individual makes contact with the service. Whenever you visit your GP because you feel unwell it is an example of self-referral. Someone who contacts social services asking for help in adapting the house to cope with a disability is using self-referral
- professional referral – where a doctor, social worker or other professional refers a client to the health or social care service. Having visited your GP, you might be referred to hospital to see a consultant. You may also be referred to social services by the GP. Both of these are examples of professional referral
- referral by others – a teacher who refers a child to the social services because of suspected abuse is demonstrating referral by others. The referral may be by a friend or neighbour and may be at the request of the client
- referral via emergency services – when a person is taken to the accident and emergency unit of a hospital as a result of a 999 call. Referral to hospital as a result of an emergency does not require the client to see a GP initially. Emergencies can also arise from heart attacks or other examples of acute ill health.

Emergency referral within a social care setting can occur as a result of:
- a dangerous breakdown in mental health
- evidence of a person (often a child) being in immediate danger.

In the previous sections we have identified the services that a person might expect to receive. However, the ideal solution may not be realistic as account must be taken of the resources available for health and social care. A number of factors have led to increased demand for health and social care resulting in pressures for higher levels of spending. These factor include higher expectations regarding care/treatment, advances in technology and also the growth in numbers requiring continuing care (e.g. growth in the population of elderly people).

Where spending is entirely 'needs-led' ways need to be found to ration the provsion of health and social care, often resulting in painful and controversial decisions having to be made. Increasingly people are expected to make some contribution towards the cost of health and social care which they receive (through 'means testing').

Cultural issues

It is essential to recognise cultural differences (for example, religion and race) when considering the needs of different client groups. This includes having an awareness of differences in attitudes towards many aspects of life. Examples of these variations can be seen in the way care for elders is achieved in different communities. In some cultures, care of elders is seen as part of the family responsibilities. Care is therefore provided within the home and demands for residential care are not made. This does not mean that support is not needed, but it does mean that care plans need to recognise the cultural issues and look to provide the support necessary.

The provision of care for elders may not meet the cultural needs of particular groups. Pakistani heritage families have traditionally cared for

---

FOCUS

Methods of referral:
- **professional referral**
- **self-referral**
- **referral by others**
- **emergency services (NHS, local services).**

▶ The Value Base and individual rights, Appendix II, page 220

▶ Accepting a society's culture, page 97

their elders in the home: this tradition continues in the UK. As a consequence, very few residential care homes cater for their particular religious and dietary needs. The implications for a Muslim requiring residential care are that provision will be offered in a home where s/he will be the only Muslim, and therefore isolated.

Without meaning to discriminate, the care services may not be able to meet the needs of individual clients and so rely on informal and family carers. You will need to consider such issues when suggesting how services for different client groups may be improved.

Other issues may relate to the provision of child-care. In areas where most families continue to live near where they were born, relatives often provide child-care, allowing parents to work and/or have some respite from the role. Where families are more widely spread, the demand for child-minders and nursery provision increases. This cultural divide may be linked to race or social class.

In the last few years there has been greater recognition of the needs of people whose mother tongue is not English. Much of the information about health and social services is now available in a variety of languages. Translators are also available in many areas to ensure that the care needs of individuals are identified and understood by all parties.

Some of these issues have been addresssed in the development of **charters**. These have made caring organisations review what they are offering and what people can expect. In doing this they have also had to identify groups who may be disadvantaged. With the charters has come increased publicity about complaints procedures. People who do not receive care that meets charter standards now have information about ways of making complaints. An example of a charter is shown in Figure 3.38.

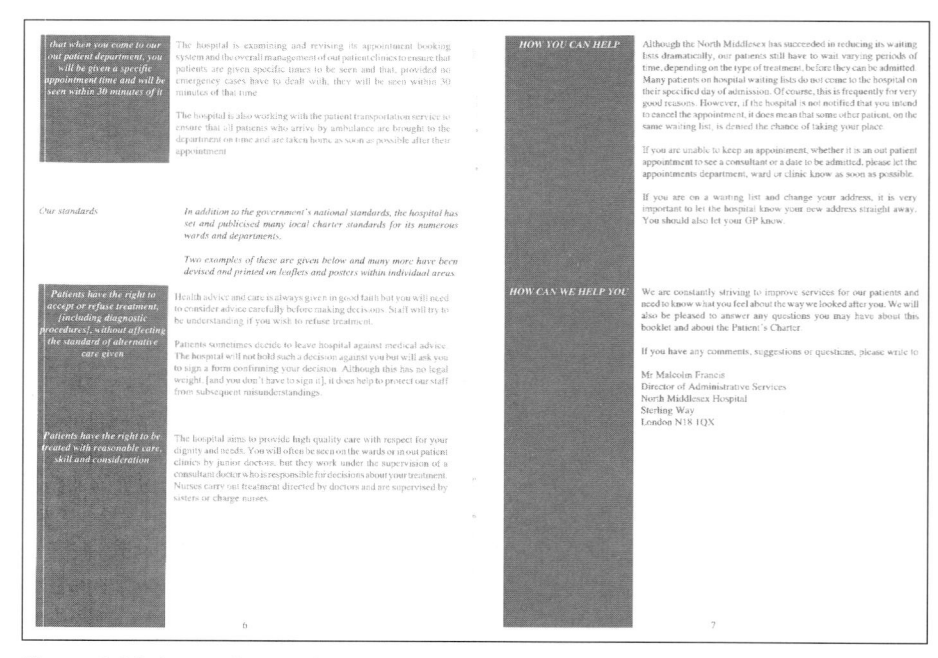

Figure 3.38 A page from a charter leaflet

Support for people with different needs

There are many people who, for whatever reason, are unable to express their needs and wishes well, possibly because of language difficulties. Information needs to be provided in a form that is understandable. Examples would be:

- provision of booklets in different languages
- use of Braille booklets
- provision of taped information for people who have difficulties with written English
- use of translators
- use of translators able to 'sign' for hearing-impaired people.

Many people who have been unable to express their wishes clearly have traditionally been cared for without being asked for their views. Care has been imposed, rather than being negotiated. People with learning difficulties are particularly vulnerable to being told what they ought to want!

A variety of organisations provide support for people who need help in achieving their rights and needs. Systems of **advocacy** have developed in which an advocate works with a person to develop an understanding of their needs and wants. This system is often referred to as Citizen's Advocacy. The advocate then works with and on behalf of the individual in discussion with the caring services. To be an advocate requires patience and understanding to identify what the client wants and not what the advocate thinks the client wants.

> **FOCUS**
>
> Support for individuals can come from:
> - provision of information
> - charters
> - use of translators
> - use of advocates.

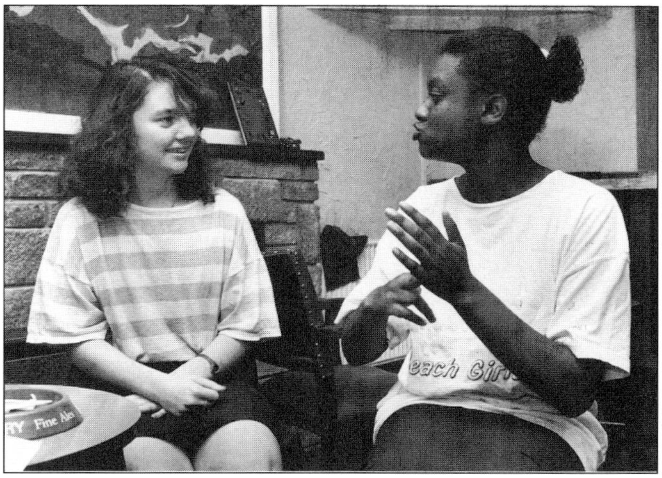

Figure 3.39 Signing information for the hearing-impaired

Who pays?

The statutory sector

When the NHS was set up it was to provide care that was free at the point of delivery. Taxes (for example, income tax), excise duties (for example, on cigarettes and petrol) and national insurance contributions (paid by people in work and employers) pay for the services. There are still some services that require payment. Most of us are aware of charges for:

- prescriptions
- eye tests
- glasses
- dental treatment.

The charges change frequently and do not apply to everyone. In most cases children do not have to pay charges. In many cases charges are not paid by people receiving certain benefits (for example, family income supplement). Pensioners are often exempt from costs. The rules do not follow a fixed pattern. People over the national pension age do not have to pay for prescriptions, but they do have to pay for eye tests.

In many cases the charges only contribute part of the cost of the service. In others the cost may be higher than the price of the service received. Many drugs cost less than the prescription charge.

> **FOCUS**
>
> Services provided:
> - which are free at the point of delivery
> - for which a basic fee may be paid
> - where ability to pay is taken into account
> - which are run on a charitable basis
> - for which individual pays
> - by family
> - by local community.

A   Who pays what?

Within your group, discuss the care **services** that you know the user may have to pay for, wholly or in part. Discuss also how you can find out what the costs are. Check with your tutor to see if you have overlooked any relevant services or client groups.

Amongst your group distribute the tasks of carrying out the research, and present your findings as a display by the whole group. Use your imagination to present the information as clearly as possible.

Individually, write a short report on your conclusions.

In social care, much of the statutory provision is free but there are increasing pressures to provide means-tested benefits.

Means-tested benefits: *a person's income and savings are taken into account and a charge determined based, in theory, on the ability to pay.*

Residential care for older people is a clear example of the client being required to contribute some or all of the costs of care provision.

The private sector

This sector generates income from the fees charged to the individual receiving care. In some cases this is paid by the individual or his/her family, or through an insurance company where appropriate insurance has been taken out. In many cases some or all of the costs are met from the statutory sector which contracts for the care.

The voluntary sector

In this sector there are a variety of services and payment regimes. Most voluntary organisations will seek to cover their costs from a variety of sources, one of which is as fees paid by or on behalf of clients. In particular, voluntary sector organisations may be contracted to supply care by the statutory sector.

Who cares?

At the start of this unit you made a list of people and organisations involved in the delivery of care. From this we described the different sectors involved in caring. This next section will address the roles of the people involved in the practical caring skills.

> **FOCUS**
>
> Jobs involve:
> - provision of care
> - support services.

Health and social care services

A Who delivers care? – 2

Look back at your list of people and organisations involved in caring. Review this and produce a list of the people involved, including those from the private and voluntary sectors which you may have overlooked when you first did this activity.

Who delivers care? – 1, page 118

Table 3.1 Health and Social Care workers

Health Care		Social Care	
Doctors	Hospital based	**Social Workers**	Field Social Workers
	General Practitioners		Education Welfare Officers
Nurses	Registered General Nurses*		Probation Officers
	Registered Mental Nurses or Psychiatric Nurses*	**Residential and Day Care Staff**	
			Care Officers
	Registered Nurses for the Mentally Handicapped*		Care Assistants
			Instructors
	Registered Sick Children's Nurse*		Nursery Nurses
	Health Visitors		Welfare Assistants
	Midwifes	**Domiciliary Support**	
	District Nurses		Community Support Workers
	School Nurses		Home Carers (extension of the home help role)
	Enrolled Nurses**		
Nursing Auxiliaries / Health Care Assistants		**Counselling Services**	
Professions Allied to Medicine			Relate (Marriage Guidance and more)
	Physiotherapists		Birth control/pregnancy
	Occupational Therapists		Drug use
	Speech Therapists		
	Radiographers		
	Paramedics		
	Ambulance Workers		
Complementary Health Care			
	Osteopaths		
	Homeopaths		

* These qualifications are being replaced with the Project 2000 training programmes. Trainee nurses undertake a common core programme followed by a branch study of one of four areas relating to the qualifications shown.

** Enrolled nursing programmes have been phased out. The re-evaluation of skill requirements on wards means that Health Care Assistants are taking over some of the roles of Enrolled Nurses (SEN)

In making your list you probably included the people mentioned in Table 3.1. You may also have included some of the many workers in the voluntary and private sectors. To a large extent these people have counterparts in the statutory sector and they undertake similar training.

What do the workers 'do'?

It is often easiest to consider what people do in the context of where they work. The **role** of a health-care assistant differs according to where he or she works. So, too, does the role of a doctor. Although it is true that some care workers tend to work on their own (for example, childminders), most tend to work as part of a team. This is equally true for people such as GPs, who may spend a large part of their working hours on their own – yet none-the-less remain key members of the Primary Health Care Team.

In looking at different roles we will break down the services into hospital-based and community-based. Where a job title (for example, social worker) applies to people in both areas, the different roles will be described separately.

FOCUS

Working roles in care involve:
- different work patterns (working on own, as part of a team with people of the same discipline) and people from other disciplines
- working with client groups (treatment, enablement)
- hours of work (daytime, nightwork, shiftwork)
- different conditions of service
- differing contracts with clients, e.g portering, administration, treatment, direct care.

FOCUS

Compare work roles in terms of:
- pay
- working conditions
- tasks.

Hospital and specialist services

We think of hospitals as places where people are taken for treatment when treatment at home is not working or is not possible. They are the places people go to for operations or for help from a specialist on an out-patient basis.

Doctors

Doctors in hospitals work as members of a team led by a consultant and normally including a registrar and 'housemen'. Most of the doctors involved are already specialists in an area of medicine or are intending to specialise. In order to specialise, many of the doctors undertake further training and many take further examinations. The specialisms include working with children (Paediatrics), working with damaged bones (Orthopaedics) and many branches of surgery.

Doctors identify what is wrong (diagnose), say what the treatment should be (prescribe) and monitor the success or otherwise of treatment. In some cases they actually administer the treatment, although this is not essential.

People are normally referred to specialist teams in hospitals by a General Practitioner (GP).

The GP provides the specialist with a report of what has been done and details of the initial diagnosis. For most people this referral means that they are given an appointment to attend an out-patient clinic where one of the specialist team reviews the situation, attempts a diagnosis and plans a course of action.

In order for the specialist to make a diagnosis they often need to call upon other specialist services. Two of the commonest are for X-ray images to be taken and for samples of blood or other material to be sent for analysis. The latter involves different specialists depending upon the analysis needed. These specialists, who are not normally doctors, have knowledge and skills which allow them to provide services to assist the doctor in diagnosis and treatment.

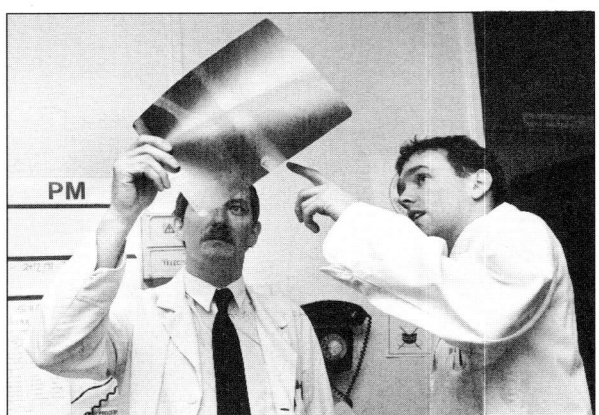

Figure 3.40 Doctors examining an X-ray

▶ General Practitioner, page 151

Nurses

Nurses are the people normally associated with hospital work alongside doctors. Nurses work as key members of the team involved in providing patient care. Traditionally nurses have worked in one area (for example, a ward or operating theatres) and have taken a general responsibility for all patients. Changes in their working practices now means that many nurses are now identified with individual patients. The nurse is involved in the care planning for the specific patient and acts as a link for all carers working with the patient.

In the past, training was provided for two levels of nurse: State Registered Nurse (SRN now RGN) training and State Enrolled Nurse (SEN) training. Recent changes have meant that training for the lower qualification (SEN) has ceased. There are still many second level nurses (SENs) currently working in health care but in future all nurses will qualify at Registered Nurse level. The second level will be taken up by Health Care Assistants.

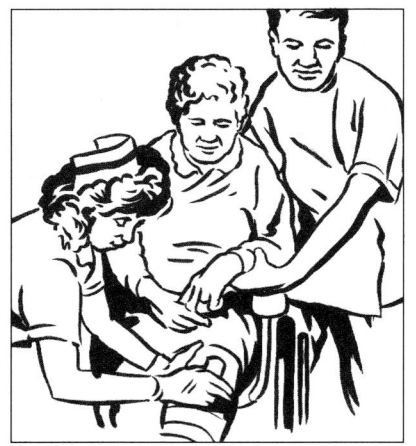

Figure 3.41 Nurses are key members of the patient-care team

Nurses have for some time been able to specialise in specific areas of care, such as sick children, mental health and mental handicap, and it was usual for these specialisms to be achieved with post-qualifying training. New training under Project 2000 means that nurses may be able to specialise at an earlier stage.

Health visitor and midwife **qualifications** are usually gained after the initial nurse training. There are training programmes leading directly to midwifery qualifications but these are not common. Both health visitors and midwives have more independence than other first-level nurses. Of the two, midwives work both in hospitals and the community, whilst health visitors are community-based.

The roles of nurses in hospitals are undergoing some changes. In the past they have been considered to be acting under instruction from the medical team, but attitudes are changing and they are now becoming increasingly recognised as members of the total team, making an important contribution to patient care. They are now taking on more roles that were at one time the province of the doctors. This recognition of their professional skills has assisted the recent reorganisation in the NHS.

The main, face-to-face delivery of care is from nurses and doctors. As we have already indicated, there is a wide range of professions allied to medicine. The roles of some are outlined briefly below.

> **FOCUS**
> Career routes:
> - academic, e.g. degrees (doctors)
> - vocational, e.g. RGN (nurses), NVQ (care assistant)
> - both! e.g. social worker
> - other requirements
> - previous jobs
> - possible future jobs
> - opportunities for job relocation.

Radiographers

Radiographers work in two different ways:

a **Diagnostic radiographers** use X-rays and ultrasound to help view internal structures. You may have needed an X-ray for a broken bone. There are few pregnant women who do not have an ultrasound scan to check on the health of their foetus.

The activities of diagnostic radiographers range from taking single X-rays and ultrasound scans to complex sequential scans (CT scans). For CT scans a sequence of images is used to build up a three-dimensional picture of the area being scanned. Computers are used to store the images and to allow the specialists to make use of the three-dimensional nature of the image.

Radiographers are now learning new techniques of magnetic resonance imaging which produces remarkably clear images of soft tissues such as tendon and muscle. These are tissues that traditional X-ray pictures do not show very well. These clearer pictures make it easier for the doctors to diagnose what is wrong.

b **Therapeutic radiographers** use focused ionising radiation (for example, X-rays and gamma rays) to destroy tissues. In particular, such treatments are used on a wide range of cancers. In these cases the treatment is called radiotherapy.

Radiographers work under instruction from a radiologist. The radiologist is a specialist doctor who interprets X-ray, ultrasound and magnetic resonance images, for example, and produces reports for the doctor requesting the image.

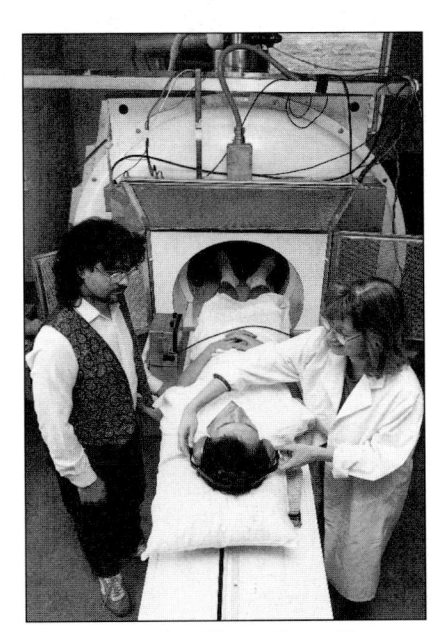

Figure 3.42 A radiographer with her patient

Health and social care services

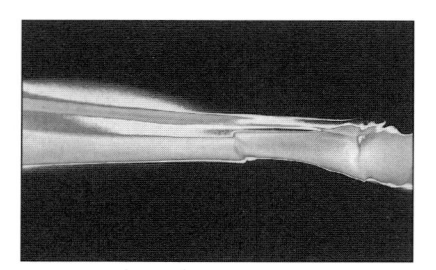

X-ray shows a fracture of the shinbone

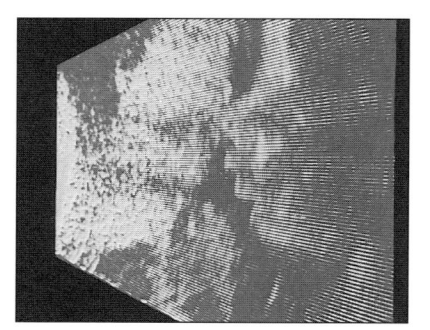

Ultrasound shows the face of a human foetus in profile

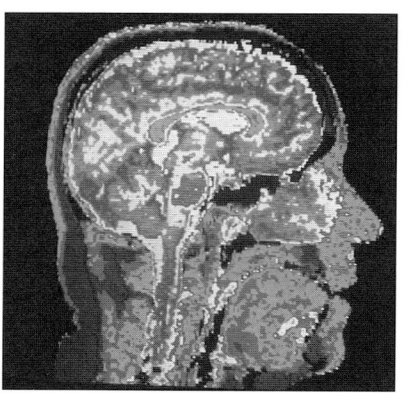

Magnetic resonance imaging (MRI) shows a section through a human head highlighting structures of a normal brain

Figure 3.43 *Radiographers use different techniques to produce pictures of the body under the skin*

Physiotherapists

Physiotherapists are involved in maintaining and improving the mobility of patients. This can be by working directly to develop joint flexibility and muscle strength. A person who has had a broken arm or leg may receive physiotherapy to help regain full use of the limb. Multiple sclerosis sufferers may be helped to maintain mobility by physiotherapists.

Physiotherapists also work to maintain physical well-being and movement of patients. People who have had pneumonia or who have cystic fibrosis accumulate mucus in their lungs. Physiotherapists work with them to help them to cough up the mucus and so improve their breathing. In many cases the physiotherapist acts as a trainer, either for the patient or a carer. The physiotherapist trains them to undertake simple activities themselves on a regular basis, in order that the therapy can continue in the absence of the physiotherapist.

As with all other caring workers, physiotherapists work as part of the team that plans and delivers care.

Occupational therapists

Occupational therapists (OTs) may be found in hospitals, social service departments or in private organisations. They work with individuals on a one-to-one basis, and with groups of people who have disabilities, to help them become more independent in their everyday lives (for example, washing and dressing). They can also give advice on the use of special equipment and adaptations in the home. The work of the OT is becoming increasingly important with Care in the Community and spending on OT services has generally increased as a result.

Speech therapists

Speech therapists work with people with speech disorders. The work is normally long-term and so only the initial stages of speech therapy are undertaken in the hospital. Much of the work takes place in the community. In hospitals the work may involve working with a person who has had facial surgery that affects speech, or supporting people recovering from a stroke.

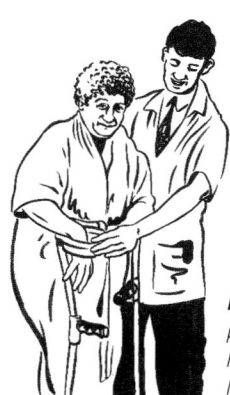

Figure 3.44 *A physiotherapist can help people regain lost mobility*

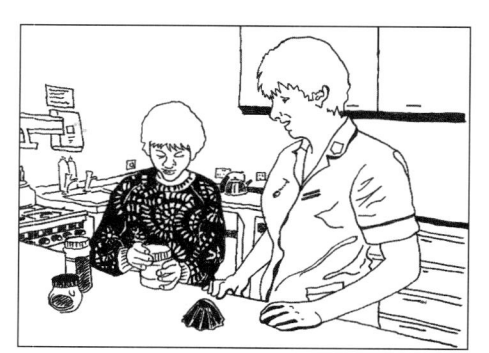

Figure 3.45 *An occupational therapist at work*

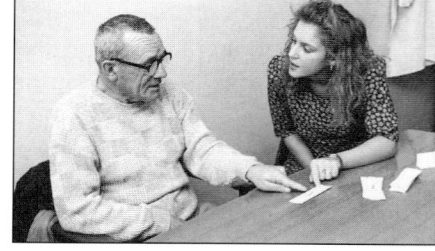

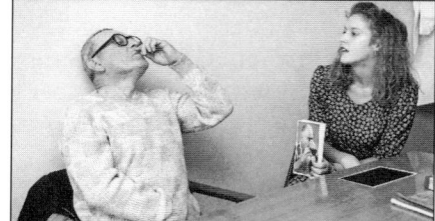

Figure 3.46 *A speech therapist working with a stroke victim*

Health and social care services

Health care assistants

Changes in nurse training (Project 2000) meant that student nurses were not counted as part of the work-force. This meant that the skills and roles of care workers had to be reappraised. It became clear that there was a need for qualified care workers to work as part of the caring team, to assist and support the more familiar professionals. It is now recognised that the previously untrained nursing auxiliaries and physiotherapy and occupational therapy assistants, need to be trained.

Their new title varies between hospitals, but they are generally recognised as Health Care Assistants. Whilst their roles include many of those previously carried out by nursing auxiliaries and 'therapy assistants', those roles have been expanded, and National Vocational Qualifications (NVQs) developed at levels 2 and 3 have been designed with them in mind. Health care assistants work in a variety of areas and the NVQs provide opportunities for people to gain qualifications appropriate to the area that they work in.

They assist the nurses and therapists to implement care plans. They undertake routine duties and in many cases provide an important link between the clients and the rest of the care team. The routine duties are often those considered less pleasant, such as assisting clients with access to toilet facilities.

Health care assistants now undertake many tasks that would not have been appropriate for the previous unqualified staff. They also have a foot on the ladder that can lead to further professional training.

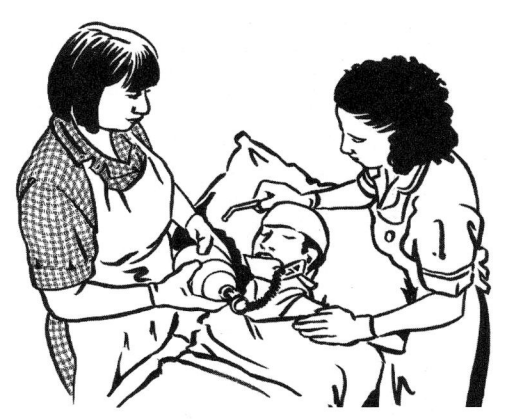

Figure 3.47 Health care assistants help nurses and therapists to implement care plans

Community-based health services

General Practitioners

The major groups of community-based doctors are General Practitioners (GPs). They are qualified as doctors and have undergone further training in general practice. It may seem strange, but their specialism is not to specialise, but to be able to cover all areas of medicine that present themselves in the community.

Everyone permanently resident or working in Britain may be registered with a GP. They may select their own GP when they are over 16 years old from the list of GPs kept by the Family Health Service Authority.

It is now common for a group of GPs to work together, each with general diagnostic skills, but also having a specialism to contribute to the practice. These group practices are often in health centres where there is also easy access to other health care specialists, who form part of the community health-care team. It is also becoming more common for the GPs to link in with hospitals and undertake minor surgery in hospitals or in appropriately equipped health centres.

Health centres are not only staffed by the GPs, but also by receptionists and possibly a nurse employed by the practice. There is very often a wide range of other Community Health services available. These usually include: health visitors, community midwives and district nurses (community nurses).

Health centres also provide a gateway to other services, for example, the schools nursing service, speech therapists, occupational therapists, physiotherapists and dentists. They may also enable people to gain access to other specialists, for example family planning, dieticians, chiropody

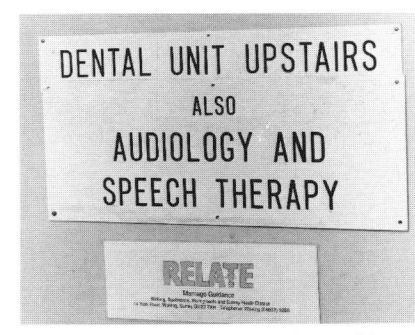

Figure 3.48 Health centres provide a variety of services in the same building. This allows teams to develop and work together

services and incontinence advisors, as well as providing a home for health promotion specialists and others such as those giving drugs/HIV/AIDS advice.

Members of the community unit provide care for people who do not need to enter hospital or who have been discharged from hospital but still need support. The members of the community units work with both the hospital-based teams and the GP practices.

Nurses in the community

Community midwives provide support for pregnant women and assist in the delivery of the baby. The mother does most of the physically hard work whilst the midwife provides the medical support necessary. Being community-based they have a role in visiting the home of the pregnant woman and also providing health care for the first ten days after birth.

Health visitors

Health visitors take over the health care of young children from the midwife. In some cases the midwife may also be a health visitor and so have an important role in working with children under five and their parents. Health visitors also have an important health-education role in their work.

Community psychiatric nurses (CPNs)

Also based in the community, and developing a more important role, following the NHS and Community Care Act, are the community psychiatric nurses and the community-based mental handicap (RNMH) nurses. These personnel provide continuing care for people who may have been receiving long-term hospital care and who have now returned to living in the community. As already mentioned, the Act requires local authorities to liaise with health authorities. On a day-to-day basis this means that there are close links between CPNs and local authority social workers.

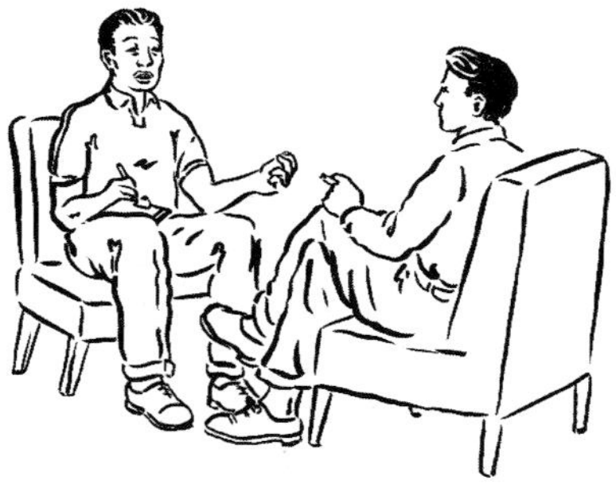

Social services personnel

The structure of the Health Services follows a clear pattern. Within the statutory personal social services the development of the organisation has been complex but the number of different types of worker is small.

If we consider only those staff directly involved in delivery of care then the number of qualifications is limited. Care can be divided into community-based care and residential care. For both areas there are qualified social workers who have taken a generic qualification covering all areas of social work, although they may specialise in one area later.

Figure 3.49 Social workers work with people, providing support and planning to meet client needs. It is important that the client is involved as much as possible

Social workers

For many years there have been two qualifications in social work. The 'field' social workers have normally achieved the Certificate of Qualification in Social Work (CQSW). Those involved in residential care have often achieved the Certificate in Social Service (CSS). Many people, particularly working in residential care, have had no qualifications related to social care.

The minumum age to become a social worker is 21, but it is useful to have had a range of experience before applying for training. This is why many trained social workers are much older than 21.

Rather like the Health sector, there has been a radical review of training needs and the qualification structures. Recent changes to training have resulted in the ending of the CQSW and CSS training and their replacement by the Diploma in Social Work (DipSW).

Care assistants

The unqualified staff supporting the social workers have always had a crucial role in residential care, providing most of the practical care.
They also work in day-care centres and as domiciliary support workers (home helps). In fact there are few areas where unqualified staff do not play an important role.

As in the case of the Health Care Assistants, NVQs at levels 2 and 3 have been developed to provide competence-based qualifications for care staff. They are based on experience, and demonstration of the ability to do the work to set standards. Thus, in many areas of social care that were traditionally filled by untrained, unqualified staff, there are now qualifications and recognition of the skills of the work force.

The roles undertaken are almost always ones which involve direct contact with people requiring care. To a large extent they involve supporting people to undertake the normal activities of daily living. This can include assisting them to dress, assisting in personal hygiene, undertaking and supporting 'housework' and assisting in obtaining and providing food and drink. In all cases care assistants work within an agreed care plan. This provides for the client's needs, but also recognises their rights and dignity.

Specialist workers in nurseries

Many Social Services departments run day nurseries for children between six weeks and five years old. The special skills required for this type of care are recognised, and nursery nurses have either National Nursery Examinations Board (NNEB) qualifications or BTEC National Diplomas or Certificates in Caring Services (Nursery Nursing). Again, there are newly developed competence-based qualifications (NVQs) at levels 2 and 3 in Child Care and Education.

Jill's route to social work, page 156

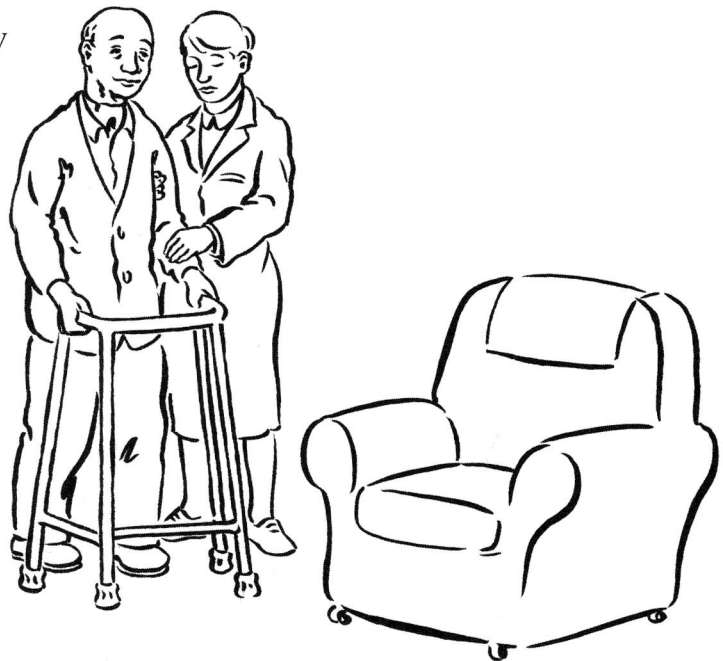

Figure 3.50 Care assistants have an important role to play in caring. NVQs provide qualifications that recognise the skills needed for this caring role

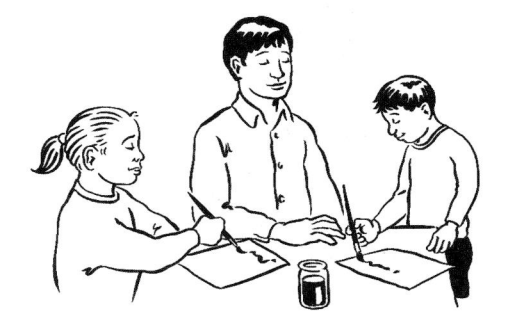

Figure 3.51 Many teenagers consider nursery nursing. This is a challenging job requiring a good understanding of children and their individual needs

Key workers

One development in caring situations is the use of a Key-Worker system. A client is allocated to an individual key worker who takes responsibility for the care. This person is the one who acts as a link between the client and other workers. The role can involve:
- being responsible for the care plan
- monitoring the implementation of the care plan
- acting as an advocate.

An advantage to the client is that they have one person who acts as a link and who is responsible for much of the care. This continuity of contact and responsibility can give the client greater confidence. The key worker also has a responsibility to the client and cannot ignore an issue, assuming that another person will pick it up.

Almost all of the professionals working in care can take on the key-worker role for a client. It is particularly noticeable in social care, where key workers can come from all groups of care worker.

Support services

In addition to those who work directly with clients, there are many who have no 'caring' contact with clients, but who provide support for the carers. Examples of these jobs are:
- clinical laboratory worker
- caterer
- clerk (for example, in medical records).

Other jobs may have some client contact and are part of the caring team:
- medical receptionist
- porter
- cleaner.

All of the support workers have a vital role to play in the running of the caring services.

A Who supports the carers?

Using a care facility you know well, identify:
- the nature and size of the facility, at least in terms of the number of clients and the average time per week spent by the client using the facility
- numbers of people in each role.

To get this information may require interviewing the officer in charge or some other member of staff to find out who is trained/qualified, who works full time/part time, and so on.

Represent this information as a diagram. Group the members of staff into those who are trained to deliver care (carers) and people who support the carers. This second group may be divided into people who work with clients and those who do not normally meet the clients.

Stereotypes

Think of a nursery nurse and you probably think of a woman. Nurses are always women. Doctors are always men. These statements reflect stereotypes for care workers. Whilst they are not accurate, they do reflect the views of many people. Part of this stereotyping comes from the view that caring roles (nurse, care assistant) are best carried out by women. Decision-making (doctor) is seen as a male province. The salaries also seem to reflect this. The male-dominated sections are well paid. The female-dominated parts are less well paid.

As long as the salaries and prejudices are biased, the stereotypes will remain. People who break the stereotypes are seen by many as 'odd'. As more break the stereotype, the situation will improve. Even when the sex stereotyping has been challenged, for example with doctors, there are still some branches that it is difficult for women to enter (for example, surgery).

When you investigate further the roles of different care workers in Assignment: Caring for Peter, try to identify any stereotypes based on:
- gender
- social class
- race.

You might find it useful to look at your original list from the Activity: Who delivers care? – 1 and think of any stereotypes that may be common for the people you have identified as being involved in care.

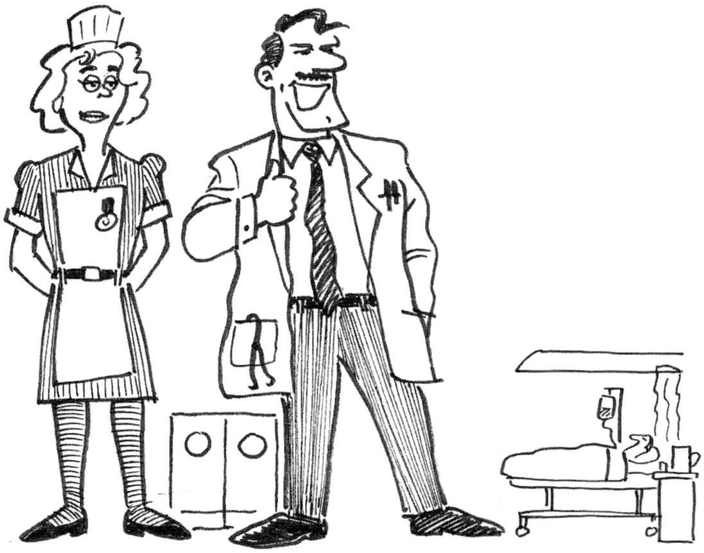

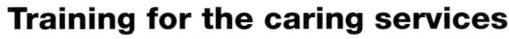

Figure 3.52 Stereotypes: Nurses are always women; doctors are always men

Training for the caring services

The range of jobs in health and social care mean that there are a wide range of entry requirements. Very good advanced level **qualifications** are required to train as a doctor. Nursing, more and more, requires advanced level qualifications. Being a care assistant often involves no qualification requirements, but an understanding of the role is important.

Your current work is leading to an Intermediate GNVQ in Health and Social Care. This will prepare you to look for work at the care assistant level. Any work experience will be useful in competing with others who may be applying for the same jobs. Your qualification will also provide you with an academic starting point to move on to advanced level qualifications. In the case study of Jill, you will see how she moves from work as a nursery nurse through to being a social worker. You, too, can aspire to entering the caring professions and moving on to further qualifications.

▶ Assignment: Caring for Peter, page 160

▶ Who delivers care? – 1, page 118

▶ Prejudices, page 190

▶ Discrimination, page 191

Becoming a care worker in health or social care

We have described many of the different health care workers and something of their roles. There are many different routes into caring and different academic requirements. Doctors, for example, have a degree from a university. The case study of Jill describes her route to social work.

Case study: Jill's route to social work

become social workers do so as mature students and have already had a significant and varied life experience. Jill is no exception to this and we include details of her route to social work. Later on we give details of a typical day's work for her.

Note. The timings for these events have not been given but the whole sequence took about twenty years. Clearly, some of the events overlap.

Left school with some GCEs and CSEs. (She was quite vague about the grades or numbers!) Jill freely admits that her school career was not totally happy, nor could it be regarded as successful from either her or her teachers' points of view.

College to study for the NNEB Certificate which she obtained after the two year course.

First job: nursery nurse in a first school working across the age range and taking responsibility for craft and play activities and the library.

Second job: nursery nurse in a school for children with special needs aged 2 – 11. She established a parent's support group and helped establish a programme to develop gross motor skills in children.

Third job: project worker for a family support worker (under 5's). The emphasis of this work was to prevent the need for children to be admitted to care.

Fourth job: community supervisor working with young people (14 –17) as a direct alternative to them being given custodial sentences. This involved a lot of group work and individual counselling.

Fifth job: co-worker in an Adolescent Sex Offenders group. This consisted of people who were under 17 and who had committed sexual offences.

For thirteen years Jill was a foster parent as well as becoming a parent herself.

Training
Whilst she was working she undertook in-service training in:
— child abuse/child protection
— therapeutic work with victims
— counselling
— partnerships with parents.

To enable her to meet the academic requirements for social work training she studied for two credits with the Open University.

In 1993 she completed her studies and gained the Diploma in Social Work and qualified as a social worker.

Jill is now a social worker in a team working with children over 11 years old.

This is a fairly typical path to social work qualifications, and Jill was in her thirties when she finally qualified as a social worker.

But what do they really 'do'?

It would be possible to provide details of a typical day for a fictional person working in the caring professions. The reality is that no two days are the same and no two workers do exactly the same things. So often the actual job done is very different from the stereotype. The only way to find out what the work involves is to experience it. The activity below is a start, but we would urge you to try to gain work experience and write your own description of what a care worker does.

To help you consider typical working days, we include outlines of the work of two care workers taken on the same day in October.

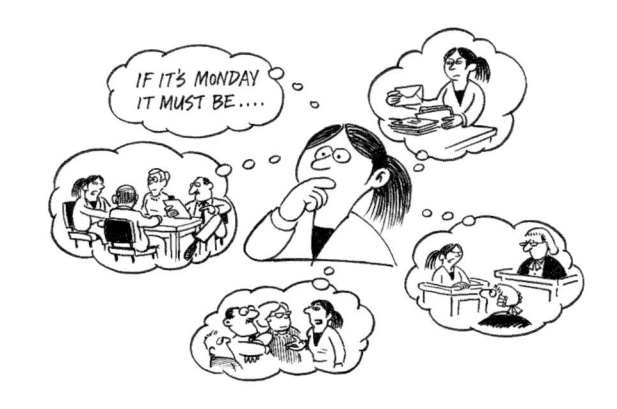

Figure 3.53 What do care workers really 'do'?

A day in the life of Jill, social worker

The following is taken from the diary of the social worker, Jill, whose route to social work was given earlier. She is a member of a team working with children over 11 years old. The comments added are those that she made when giving the details.

9.00   Resource allocation meeting. Request a placement and outreach support for a young person. This means that accommodation needs to be found for a young person and specific support allocated.

9.45   Pick up messages and deal with the post. This usually means more requests for information and reports.

10.15   Visit the young person (see 9.00) at emergency foster parents and develop plans to help the move to independence.

11.30   Meeting to plan family therapy sessions. Together with two other social workers we try to plan family therapy for the next two weeks.

12.30   Lunch. The Social Services department blocks all phone calls to enable a quiet lunch period. (Emergency calls have a manned phone at all times.)

13.30   Liaise with a colleague to produce a joint report.

13.50   Attend court with a young person. The length of time needed for this is difficult to predict. It is almost always longer than you expect.

15.30   Office. Returning phone calls. (Jill's actual comment was 'What, out already!')

16.00   Visit a parent and adolescent child in their home. There is conflict between parent and child and they need help.

17.15   Home. When will I find time to write up the reports?!

Health and social care services

A day in the life of Sofia, Nursery Nurse
Sofia is a Nursery Nurse working in an education nursery which is resourced to take one in eight children with special needs. She qualified with an NNEB certificate and this is her first full time post.

8.45   Start work: prepare the room and resources for the children. Check which area I will be supervising. Brief team meeting to confirm the plans for the day and which children are targeted for observation.

9.00   Children and parents start to come in. Talk with parents about their children, in particular those that have just started. Direct children to particular activities.

9.10   Supervise wet area (painting and water play), working alongside the children and facilitating. Observe target child and make a brief note of activity.

9.40   Assist children who are on a toileting programme. Record results so that the programme can be monitored by the special needs teacher.

9.50   Assist children to tidy up before going to the hall.

9.55   Supervise children waiting to go to the hall. It is important to check their footwear for hall use. Some of the newer children need reassurance.

10.00   Help supervise children through the school to the hall and then assist the teachers in charge of the activity in the hall.

10.20   Return to the nursery and help the children to change shoes and put on coats for outside play.

10.30   Supervise the small group of children on outside play. This is a good opportunity to observe some really good cooperative play and role play as fire-fighters.

10.55   Bring the children in from outside and help them change to indoor clothes. Ask some of the children to start tidying up.

11.00   Settle the children for a group session, and assist the teacher telling the story. About once a week I take the group, this time being helped by the teachers.

11.15   Children are collected by their parents. This is the time we need to pass on information, help the children dress themselves for going home. We also need to sort out pictures, letters, mislaid and soiled clothes to go home. As the rush dies down, move to tidy up my area and prepare for the afternoon children.

11.30   Break and time for a cup of tea.

11.45   Team meeting starts over the last of the tea. The special *needs teacher is outlining some of the recording systems that will help with the statementing process for one of the children. About twice a week we review the observations on the targeted children and agree their progress on their records of achievement.*

12.05 Lunch break. Sometimes we go out as a team but normally we eat in school.

13.00 It all starts again with the afternoon children.

Notice how Sofia works as a member of a team. All of the time she is responsible to the teachers for her work. However, she does take responsibility for her own area and sometimes takes the whole group. As a team member she contributes fully to the activities of the nursery, including using her observations to contribute to the children's individual records of achievement. Also note that what Sofia actually does is not quite the same as the stereotypical nursery worker.

A Now who delivers care?

1. Review the list you made at the start of this unit. In the light of your increased knowledge, make a list of all of the key personnel involved in delivering care, both health and social care. Find out some of the places where they work in your local region.
2. Using your school or college library, careers adviser and careers information publications find out what qualifications are needed for each of the work roles. Arrange to interview people already working in that area locally.

Note. You should try to co-ordinate your work with other members of your group so that you can share information or invite people in to talk to your group.

3. Within your class or group of colleagues share your information and produce a chart indicating the routes to qualification and working in the care professions.
4. Each of you should write up the descriptions of the qualifications, daily work and career prospects for three people. In doing so you must describe at least one person from health care and one from social care.

Describe how the various professionals reached the position they have and what their career progression might be. Describe the roles undertaken by your chosen professional. Describe a typical day's work for the person interviewed.

You should also say how your views of the work have changed following your research. Being a nurse is not like the television programmes!

Who delivers care? – 1, page 118

Health and social care services

Case Study: Peter's story, page 134

Assignment

CARING FOR PETER

Setting the scene
Care is provided by a variety of organisations. In this assignment you will investigate the provision of care for an individual throughout his life. In doing so you will produce a report that would help guide someone through the maze of services that are available. Your work will be based on Peter's story, and also it will reflect your local services.

The product of this assignment should be a report that identifies services for people like Peter and his mother. The report should identify:
- the name of the organisation and its national and local addresses
- the support that the organisation offers
- the way the organisation is funded.

Task 1
Describe the structure of the statutory health and social services available in your locality. Use the information to provide a diagram showing how the local structures fit into the national organisation.

Task 2
In Peter's story it is clear that both Peter and his mother could have benefitted from some voluntary sector support. Identify two voluntary sector organisations that could have provided support.
Draw a pie chart for one of the organisations to show the different sources of funding.

Task 3
Both Peter and his mother eventually needed to enter private residential care. Identify private sector organisations that provide this type of care. Describe how these organisations are funded.

Task 4
Imagine what it might be like to be Peter's mother. Peter cannot be left alone, and you have little time for yourself. His regular visits to the hospital mean that you have to catch two buses and have a long walk from the bus station.
What difficulties would there be and how might informal carers be involved in providing support and care for Peter and his mother?
Describe two situations and say how the carers might help.

Opportunites to collect evidence
On completing these tasks you will have the opportunity to meet the following requirements for Intermediate GNVQ Health and Social Care.
Unit 3
Element 3.1 PCs 1,2,3,4

Health and social care services

Core skills
Written communication skills are developed in this assignment.
Application of number will be involved in producing graphs to indicate sources of funding in the voluntary sector.
Information technology may be used to prepare the written documents.

Grading
The grading theme: Planning, information seeking and information handling will be available in the tasks. Quality of outcomes will be available in your report.

Assignment

MEETING THE NEEDS OF CLIENTS

Setting the scene
Many people need to obtain care for varying periods of time. In this assignment you should make use of Peter's story as one of the examples, together with that given below.

Note. This element needs to be achieved by working in your local environment and carrying out a survey of the needs of local people and how they are met. You should also identify how individuals have been able to gain access to the services. You will produce case studies for three people. In doing this you must gain permission from them to use the information. You must also do everything possible to maintain confidentiality.

A child in torment
Jane had been taken from her home by social workers because she was being abused. She was two years old. With her five brothers and sisters she was moved to an emergency foster home where she lived for two weeks. The family was then split up, with Jane going to a second foster home for two months with her younger sister. Before she was five she moved from foster carer to foster carer seven times. Sometimes she was with a brother or sister; many times she was not.

Eventually Jane was placed with a family who were asked to provide long-term care. This happened just before her fifth birthday.

In this new home Jane started to settle with the family which included two older boys who were not her brothers. Her behaviour was quite odd. She would walk out of the room whenever her foster mother walked into it. She would, however, go up to strange women and try to hold hands with them. Jane also regularly deliberately broke her glasses that she needed to correct her pronounced squint.

It appeared from her behaviour that Jane was provoking rejection: she was looking to move on to her next foster home. After all, she had already had eight sets of foster parents. Jane's foster mother thought that help from a psychologist would be useful. At the same time, the foster mother felt that she needed a break from the strain of caring for an unresponsive child.

Case study: Peter's story, page 134

Task 1
From the two case studies (Peter's and Jane's) select three individuals, one of whom needs the services of the NHS and at least one requiring a different service. Identify the needs of the three different people and the caring services that could be provided to meet the needs. At the start, the task may be discussed as a group.

How would the services provided meet the needs of the people involved?

Task 2
From the case studies, identify how the people involved could have been referred to the services required. What support might be needed to make best use of the services provided?

Find out how your local services would have provided for the needs of the people involved. Find out how they provide information (about services available, how to access services, and rights within the service).

Task 3
Using the information collected, produce a report that identifies the needs of the different people involved and how services provided could meet their needs. For each person describe how referral to the caring service can occur and use your local information to describe the support from the services (in terms of information about services available, how to access services, and rights within the service).

Opportunities to collect evidence
On completing these tasks you will have the opportunity to meet the following requirements for Intermediate GNVQ Health and Social Care.
Unit 3
Element 3.2 PCs 1,2,3,4

Core skills
Communication core skill is developed.
If the report is produced using IT then there will be evidence for this core skill.

Grading
Action planning and information seeking are both important. You will need to identify from the clues in the case studies the services that were used (there are at least seven). You will then need to find out more information about them.

Evaluation of the information you gather against the performance criteria and selection of appropriate material will contribute to the evaluation grading theme.

Quality of outcomes will be demonstrated by the report, which will require a careful analysis of the case studies to provide the initial information.

Assignment

WHERE DO I GO FROM HERE?

Setting the scene
Within this assignment you will have the opportunity to investigate different jobs in health and social care. On completion you will have developed a resource that will provide information about the range of jobs available and a realistic understanding of what they each involve.

Task 1
Review the list that you made at the start of the unit. In the light of your increased knowledge, make a list of all of the key personnel involved in delivering care, both health and social care. Divide the list into two parts:
- those people who provide care
- those people who provide support services.

Task 2
Find out where the key personnel work in your local region. Using your school or college library, careers adviser and careers information publications and databases, find out what qualifications are needed for each of the work roles.

▶ Provision in your local area, page 130

Task 3
Select three of the roles that interest you and arrange to interview people already working in these roles locally.
You should interview one person from each of the following areas:
- support services
- health and medical care
- social care.

Note. You should try to co-ordinate your work with other members of your group so that you can share information or invite people in to talk to your group.

Task 4
Within your class or group share your information and individually produce a chart indicating the routes to qualification and working in the care professions.
Describe how they reached the position they have and what their career progression might be. Also find out what would be a typical working day for them. Decide how the roles undertaken by your chosen professionals compare with the stereotypes of these roles, for example on television programmes.

Task 5
Individually, write up a job description to include the qualifications required, daily work and career prospects for the three people. Remember, in doing so to describe at least one person from support services, one from health care and one from social care. You should also show how your views of the work involved have changed following your research. Being a nurse is not like the television programmes!

Opportunities to collect evidence
On completing these tasks you will have the opportunity to meet the following requirements for Intermediate GNVQ Health and Social Care.
Unit 3
Element 3.3 Pcs 1,2,3,4

Core skills
Core skills in communication (both written and oral) are particularly well developed.

Grading
All grading themes, particularly planning (in organising the interviews), information seeking and information handling (in dealing with the information gathered and presenting it as job descriptions), will be available.

Health and social care services

Questions

Each question shows more than one possible answer, a,b,c and d; only **one** is correct.

1. Organisations established and financed by the government are known as:
   a public organisations
   b voluntary organisations
   c private organisations
   d statutory organisations.

2. The role of voluntary organisations could best be described as:
   a providing better standards of care
   b filling any gap in statutory provision
   c providing competition
   d making a profit.

3. Social services can sometimes offer a carer or their charge a short break. This is referred to as:
   a respite care
   b residential care
   c family care
   d community care.

4. Which organisation is responsible for the registration of childminders, playgroups and nurseries?
   a District Council
   b Health Department
   c Education Department
   d Social Services.

5. Homes which provide for people who can no longer live in their own home and who are ill and in need of professional nursing care are called:
   a residential care homes
   b sheltered housing
   c community care
   d nursing homes.

6. 'Which one of the following professionals offers help and advice about the care and development of children?
   a the chiropodist
   b the optician
   c the health visitor
   d the physiotherapist.

7. Private, voluntary, charitable and non-profit making organisations are referred to as:
   a the independent sector
   b the statutory sector
   c the public sector
   d the other sector.

8. Many hospitals now have trust status. This means that they are:
   a self-governing
   b governed by the local authority
   c governed by district health authorities
   d governed by regional health authorities.

9. Which one of the following is an 'informal' care provider?
   a the Health Service
   b voluntary organisations
   c the family
   d Social Services.

10. Reference is often made to the new structure of the NHS. The initials NHS stand for:
    a New Heart Service
    b New Health Service
    c National Health Service
    d National Heart Service.

11. The purchasing of hospital and community health services for the local population of a given area is the responsibility of:
    a Parliament
    b District Health Authorities
    c GPs.
    d Family Health Services Authorities.

12. The services provided by Social Services Departments for a wide range of different client groups are called the:
    a personal social services
    b public social services
    c voluntary services
    d preventive social services.

13. Which one of the following professionals operates as part of a primary health care team?
    a a practice nurse
    b a consultant paediatrician
    c a psychiatrist
    d a hospital consultant.

14. Which of the following groups of people provide informal care?
    a GPs, district nurses, health visitors
    b GPs, practice nurses, community midwives
    c social workers, chiropodists, speech therapists
    d children, parents, friends, neighbours.

15 Which one of the following services is provided by the Local Authority Social Services Department?
a opticians
b home help
c pharmacists
d Ambulance Service.

16 Providing physical support, for example adaptations to the home which allow a person with a disability to live independently, is part of a process called:
a patronising the client
b personalising the client
c marginalising the client
d empowerment of the client.

17 An illness which comes rapidly to a crisis and is of short duration is called:
a an acute illness
b a chronic illness
c a long term illness
d an ongoing illness.

18 Which one of the following services is an example of secondary care provision?
a GP services
b hospital services
c pharmacists
d dentists.

19 Private Health Care Services are available to:
a all members of the population
b those members of the population who pay the full cost of the services
c all elderly members of the population
d professional members of the population.

20 Residential homes are provided by the Local Authority or by a private (or voluntary) agency, or both. All private and voluntary homes must be registered with:
a the Social Security Office
b the National Health Service
c the Housing Office
d the Local Social Services.

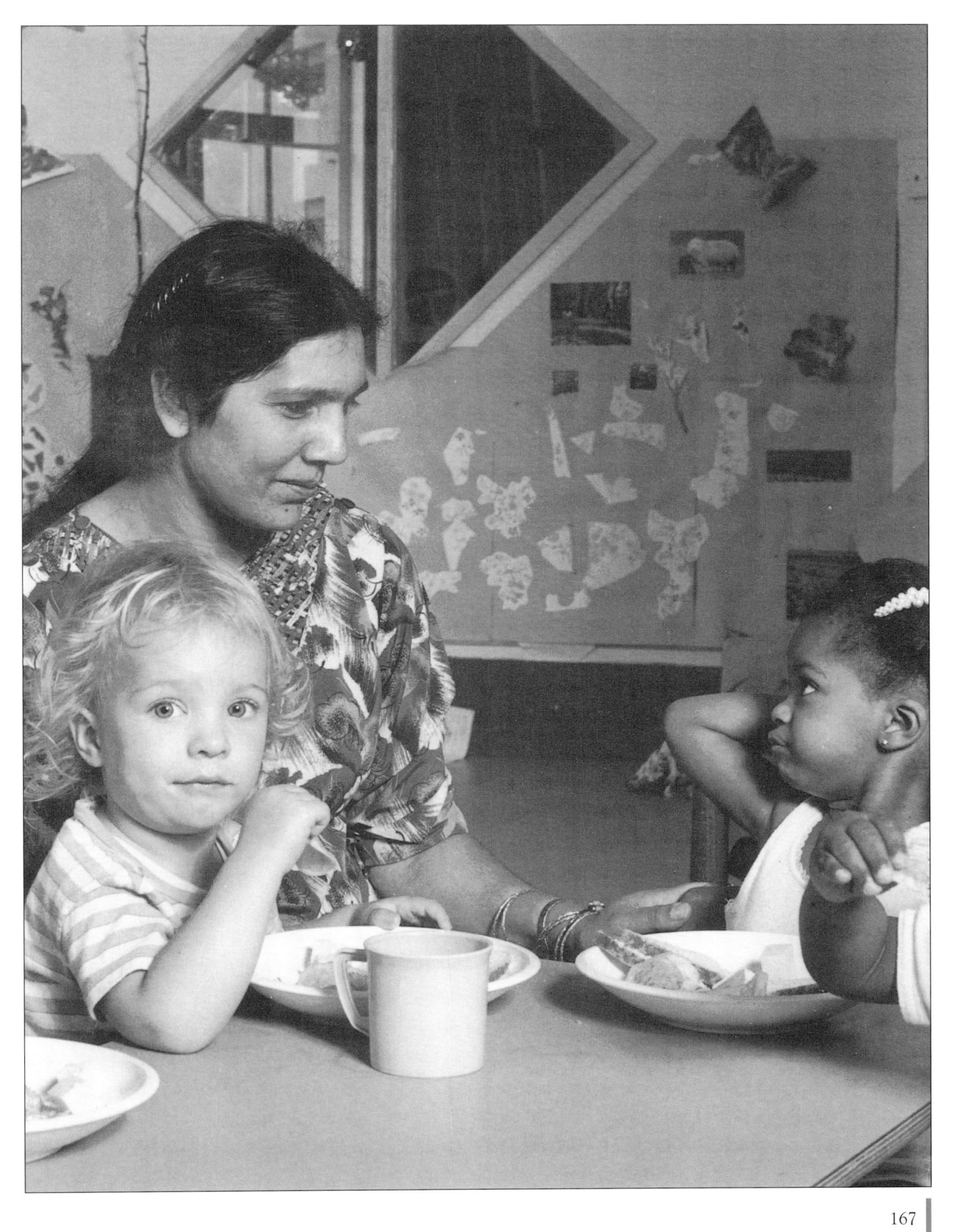

Health and social care services

4 | Communication and interpersonal relationships in health and social care

Every day many people spend time looking after someone else. Many of them are working in the caring professions where their skills of listening and responding are so important. They have the ability to work with a range of people and understand something of their individual needs. They can mentally place themselves in situations similar to those of the people they are caring for, and in doing so they can help provide the support needed.

These people have the ability to communicate not only with individuals but also in groups. They understand how to communicate both verbally and non-verbally (without words). They recognise people as individuals and can provide them with emotional support. This unit describes these skills and assists you to develop them for yourself.

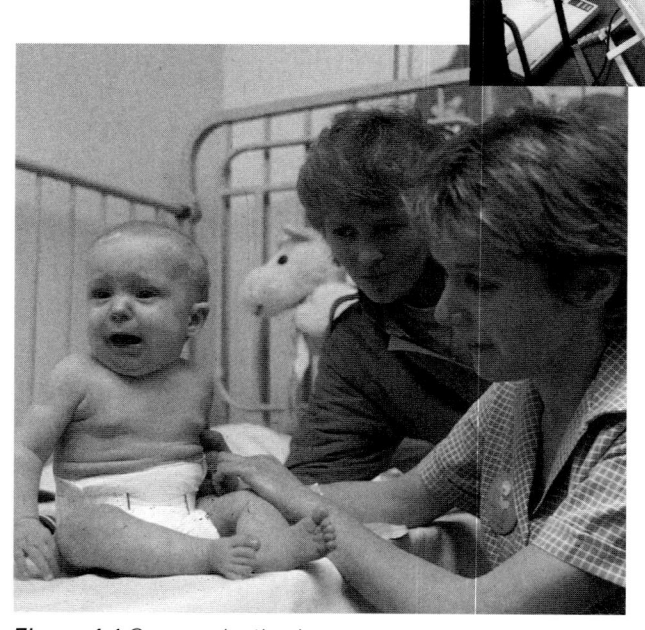

Figure 4.1 Communicating in care environments

The Elements

Develop communication skills
- explain why it is important for individuals, families and groups to communicate
- demonstrate listening and responding skills to encourage communication with individuals in different contexts
- demonstrate observational skills to encourage communication with individuals in different contexts
- identify obstacles to effective communication
- evaluate one's own communication skills and make suggestions for their improvement.

This involves developing the skills of conversation, listening and questioning, whilst using non-verbal messages and recognising a person's individuality.

▶ Why communicate? page 170

Explore how interpersonal relationships may be affected by discriminatory behaviour
- provide examples of the different forms which discrimination may take
- describe behaviours which may indicate discrimination
- describe how stereotyping individuals and groups can lead to discriminatory behaviour
- describe the possible effects of discrimination
- identify the rights which all individuals have under current equality of opportunity legislation

Taking the recognition of individuality a stage further: showing how prejudice, and types of discrimination affect the ways people work together.

▶ Individuality, page 189

Investigate aspects of working with clients in health and social care
- describe how the caring relationship may differ in nature from other forms of relationship
- explain the ways in which clients may respond to being in receipt of care
- describe how different types of support may affect inter-personal relationships between clients and carers
- describe the role of effective interaction in caring relationships
- explain why confidentiality is of critical importance in health and social care settings
- explain the ethical issues which individuals may face in relation to maintaining confidentiality.

Looking at the nature of caring relationships and the types of support needed. Developing an understanding of the importance and the need for the value base in care.

▶ Working with people in health and social care, page 194

Communication and relationships

Why communicate?

A   Life without communication

Imagine that communication did not exist. Imagine that there was no way in which you could express your needs and ideas to others.

1. What different methods of communication do we use? What would happen if each of these methods did not exist?

In small groups record your ideas as a spidergram so that you can share them easily with the full group. Discuss the effects of not having:
- radio and television
- written communication
- spoken language
- signs and signals (non-verbal language).

2. What equipment is available to assist people with communication difficulties to communicate? You might investigate phonic ears, Lightwriters and Touch talkers.

We often consider that **communication** involves mainly using words, either written down or spoken. This is one of the major achievements of mankind, but it is clearly not the only method. Language is used to communicate needs, ideas, emotions and beliefs.

At the level of the individual, communication supports development. A baby crying because of hunger communicates this and is fed. The parent communicates love and affection, providing support for emotional development. Later, language is used to help promote learning and intellectual development.

Communication is used to explain personal beliefs and preferences. People may develop forms of communication (for example, language) to help them share with others their beliefs, religion or politics. We often use words that have a specific meaning for the people we are with. In terms of GNVQ an element describes part of a unit; in chemistry it defines a substance made up of similar atoms with the same chemical properties (carbon and hydrogen are elements).

Communication, therefore, has many roles: developing individuals, acknowledging beliefs and developing groups. One of its greatest features is to enable people to share ideas and understanding. This helps to promote co-operative development and can reduce the risk of conflict. In the rest of this unit you will be able to explore some of the various aspects of communication and the ways in which they can be used in providing health and social care.

Supportive communication

Who can you talk to? Why are they easy to talk to? If you were worried or in trouble, who would you go to?

The answer to the last question in particular may well be someone who can provide you with emotional support. The skill of providing emotional support is one that you will need to develop if you want to work in the caring professions.

Emotional support: support and respect for feelings, needs and beliefs.

A   Relationships

Make a list of the things you like about your relationship with a particular person.

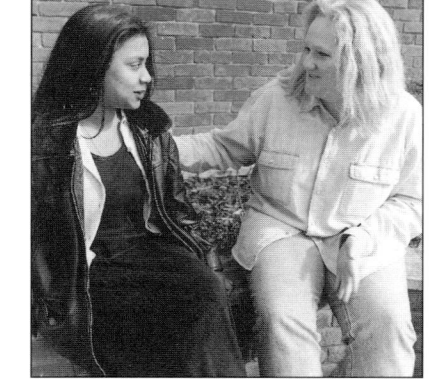

Figure 4.2 Most of us have someone we can confide in

Most of us have someone in whom we can confide; someone who is easy to talk to; someone who listens. It may be a best friend, a parent, teacher, or relative. What is it that these people do that makes them your friend? It is possible that your list contains:
- they listen to what I want to say
- they seem to understand, even when I can't really say what I mean
- we seem to be able to pick up where we left off even if we have not seen each other for a while
- we agree about most things, and even when we don't it doesn't create problems. We agree to differ
- it's as if they can read my mind and know what I'm going to say.

All of these characteristics indicate someone who has developed skills in **conversation** and can use them to help understand others' needs. A word that describes this skill is empathy.

Empathy: *understanding and experiencing how a person is feeling – putting yourself in their place.*

This can involve using your own experiences and feelings in similar situations to help you to understand what a person is really saying. Developing these skills will help you in providing support for other people. These skills are particularly useful when working in caring situations with people who have difficulty expressing themselves.

The main skill areas are:
- conversing (listening, in various ways, and talking)
- interpreting what has been said
- supporting and respecting.

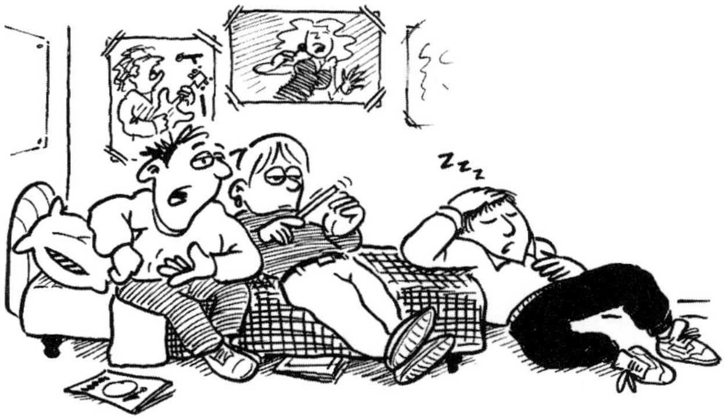

Conversation

We often think that conversation is about being able to talk. In fact, two essential aspects are listening and knowing when not to talk. It is very easy to hog a conversation or treat it as a competition. You may think that you are showing you are listening by capping every story with one showing how you have 'done it faster, got a bigger one or suffered more pain'. These are forms of 'I strain' where you overuse the word 'I' and show little respect for the person talking with you.

In caring situations conversation is very important. It encourages people to talk about themselves. Such conversations are often difficult for the person receiving care if they lack self confidence. They are essential as a way of gaining understanding and assisting the care processes. Whenever you are involved in a conversation it is important to consider the needs of the other person involved. The many pitfalls associated with conversation failure include:
- failing to use language that you both understand
- taking the conversation into areas that the other person does not want to talk about
- failing to check that the message you are trying to put over is being understood as you intended it
- being insensitive to the other persons' beliefs, preferences and feelings
- talking when you should have been listening.

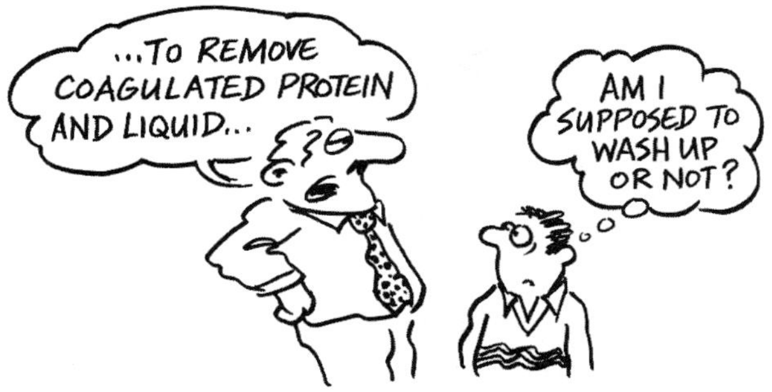

Figure 4.3 Some ways of recognising 'I' strain

Figure 4.4 It is important to use language that the listener understands

Communication and relationships

A | Identifying pitfalls

On your own, compile a list of suggestions as to why you think your 'failed conversations' were not successful. Share your list orally with the others in the group. Check with others as necessary to make sure you understand all the items on their lists, and revise your own list if appropriate. See how far it is possible to produce a single list with which you can all agree.

Listening and talking

Those of us who can hear also think we can listen. The two are not the same. Hearing means detecting the sounds. Listening involves concentrating on understanding what is being said and not being said. The following activity provides an example of the difference between the two.

A | Listening

Read out this passage to a person outside your group, saying that you will want to ask a question about it at the end.

'Imagine you're driving a bus. At the start of the journey there are ten of each type of coin in the cash box. That is, ten £1 coins, ten 50 pences, ten twenties, ten tens, ten fives, ten twos and ten pennies. That makes a total of £18.80.

At the first stop four people get on. The one with the red hat pays for a fifty pence ticket with a pound coin. The person with the white scarf shows a season ticket. The woman with the grey coat hands over three ten pence coins for a twenty-five pence journey and the last, a school-girl with plaits, pays her fifteen pence half fare with two coins giving the correct amount.'

Now ask the other person, 'How old is the bus driver?'
(You need to read the first sentence carefully to work it out!)

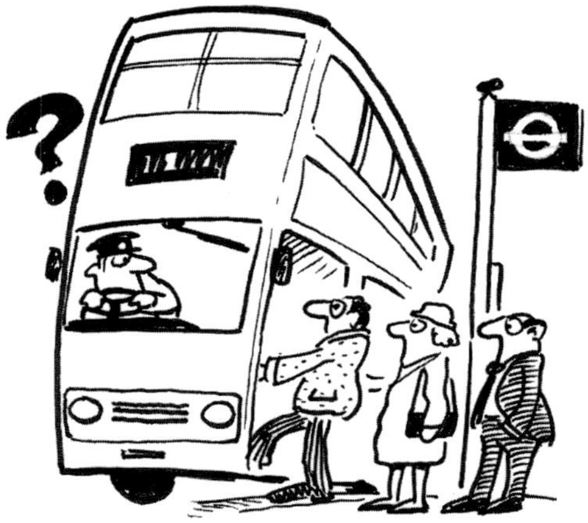

Figure 4.5

It is probable that your neighbour did not immediately know the answer. Even if you just read the passage to yourself it is likely that you had to re-read it to find the answer. You had given so much information that whilst what you said was heard, it was not understood: there was too much to concentrate on at once. You had set up a situation that could lead to hearing overload. Listening and understanding are hard work!

Listening skills

We all have a tendency to hear what we want to hear or what we expect to hear. Have you ever been in the situation where you have asked for something expecting one answer only to be given a different answer? It can be very embarrassing to launch into the arguments, only to realise that the answer you were given was not the one expected. You heard the sounds but did not listen.

Where the words are unfamiliar or complicated or not spoken clearly we can mishear what is being said and interpret the sounds as familiar words and phrases. This is often true over a poor telephone line.

This hearing 'defect' is used in the game Chinese whispers. In this game a group of people sit in a circle and pass on a message by whispering it to their neighbour. At the end of the circuit the last person repeats the message and it is compared with the original. The more complex the original message, the more likely it is to be corrupted and the meaning changed.

Communication and relationships

There is a story that tells of a general who sent a verbal message by a series of runners to the headquarters. The original message was: Send reinforcements the general is going to advance. It arrived as: Send three and fourpence the general's going to a dance.

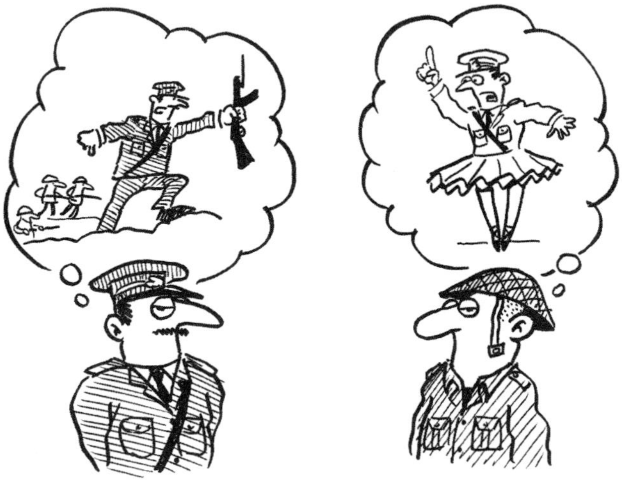

A   Chinese whispers

Try playing Chinese whispers with the whole of your group. Try to use one or two long sentences read initially from a newspaper or magazine. Were the messages passed on accurately?
It is important to develop systems for checking what you have heard and understood.

Figure 4.6 It is easy for messages to be confused if they are passed by several people

How to listen

Wherever you work in the caring professions, one of the crucial skills is to be able to encourage clients to communicate with you. Active listening is one of the first skills to learn in order to support your work. The next activity shows how powerful this is, and how difficult it is not to do some active listening.

A   Effects of different listening styles

In this activity you need to work with two neighbours. Take it in turns to be either the speaker, the listener or the observer.
The speaker should talk about something of interest for up to five minutes. The listener should do one of three things:
- sit, concentrating on listening in silence, making absolutely no movements. If something funny is said, do not even smile!
- look out of the window. Play with your pen. Think about how boring this activity is. Do almost anything but do not concentrate on what is being said.
- listen and concentrate hard on understanding what is being said. Try to pick the natural gaps in the flow of words to indicate that you are still listening by nodding your head or making 'encouraging noises'.

The observer should watch the speaker and listener and make notes on how they each reacted to the situation. Pay particular attention to the ways they sat and behaved.
When you have finished discuss how it felt to be the speaker. What did it feel like to get no response? How easy was it to listen without responding? How much can the listener recall of what was being said? What were the differences when a clear effort was made to show that the listener was listening and understanding? What reactions did the observer notice?
You may prefer to practice your listening styles on unsuspecting family or friends – as long as you're sure they won't be upset if they realise what you are doing.
Note. The observers' notes will be useful when we look at non-verbal communication.

▶ Role play – debriefing, confidentiality, page xxi

▶ Non-verbal communication, page 182

173

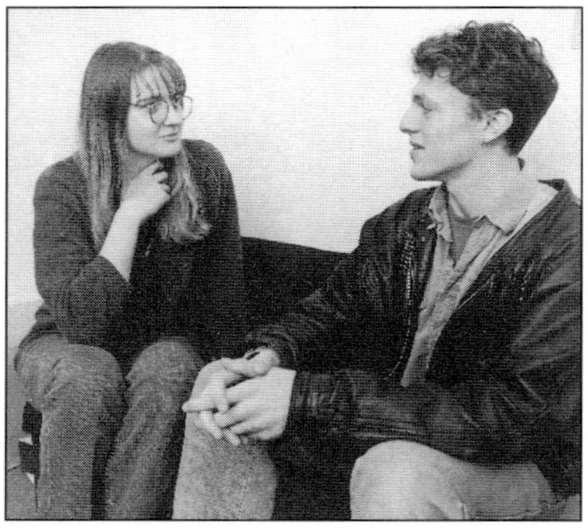

Communication and relationships

Figure 4.7 You have to concentrate on listening

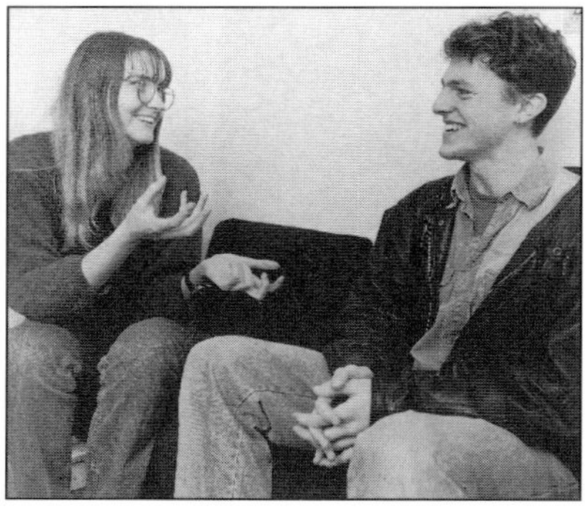

Figure 4.8 Summarising helps to confirm that you are getting the right message

The activity clearly demonstrates how conversations require feedback from the listener. Without feedback we feel uncomfortable. The simplest aid to listening is to respond to what is being said.

Responding can mean nodding your head or saying things like 'Uh-huh' or 'Yes, I see what you mean' at appropriate points. You have to concentrate on what is being said to know when to join in. This active feedback technique helps the person talking to know that you are listening and that you are interested enough to want to hear more. By interrupting at appropriate points, without stopping the flow of what is being said, you are also demonstrating basic empathy with the speaker. It takes time and practice to develop this basic skill.

The barriers to listening

So far we have not considered your surroundings, where much of your listening and talking takes place. If you carry out many of the activities in this unit in a cramped classroom where you can be overheard, then you may feel embarrassed. Think about what it would be like to talk about something very private with other people listening.

Where you carry on a conversation is important. You need to consider the comfort of both people involved. This may be provided by:
- comfortable chairs
- a quiet area away from where you can be overheard.

You also need to consider the best place to talk. It may be better to talk in a client's room than in an office. A common room may be noisy and people may overhear. If the right environment is set up, then the people involved in a conversation will be better able to talk freely and communication will be improved.

A | Active listening

In a small group, try to agree a summary of do's and don'ts for active listening, and present it in the form of a checklist. Remember to listen actively to one another during your discussion. We suggest you do this before reading further.

Reflecting and summarising

Two important ways of checking what you have heard are to repeat important words and to summarise what has been said. In repeating important words it confirms to the speaker that you hear them as important: it helps the speaker to monitor that the message is getting across.

When you listen to someone you should be prepared to stop and confirm what you have heard. This helps your understanding of what is being said. It also sends the message, 'I'm interested. Would you like to talk about that a bit more?'

A | Reflecting and summarising

Health warning

These activities can be very powerful counselling techniques used to enable a person to talk about deep feelings. It is possible that you would not be able to deal with such a situation in a way that fully supported the speaker. Stick to safe areas for conversations and do not try to counsel/interpret your friends without full and proper training. Use the techniques with great care.

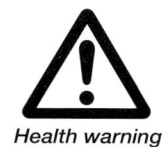

Within this course you are not expected to become counsellors and it is important to know some of the techniques so that you are aware of the dangers.

In order to practise your listening skills it is important for all people involved to agree to the exercise. It is also important to agree about confidentiality. When somebody tells you something you must not repeat it to anybody else without permission. For example, you must both agree if you wish to use a record (audio, video or written) for your GNVQ portfolio.

1 Working with a partner, one of you describe the journey from home to school. The other should use direct repetition of important words as often as possible.

For example:
Speaker: I live at 39 Smith Street, and …
Listener: 39 Smith Street?
Speaker: Yes … and I leave at quarter past eight every college day.
Listener: Quarter past eight?
Speaker: Yes …

Change roles of speaker and listener and repeat the activity, but this time the listener should only interrupt where necessary to encourage the speaker or to confirm things that are misheard.

2 At the end, each person should summarise what they heard. Discuss how you both felt to be the speaker and listener in each case and how accurate the summaries were.

The simple repetition of a few words can help a conversation to flow. It also helps to stop you, the listener, from missing important details. Of course, you have to think about what you want to repeat. The examples in the exercise demonstrate something about reflective listening and summarising.

Reflective listening: *a technique in which important things that are being said to the listener are repeated in order to encourage the speaker to say more. It involves a combination of skills.*

Reflective listening can be done badly. The first part of the Activity: Reflecting and summarising, showed how it can interrupt and stop conversation. Both people involved were probably a little frustrated and uncomfortable with the way they felt.

In the second part the listener concentrated on what was being said and interrupted in ways that displayed interest. This encouraged the speaker to talk. The act of summarising what has been said helps to confirm that the important information has been understood, and can also be called thinking aloud.

Summarising: *restating in your own words what you have heard. In doing so you should identify what you think is important in what has been said. It helps to confirm to the speaker that you have understood what was said.*

In this case both people should have felt more satisfied. The speaker said what s/he wanted to say. The listener showed s/he had been listening and valued what had been said.

For both techniques you need to be able to:
- concentrate on what is being said
- identify important words and phrases to:
  - show you are listening
  - ask for more information
  - help you to understand
  - check you have understood the message.

This assists you in maintaining the conversation and providing emotional support by:
- encouraging the speaker to make clear what they want to say
- helping you to respond in an appropriate way
- showing the speaker that what is being said is important and valued by you
- allowing the conversation to flow and continue.

It is important to use reflective listening and summarising to enable the person speaking to continue to talk.

Reflective listening and summarising are very powerful skills to develop. Done well they support conversation: done badly they destroy it. One of the crucial skills is to be able to stay silent rather than interrupt. Quite often a person will make long pauses in the conversation, especially where there is a great deal of emotion involved. These can appear to be opportunities to reflect back on what has been said, but if the person needs time to think, then to interrupt would be wrong. It is important to know when to speak: you can learn to understand the non-verbal cues given by the speaker.

> Reading or sending non-verbal messages, page 182

Advanced listening skills

We have already seen that conversation requires more than just people talking to each other. There is the skill of reflective listening. There are also the questioning skills that can make a conversation flow, or stop it dead.

In starting a conversation it is more likely to succeed if there is an invitation to talk, rather than a series of questions. The invitation to speak may come from non-verbal clues rather than a verbal request. For the conversation to continue, it is important to use verbal and non-verbal clues that help you to know that things are progressing. There are complex 'rules' about who is to talk and when someone else can start. To a large extent these rules involve non-verbal communication.

Verbal clues that help a conversation

We have spent some time looking at ways to improve listening skills. It may seem odd to write about looking at listening: reading or hearing about listening would seem to be more appropriate. However, sight is the major sense and so affects the way we apply language.

Communication and relationships

A Just imagine

Think about what it would be like to visit Eurodisney. Write down the first five things you imagine.

High on most people's lists from the activity above would have been visual images of Eurodisney. This is because most of us use pictures to help us remember or stimulate imagination. Some people would have had initial thoughts relating to sounds, whilst a smaller group would have first thought of feelings or smells. The way each person remembers is expressed in the language used:
- people who remember using visual images may '...see what you mean'
- people who remember using sounds may '...hear what you say'
- people who recall feelings first may '...know how you feel'.

By listening to the words a person uses it is possible to get an idea of how they think. If you are able to match your words to the way they access memory then you have a better chance being fully understood and of maintaining a conversation.

Asking questions

Most young children seem to be one big question. They constantly ask questions in order to help them learn. If you are to be successful in caring you will need to learn how to ask questions.

Questioning can be used to gather information. It helps you to understand the people you are working with, both clients and colleagues. You can use questions to obtain sufficient information to help you develop a level of trust and empathy. Incorrect use of questions can lead to a breakdown in communication.

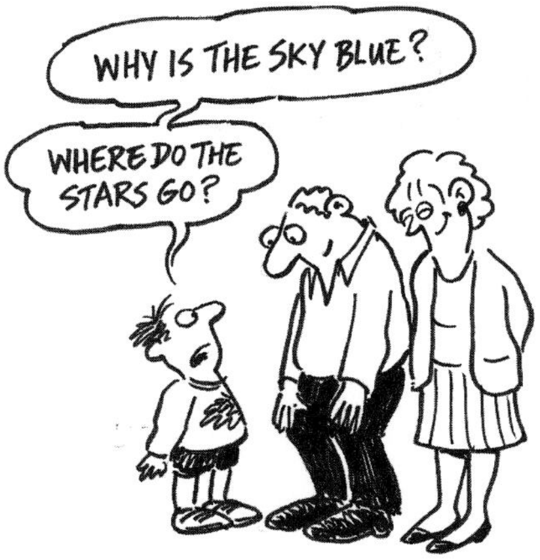

Question types

What is the difference between these questions?

What is your favourite drink?
Is coffee your favourite drink?

Both are questions about drinks but the first gives an opportunity for any response whilst the second requires the answers 'Yes' or 'No'. The first is an **open question** which encourages the person answering to expand on the answer. The second is a **closed question** which demands a response from a limited range.

Both types of question have a use in conversation. Skilled use of both types can help to maintain the flow of conversation. They can support and help develop a relationship.

Figure 4.9 Young children are always full of questions

A Using open and closed questions

With a partner, take it in turns to find out about your partner's favourite foods, pastimes, rock group, etc.
You may ask only five closed questions that can be answered with a fixed range of responses. You may not ask directly, 'What is your favourite ...?'
After five questions write down what you think is your partner's favourite ...
Now ask five open questions about the same area.
How much more information about your partner's likes have you discovered?
(Think of the difference between the information gained from:
Do you like curries?
and
If you were going out for a meal what sort of restaurant would you choose?)

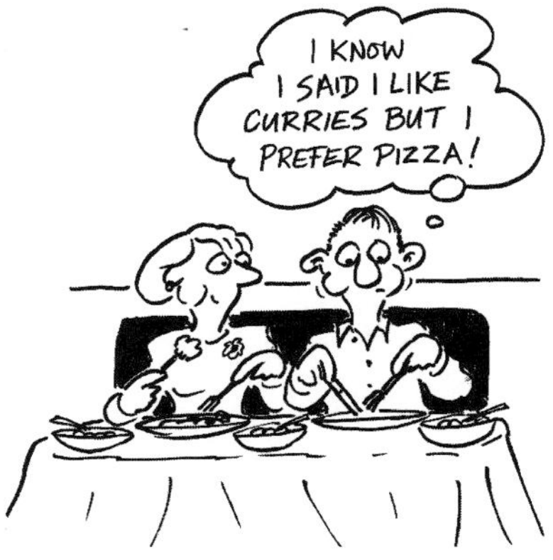

Figure 4.10 Closed questions don't always give you the information you are looking for

177

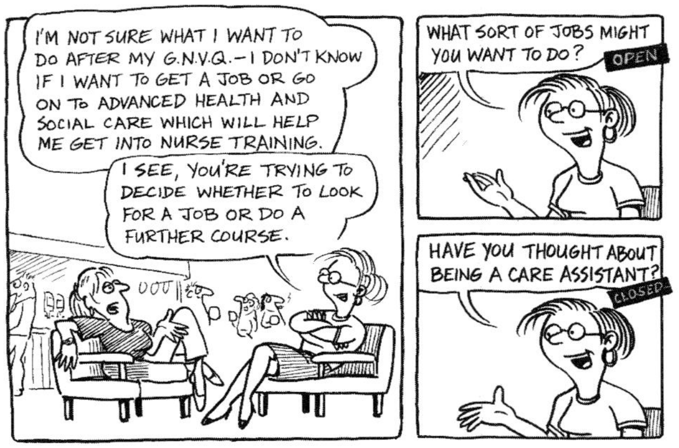

Figure 4.11 Using open questioning and summarising

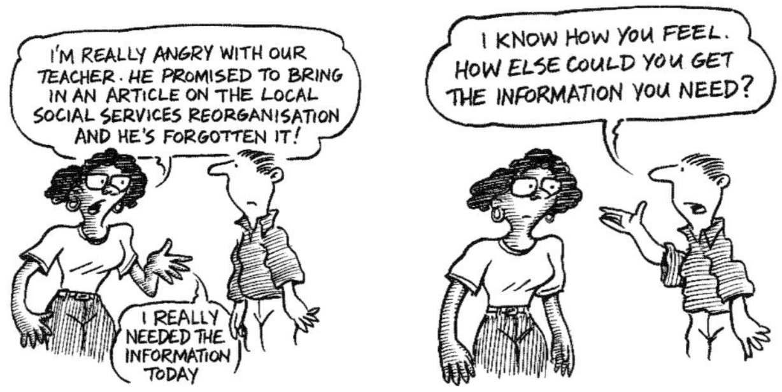

Figure 4.12 Using an open question to refocus a conversation

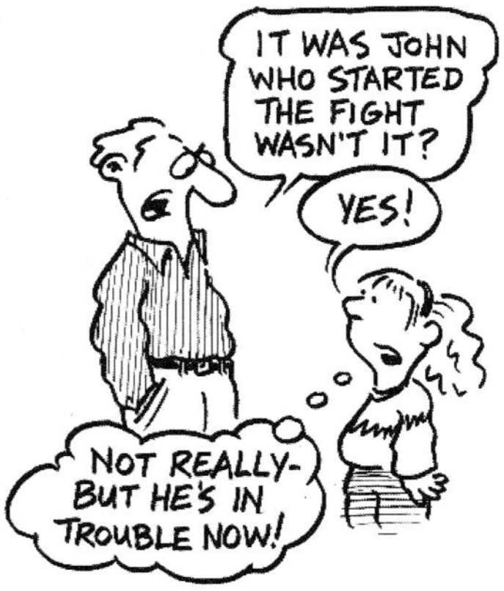

Figure 4.13 Leading questions must be carefully thought out

When to ask questions

Questions have a role in helping the speaker to provide more information. Early on in a relationship there is a need to gather information. Some of this is factual information that can be gathered by using closed questions.

As a conversation develops the information required can become more about feelings and emotions. At these times open questions should be used, supported by reflective listening and summarising. In other words use the skills of identifying when to speak and when to ask an open question.

In open questioning the speaker needs to think about the answer but has free response. The listener has said, 'Tell me more.'

With the closed question the speaker needs to think very little and can answer simply 'Yes' or 'No'. The listener has effectively said, 'I want some specific information.'

Open questions: these ask the speaker to think about the answer and expand upon it. They give more opportunity to explore the detail of what is being talked about, and enable the speaker to think further about the subject. In many cases open questions help the speaker to gain a new perspective on the situation.

Use of closed questions

Closed questions: these allow a limited fixed range of responses.

Closed questions can be used to gain basic factual information such as forenames, surname, age, date of birth. They can also be used to direct the conversation.

Closed questions are used when following one clear route with a need to get basic information. They allow the questioner to maintain control of the flow of the discussion. They can be especially useful when the speaker regularly goes off the subject. Care needs to be taken, however, as going off the subject can indicate distress or a need to talk about an area that has been missed.

Closed questions can also be used to bring a conversation to an end. They can be used to confirm a summary statement and agree an action plan. Again, care needs to be taken to ensure that the closed questions are not stopping the speaker from saying what he or she wants to. In this situation they can also be used where you as a listener do not feel confident about your ability to cope with things that a client is saying. You take control, and either end the discussion or move to a safer area.

Leading questions

Leading questions: questions phrased in such a way as to give the respondent information about the expected answer. This can be achieved both in the words used and the tone and pitch of the voice.

It can be very easy to ask questions that lead people to an answer. The question can suggest an answer that will meet the needs of the questioner.

Sometimes it is useful to use leading questions. If a person lacks confidence, a leading question may give a clue as to the expected answer and so encourage a response. This may then be the start of a useful communication. By hinting at the expected answer, the questioner can give the respondents the confidence to answer. There are dangers in leading questions. Because they lead a person to the expected answer they can be used to influence a person's decision. Care must always be taken to ensure that any information gained from using leading questions really does reflect what the respondent wanted to say.

Organised question sequences

Quite often it is important to use questions to follow up an idea or feeling. You could, for example, focus on an older person in a residential home and talk about what they do or don't like about the meals, and what changes they would like to the menu.

It would be easy to ask, 'What changes would you like to the menu?' This would give a chance for a free response but would not always get one. It would be easier to say, 'I do not want any changes', than to try to look at all the possible foods that could be changed.

It would be better to 'work round' to an answer by asking a question sequence.

In the conversation in figure 4.14 a series of questions has been used to establish a supportive relationship with Mr Jones. In doing this, information about the foods he likes has been obtained.

A good listener would also have picked up that Mr Jones and his wife shared the cooking and that Mr Jones cooked the toad in the hole. There was also information about Mr Jones 'not being able to do it any more'. It would be reasonable for the carer (with Mr Jones' permission) to talk to the officer in charge and the cook about the possibility of involving Mr Jones in the cooking. The officer in charge should also follow up on Mr Jones' problems with his hands. He may have arthritis and might welcome some support with, for example, adapted cutlery.

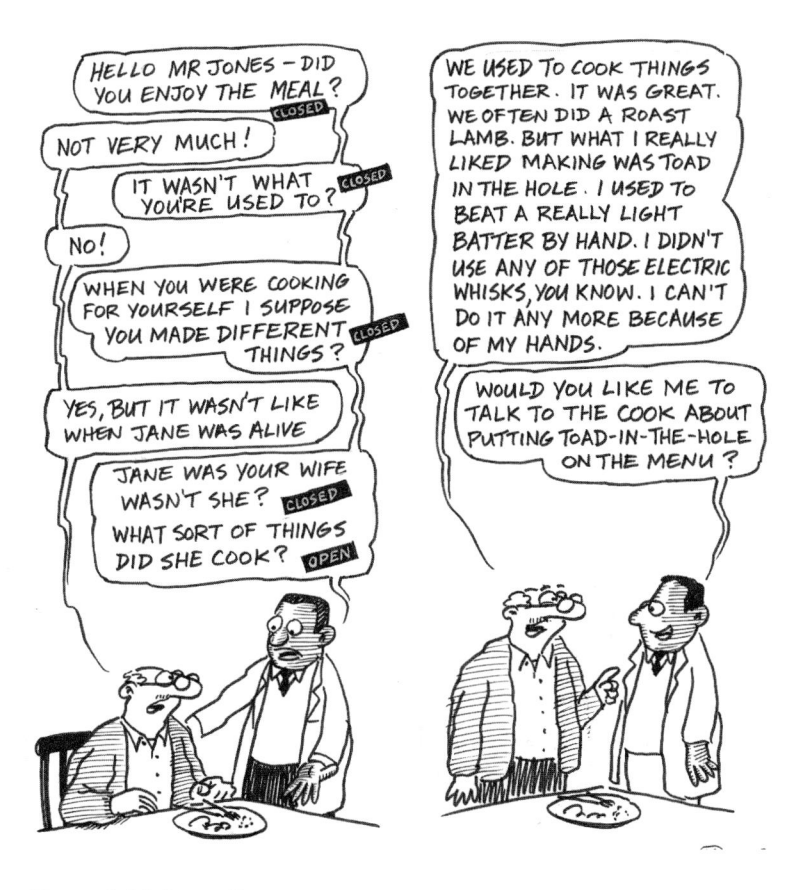

Figure 4.14 A question sequence

Communication and relationships

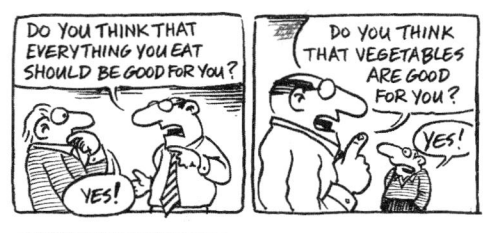

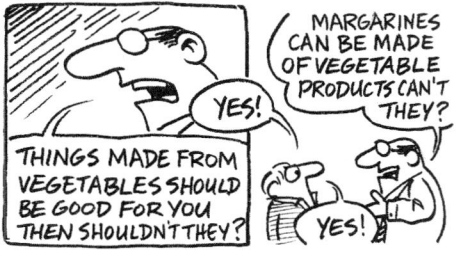

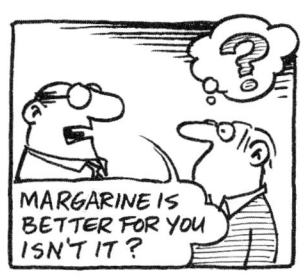

Figure 4.15 Leading questions and careful sequencing

A more common version of this poem, page 231

Complexity of questions

Question sequences can also be used for different purposes. A combination of leading questions and careful sequencing can bring about the response that you want, which may not be the one wanted by the person being questioned (see figure 4.15).

The temptation is to continue answering 'yes'. But the last question does not mean anything. 'Better than ...' what?

Question sequences like the one in figure 4.15 can be used to show that people think that margarine is better than butter. However, changing the questions to include some questions about chemically processed food and the fact that margarine is chemically processed could give a result that people think that butter is better than margarine.

It is important for the language used to be understood by the person being questioned. People working in any area tend to develop a language associated with the work. Whilst care assistants may talk about the need to toilet Mrs Jones it would not readily be understood by Mrs Jones. One of the many criticisms of doctors is that they use 'medical words' and do not explain things to their patients in ways that can be understood.

Below is a well known poem in complex language. Try to work out the common form of this poem.

Scintillate, scintillate globule vivific.
Fain would I fathom thy nature specific.
Loft'ly suspended in ether capacious
Strongly resembling a gem carbonaceous.

Complexity can also be as a result of unusual and difficult-to-follow sentence structures. For example, The question below could lead to odd answers: ask your friends.

'If you were asked if heart attacks were always fatal, would your answer be no?'

The answer 'no' to this question means the respondent is saying that heart attacks are always fatal. Of course, this is not the case.

Questions need to be phrased so that the intended audience understands. It is no use asking complex questions of young children; the answers will probably be worthless. Similarly, to use language appropriate to a three-year-old might seem patronising to a teenager. It is very easy to assume that because people are in a care environment they all need to be asked very simple questions.

Questions need to be:
- clear
- at the right level for the listener
- checked to see the response is reasonable.

You should always check if the answer you get seems out of place. A simple example of this would be if a person was asked, 'Would you feel more comfortable in bed or sitting in a chair?' A response of 'yes' is not a valid answer to the question. The person may not have realised that a choice was being offered.

A What does this mean

Put together, in small groups, a guide to hard-to-understand phrases you have had to struggle with. Identify them in the expressions of parents, teachers, in textbooks, in forms you have to fill in, and guidance notes that go with them, for example evacuation procedures. Set them out in the first of two columns. In the second column offer a translation. Try to make sure everyone's contribution is heard and considered. Have a chairperson and secretary for each group.

Probes and prompts

As you develop conversational techniques, it will become clear that you need further skills to help you to provide support. This is particularly true when you are working in caring situations where conversation with clients may need to be focused on their needs.

Your listening skills and interpretation of non-verbal messages may tell you that there is more to be said. The speaker may be waiting for 'permission' to say more. You may think that something that has been said needs further investigation.

Open questions can be used to start exploring an area. The response can be followed up with a short probe question to test if there is any more that the speaker wishes to say.

Probe: *a short question used to help a person expand on a previous answer. Probes can help bring out issues that a client needs to talk about, but is afraid to do so. A probe is used to reveal what a person is concealing.*

Example

Asking a boy about his birthday party you get the response, 'It was good. The presents were great. The food was OK, I suppose.'

If your interest was the food, because you were planning a nursery party for the boy, you might probe for more information with 'What food did you have?'. You might need to follow up with another probe, 'What food did you like?'

The two probe questions would help to establish what foods had been available at the party, and what was liked. A skilled listener might note the difference between the lists and check if this suggested food that he did not like as well as those he did.

It is also possible to encourage a person to talk by using prompts. These questions often lead the person by suggesting something about the answer. They lead the person towards giving more information. Prompts can be particularly useful in bringing a person back to the subject.

Prompt: *a short question or statement used to focus on an area. Prompt can help lead a conversation. They can also refocus a rambling conversation. A prompt is an invitation to elaborate on what has been said.*

Example

What did you like about the red jumper?
Did it feel warm?

Both questions would help prompt a person to concentrate on the red jumper and then on a specific feature – its warmth.

The Health Warning about counselling still applies!

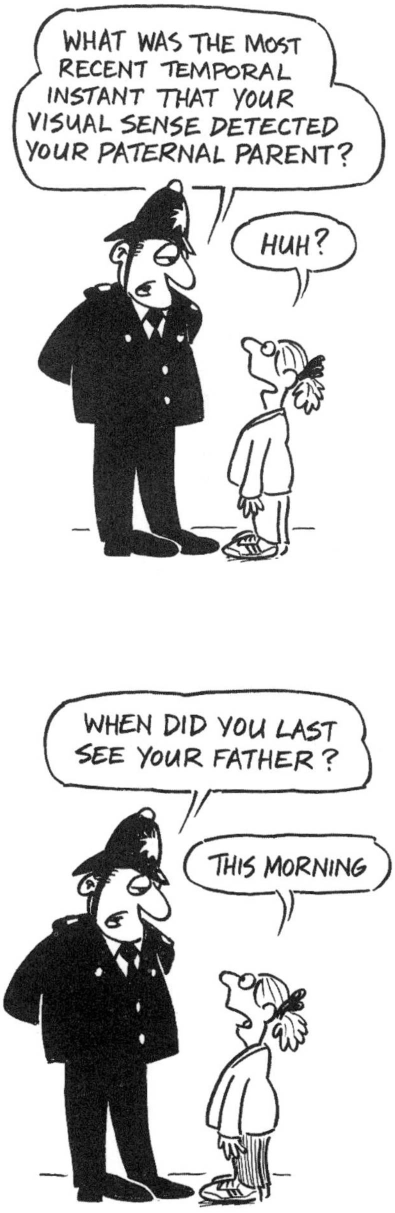

Figure 4.16 Language level is very important in questioning

▶ Health warning, page 174

Communication and relationships

Both prompts and probes can be used to check out a hunch. They help stimulate conversation where you think the person speaking is avoiding an issue, or wants to say more, but does not feel able to. Unskilled use can get you into areas in which you may be unable to cope.

A What generation gap?

Probes and prompts don't always have to be verbal. Explore with a willing older person – someone of your parents' or grandparents' generation – a topic with which you both feel comfortable and of which you both have experience. Appropriate topics could be: getting prizes or detentions at school; favourite childhood toys, sports stars, comics, seaside holidays, pets. Bring to the conversation items that might stimulate conversation, and covering information, such as photographs ('my friends, Pearl, Joe and Kanajit', 'our depressing school buildings', 'the second eleven when I was in it', ' how ridiculous I looked in my gym kit!') and other images such as certificates, rosettes and results sheets.

Non-verbal communication

In one of the activities you were asked to note how people reacted. There have also been references to non-verbal communication without explanation. In this section we will explain more, and help you to develop the skills of understanding non-verbal communication.

About 80% of communication is without words and comes from the way you use your body whilst talking and listening. This non-verbal communication is often described as body language. To a large extent we are all able to interpret some visual clues. Learning to read the language of non-verbal communication is an important part of being a good communicator.

Reading or sending non-verbal messages

A Charades

▶ Building a non-verbal dictionary, page 184

Do this in pairs or larger groups. One person should act out a feeling or emotion. The actor should show an emotion such as looking shy, angry, happy or any other emotion, but he or she must not make a sound. The other person, or persons should observe and write down what the emotion or feeling appears to be.
The observer(s) should also make notes about how the person looks – eyes, hands, body position, anything that helps to understand the feeling being expressed.

Most people are aware of how emotion is shown by facial expression. In fact, we use facial expressions to send messages we don't always mean. Very early in life we learn to 'hide' the disappointment of an unwanted present and smile whilst saying thank you. However, the basic smile does not mean that the real message is not getting across. It is very difficult not to show your feelings with all your other small gestures.

Communication and relationships

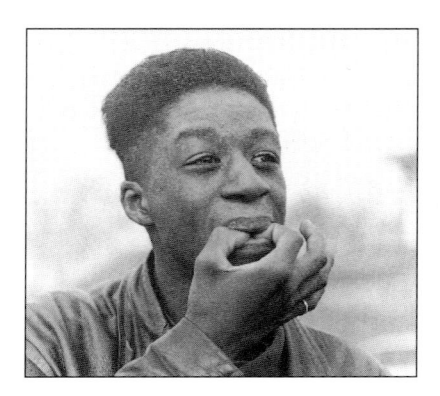

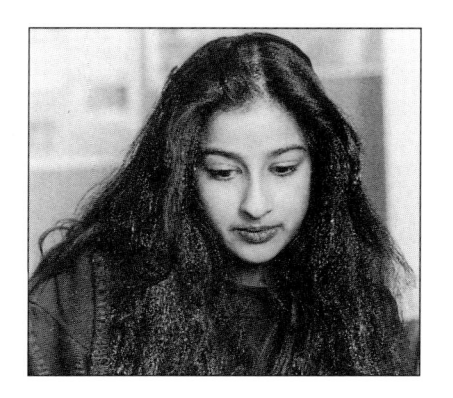

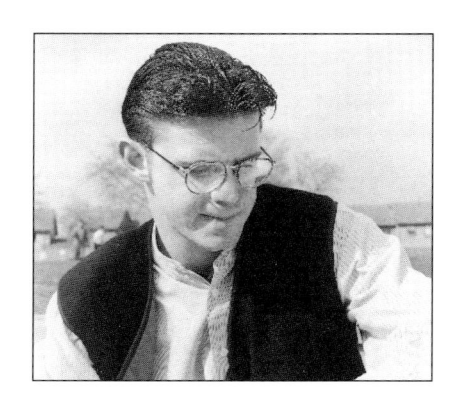

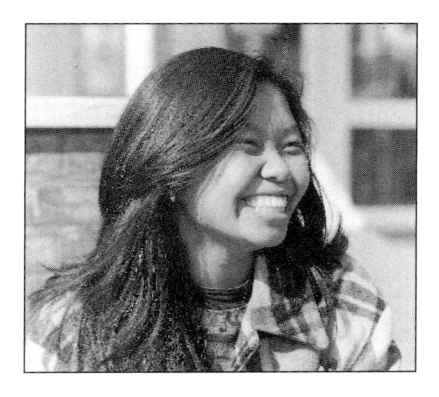

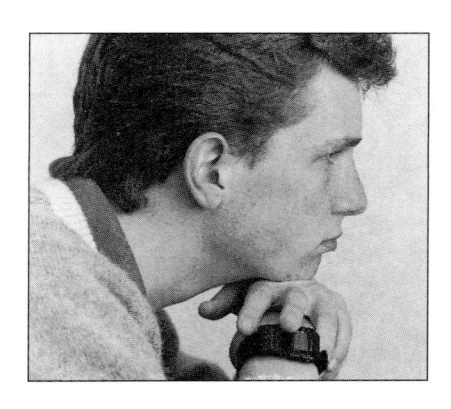

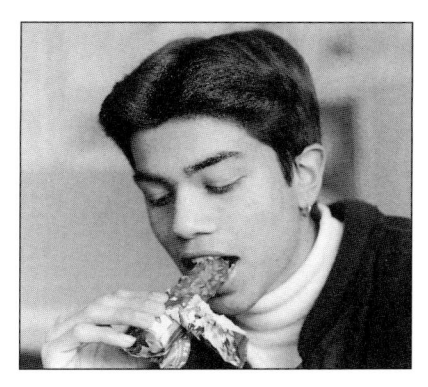

Figure 4.17 We can learn about people from the expressions on their faces, the clothes they wear, the way they stand and so on. What do these expressions mean to you?

One of the most interesting things about non-verbal communication is that we all learn to use it. It is learnt even before spoken language and even very young babies demonstrate a good understanding of non-verbal clues. Rather like listening, it is not so easy to consciously 'read' it: you need to develop a dictionary of the language and appreciate where the 'words' come from.

Facial expression is important. This list shows the most important areas involved:

- facial expression   forehead
  eyes
  mouth and cheeks
  nose – breathing movements

- body movements   arms – hands, fingers, gestures
  legs
  rocking, rigid
  breathing rate and depth

- posture   head position
  muscle tension/relaxation
  sitting or standing

- voice   tone of voice
  speed of speaking

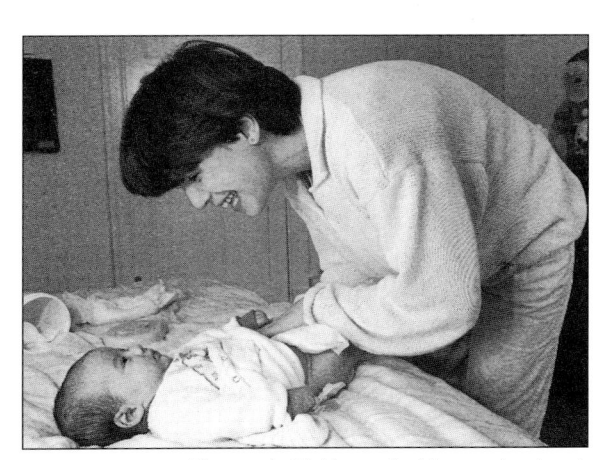

Figure 4.18 Young babies understand non-verbal clues

Also important are touching, closeness and sharing or mirroring of body position.

All non-verbal communication is much more important when caring for people with communication difficulties. It is, however, important to recognise that communication difficulties do not necessarily mean that the person cannot hear and understand. Somebody with severe cerebral palsy may be unable to talk clearly or to write, but can hear and understand. You may need to take time learning how to understand that person's non-verbal communication.

A Building a non-verbal dictionary

Note. This activity can form part of the previous activity, Charades.

This activity is made up of a series of role plays. The examples given should be seen as starting points. You should make up some for yourself. For each role play there should be participants and observers: the participants should try to act out the role play, and experience the emotions involved.

The observers should note carefully details of things like: eyes, mouth, hands and arms, body position and movements.

After the exercises create a table like this – you might even include stick drawings and face shapes.

Situation	Eyes	Mouth	Hands	Body
Fear	wide open			
Anger	wide open	lips taut teeth clenched	fists tense	tense muscles

▶ Role play – debriefing, page xxi

Role play 1
Anger: You have just been told that someone has deliberately destroyed your last assignment.

Role play 2
Fear: You are being threatened by someone with a knife.

Role play 3
Depression: Everything has gone wrong. You can't do anything right – even your dog has left home!

Role play 4
Happy: You have won a crossword competition, it is your birthday and you did get that present you have always wanted.

Role play 5
Puzzled: Your tutor has explained the requirements for GNVQ grading. It might as well have been a foreign language.

Role Play 6
Concerned: Your best friend has failed to meet you. You know her car is unreliable and may have broken down.

The list of roles is enormous. Add some more of your own. You could for example, as many students do, identify how a new teacher shows that he or she is nervous.

At the end of the exercise you should have produced your own dictionary (table) of non-verbal language. To test out your understanding, produce your own 'silent movie' of a situation in a care environment. Several people should agree a complex charade and ask the observers to explain what is happening.

Using verbal and non-verbal language in conversations

When you are talking with somebody how do you know whose turn it is to speak? In a meeting the chairperson should ensure that each individual is given the opportunity to speak. To do this they need to be able to see who wants to speak next, and also identify people who are unsure about speaking. This is often a formal process. However, there are rules even in informal situations.

Whose turn is it to speak?

Non-verbal communication is important in controlling conversations. A good listener may well be someone who encourages someone to continue talking by 'handing back' the permission to talk with simple gestures.

When two people are talking together there is some eye contact. In normal conversations the speaker starts talking and at the same time makes brief eye contact with the listener. The speaker looks away and continues to do so. As the speaker is coming to the end of what is being said he looks at the listener. At this point the listener is being invited to take over and speak. This is also an important time for helping the conversation to flow. When the eye contact is made, offering to let the listener speak, the listener can just nod or say something like 'I see' or 'Go on'. All of these give the permission for the speaker to continue talking.

Eye contact is also useful in showing somebody that you care. It can be an indication of the development of a good caring relationship. However, eye contact can be threatening. If a person makes eye contact, and then maintains it as a stare this can be seen as an aggressive act. By maintaining eye contact the starer is trying to dominate the other person.

A   Permission to speak

Video two people in conversation. Watch the eye movements and look for any small gestures that show how 'permission to speak' is given or requested. Replay the video and note down the non-verbal messages that were used. If you are going to use this as evidence for your portfolio you will need to use the video counter to identify where on the tape the communication occurred.

These small signs can be exaggerated in order to attract attention. Think of situations where this happens, for example where someone is trying to join in a conversation after it has started.

Other non-verbal messages

While working on the activities in this unit you may have noticed other non-verbal signals. Breathing depth and rate vary under stress. Skin colour and sweating are also important non-verbal clues that help communication. To concentrate on all of these is very difficult, but being aware of them can help you to understand communication.

The total body position

We started this discussion of non-verbal communication looking at an individual's small movements and expressions. It is also important to look at their position in relation to others. This can say a lot about how people are reacting to each other.

A Matching pairs

In pairs with an overall observer:
Find someone to talk to: make sure you are comfortable, and talk about something that interests you both.

Observer: After about five minutes, when all pairs are talking in a relaxed way, tell everyone to stop talking and freeze in the position they are in.
Ask each pair to look at similarities in their position/postures. Ask each pair to comment on their positions to the rest of the group, and add any comments of your own.
Are there any general observations that the group can make about body positions?

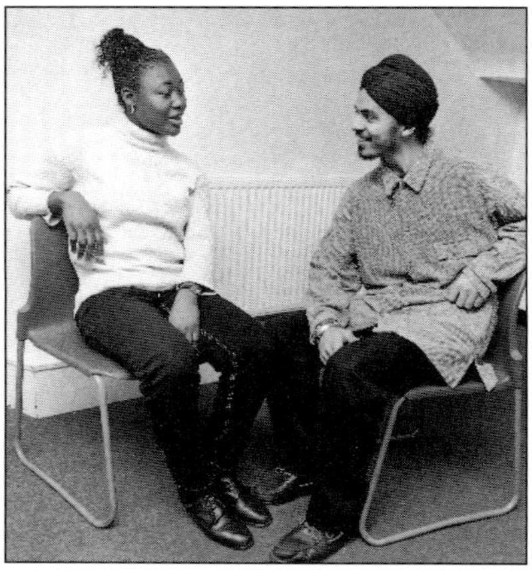

Figure 4.19 Mirrroring: note positions of head, arms and legs are similar

In the the last activity it is probable that the members of each pair were adopting similar positions, for example, feet up, head angle, arm positions. It could be possible to imagine a mirror between the individuals, each person being a reflection of the other. This non-verbal signal, mirroring, shows that the two people are sharing and communicating comfortably and are broadly in agreement.

Sales people are often trained to consciously mirror a client in order to develop a strong rapport so that a sale may be more successfully concluded. When you know it is being done it is possible to observe a salesperson's technique.

Personal space

If you watch people talking, it is often possible to guess how friendly they are by how close they get to each other. Two strangers may stand 50cm or more apart, not touching in any way. Two people in love may be standing so close that they touch in many places. Close friends, sharing a book to read, may touch heads whilst maintaining gaps elsewhere.

Think about how you feel as people move physically closer to you. It is almost as if there is a barrier forming a circle round your body, that only some people are allowed to pass through. If someone comes too close then you will step away rather than letting them cross the barrier.

There are situations where this personal space has to be breached. On a crowded bus or train or in a queue people who don't know each other often have to stand inside personal space. Where this happens people try to avoid eye contact and stand back-to-back or present their sides to each other.

The size of personal space varies according to emotional closeness and trust between the people involved. It can also vary with different cultures. For example, many middle eastern men stand much closer, and have smaller areas of personal space than their British counterparts. Thus a normal 'distance' for one person can be thought to be aggressively close by another.

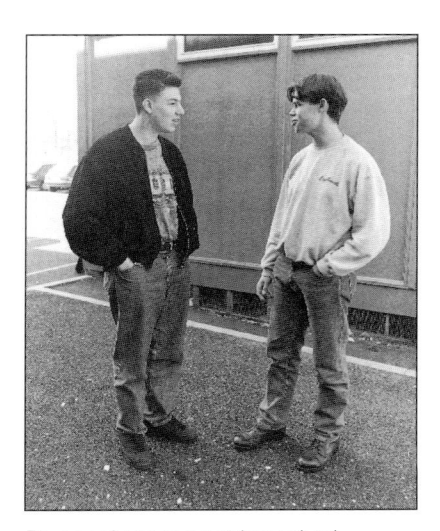

Personal spaces not breached – normal communication

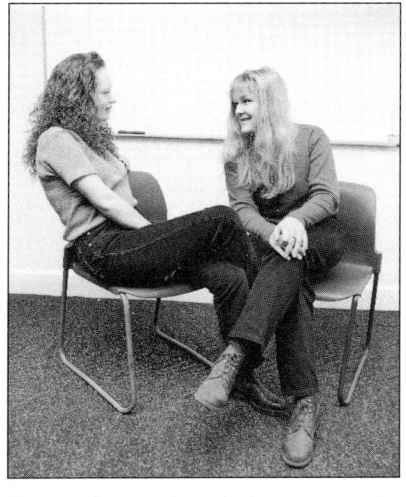

Personal space invaded – movement to re-establish space

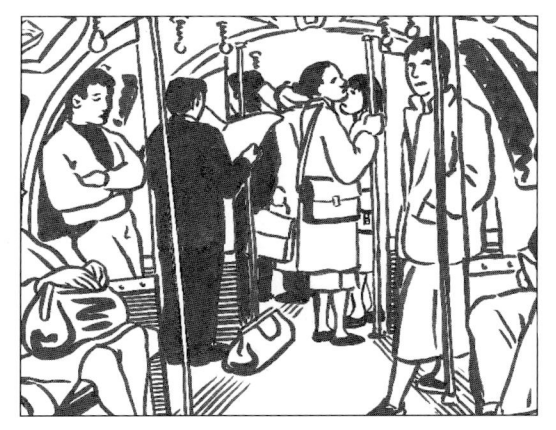

Personal space invaded – eye contact avoided

Figure 4.20 *Maintaining personal space is important*

Crossing the barriers

Working in caring professions it is often important to be able to enter someone's personal space – for example, assisting an older person to dress or working alongside a child in a nursery. To make this contact appropriate, it is essential that permission to breach the barrier is obtained and it is done in a non-threatening way.

A Give me space

Working in small groups, preferably not with close friends, try to establish what sort of approaches feel comfortable and what less so. Use the following situations to help you.

Situation 1
One person sitting down reading. Another approaches and stands behind, looking over the reader's shoulder. Think of times you were working in school and the teacher stood just behind you. How did you feel?

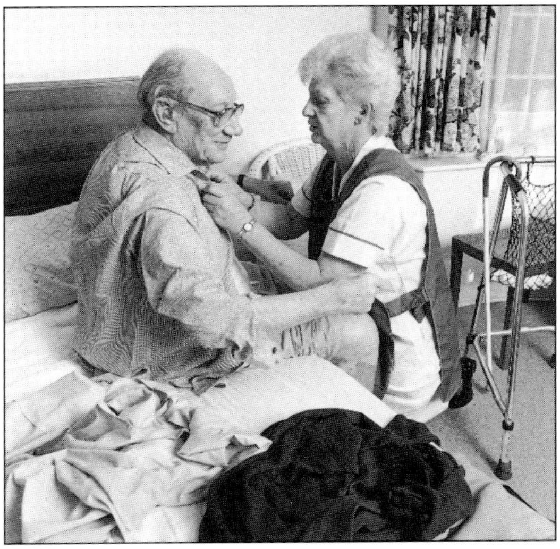

Figure 4.21 *Sometimes it is necessary to enter someone's personal space*

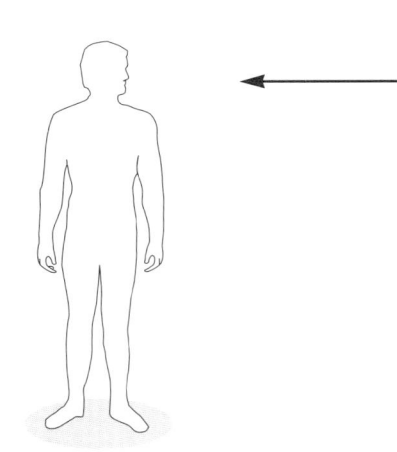

Communication and relationships

Situation 2
Draw a body in outline – like this.
Mark on it the areas that you would feel happy about touching on:
- a comparative stranger
- a close friend
- a young child.

As a larger group come together and discuss your findings.
Are their areas:
- acceptable for all to touch
- unacceptable for anyone to touch
- dependent on who is touching?

What determines who has access to which areas? How do you determine who can touch you? In general, do these areas vary with the age of the person? Think about how and where we touch babies and young children in the normal course of working with them.

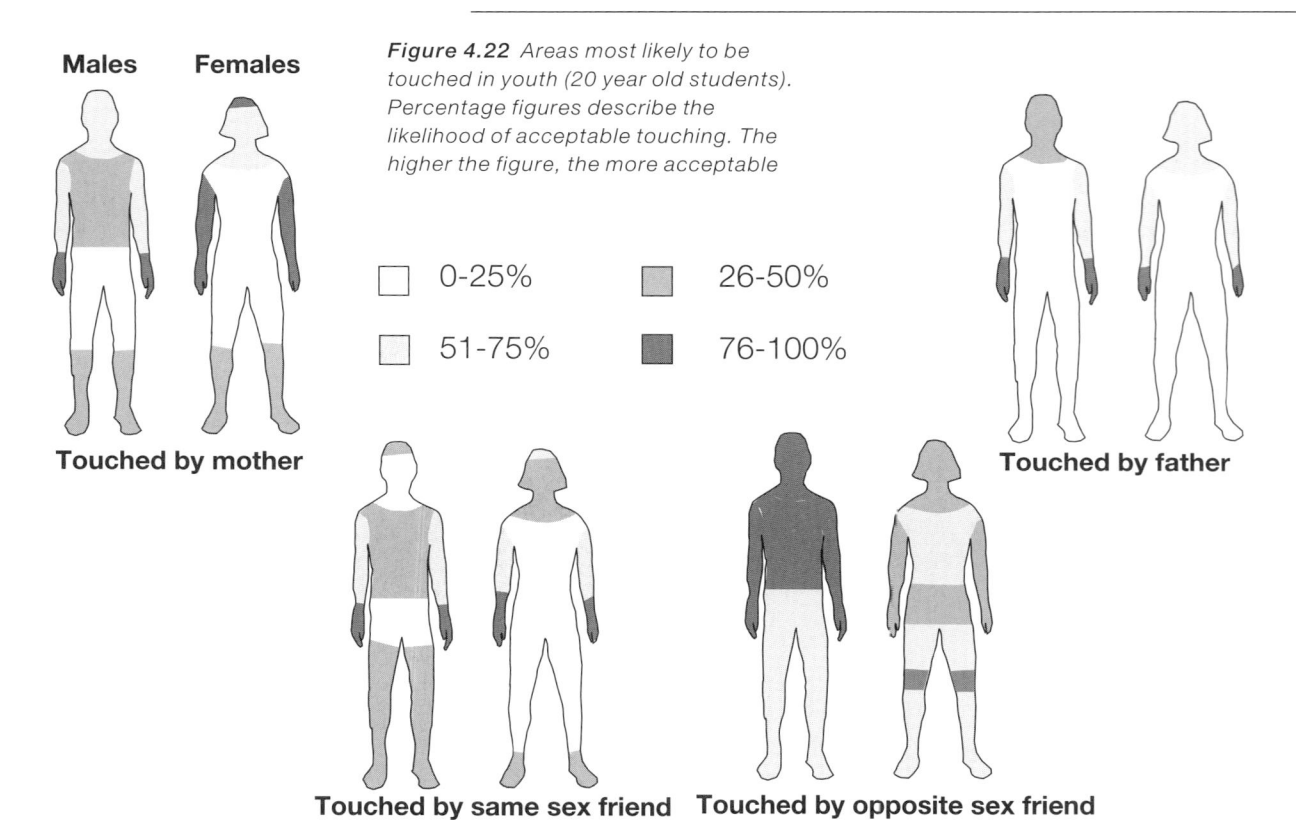

Figure 4.22 Areas most likely to be touched in youth (20 year old students). Percentage figures describe the likelihood of acceptable touching. The higher the figure, the more acceptable

- ☐ 0-25%
- ▨ 26-50%
- ☐ 51-75%
- ■ 76-100%

Touched by mother

Touched by father

Touched by same sex friend

Touched by opposite sex friend

Working in care organisations

People whose work is caring for others have a great responsibility. They are in a very powerful position over those they care for. Most of those people needing care are vulnerable in some way and it is easy for the carer to forget to treat them as individuals and deprive them of their rights. These rights are the rights of all people and form the values which underpin all caring practice.

Individuality

Everybody is an individual. Even identical twins, who have so much in common, are individuals. We all have our own likes or dislikes.

People are identified in different ways: often they are stereotyped because of the group characteristics. Women have for centuries been seen as less strong and less scientifically minded than men. If you have these prejudices, and we all have many, then they can reduce your ability to communicate. The next activity is designed to help you to identify some of these prejudices in yourself. In doing so it gives you the opportunity to review and challenge them.

In any conversation you must be aware of your prejudices, and also recognise that the person you are talking to will have some prejudices and stereotype models. You must try to ensure that you do not use your pre-formed views,rather than reality, to affect your conversation.

A — Time to think

Is there anybody on your course with whom you seem to have very little in common? Try to work out what makes you different. Consider obvious differences like race, gender, the way they speak, and less obvious ones like their likes and dislikes, their hobbies.

Can you also think of someone you took an instant liking or dislike to – why do you think this was?

Were your first thoughts about them right?

Before you can consider providing emotional support to strangers it is important to identify any areas that you might be uncomfortable about. Complete the following table for yourself, ranking each of the groups of people both for how much you know about them and how you feel about being with them. Use different colours – one to produce your profile for knowledge, the other to produce your profile on feelings.

| A: Knowledge | 1 Very little ⟶ A lot 6 |
B: Feelings	1 Uncomfortable ⟶ Comfortable 6
People of the opposite sex	1 2 3 4 5 6
Elderly people	1 2 3 4 5 6
People in wheelchairs	1 2 3 4 5 6
Children	1 2 3 4 5 6
Drug takers	1 2 3 4 5 6
Child abusers	1 2 3 4 5 6
People with	
– Alzheimer's Disease	1 2 3 4 5 6
– HIV	1 2 3 4 5 6
– different mental abilities	1 2 3 4 5 6
Afro-Caribbean people	1 2 3 4 5 6
Sikhs	1 2 3 4 5 6
Hindus	1 2 3 4 5 6
Moslems	1 2 3 4 5 6
Christians	1 2 3 4 5 6
Atheists	1 2 3 4 5 6
Homosexual men	1 2 3 4 5 6
Homosexual women	1 2 3 4 5 6

From the results of your work identify three groups where your lack of knowledge or your own views could affect the way you communicate with them or where you have possible prejudice. Spend some time finding more information about the three groups. Use the library, talk to teachers and anybody who knows the group well. If you are uncomfortable about the group, try to work out what makes you feel uncomfortable.

If you were working in a caring situation how would you react to working with people from these groups as colleagues or clients?

Prejudice

In the Activity: Time to think, we put people into groups. In putting people into groups we tend to view them not as individuals but as a stereotype member of the group, in particular when we have little knowledge of the group. Putting individuals into groups enables us to create a language framework that determines attitudes. The language emphasises the differences and disabilities, rather than the normality, abilities and potentiality of a person. It fuels stereotyping and encourages prejudice.

Prejudice: this is not an easy concept to define. The dictionary offers – a judgement or opinion formed beforehand or without due examination; bias; injury or hurt; disadvantage.

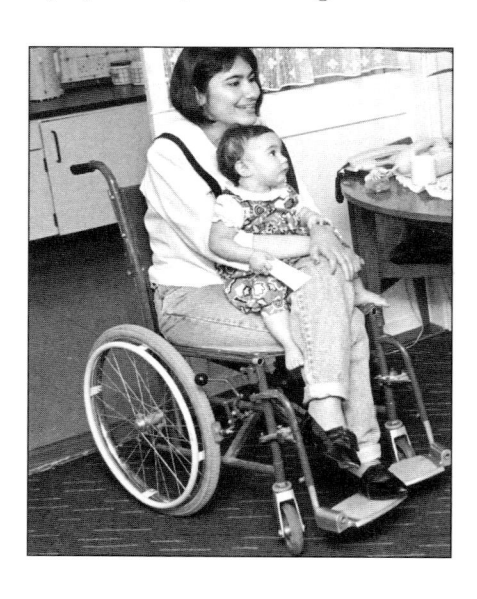

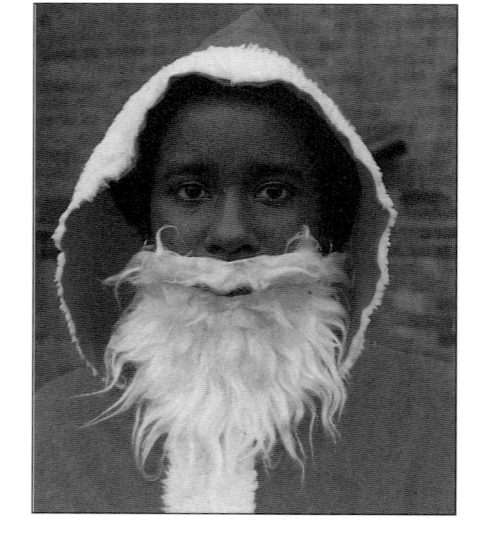

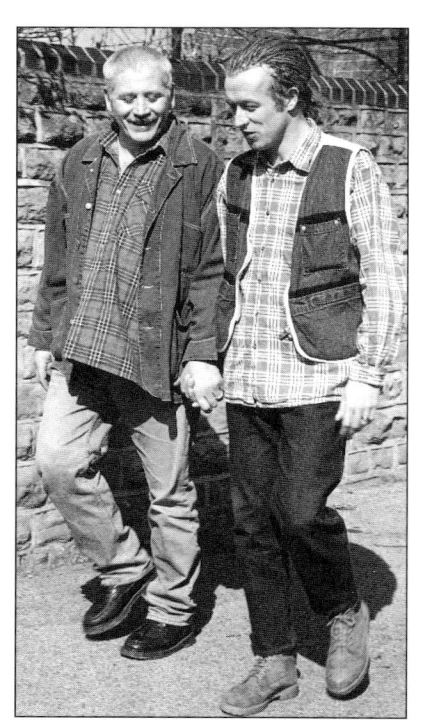

Figure 4.23 Stereotypes make these photographs unusual – the start of prejudice

Prejudice then, is the pre-judging of people or groups of people. This is not based on any evidence or factual knowledge but on ignorance and fear. These prejudicial attitudes can be expressed either consciously or unconsciously in a person's behaviour, when some people are treated less favourably than others. This unequal treatment is discrimination. Many people suffer **discrimination** on the grounds of:
- race, and/or ethnic group
- age – for example, youth, old age
- sex
- sexual orientation – for example, gay, lesbian, bisexual
- disability – for example, physical, sensory, learning
- religion – for example, Catholic, Protestant, Jew, Moslem.

The Value Base and individual rights, Appendix II, page 220

Discrimination

Discrimination comes in three forms:
- **open and valid**
- **direct**
- **indirect.**

Open and valid discrimination

Open and valid discrimination describes the type of discrimination that takes place when seeking to appoint somebody to a job. The criteria by which an applicant is to be judged are made clear and can be justified because of the work role. By publishing the criteria to the candidates it is possible for them to identify their own strengths in relation to the job. In such situations the interviewers are usually prepared to explain their decisions to the candidates. In delivering care there will be occasions where such discrimination has to be made but it must always be with the full knowledge and understanding of all people involved.

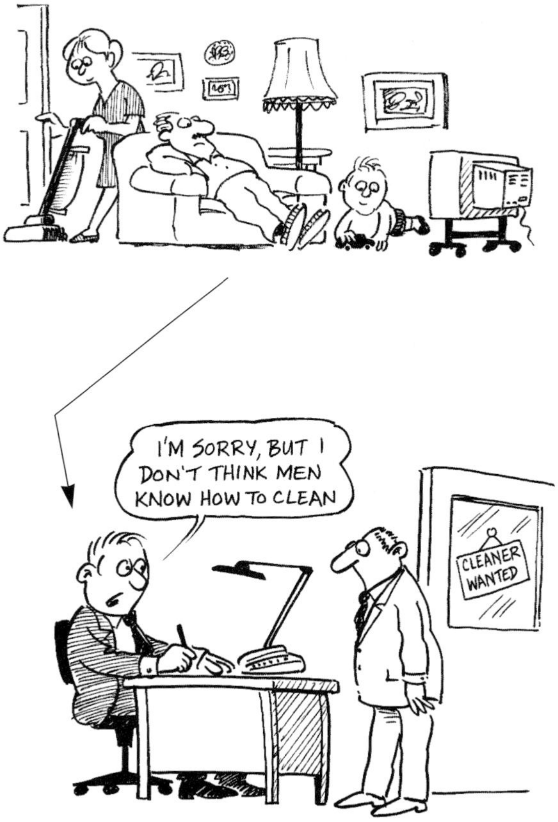

Direct covert discrimination (open and invalid)

Direct discrimination involves saying and doing things which clearly demonstrate prejudice against a specific group. Name calling and reduced access to services are clear examples of direct discrimination. In employment, the direct indication that only white women should apply for a job demonstrates direct discrimination on the grounds of race and gender. It is normally easy to detect direct discrimination and so it may be easier to challenge than indirect discrimination. However, direct discrimination is often a product of strongly-held views that have formed part of early socialisation.

Socialisation: *the attitudes and beliefs learned as a member of a group within society.*

Direct discrimination can be demonstrated by:
- the use of abusive language
- name calling
- avoiding physical contact because of unfounded prejudices. You do not catch HIV from shaking hands!

Figure 4.24 Discrimination may start with early socialisation

Communication and relationships

- telling racist or sexist jokes or jokes about people with different abilities
- talking to the carer not the client when the client is perfectly able to respond. BBC radio produces a programme called 'Does He Take Sugar?'. The title highlights this form of discrimination.

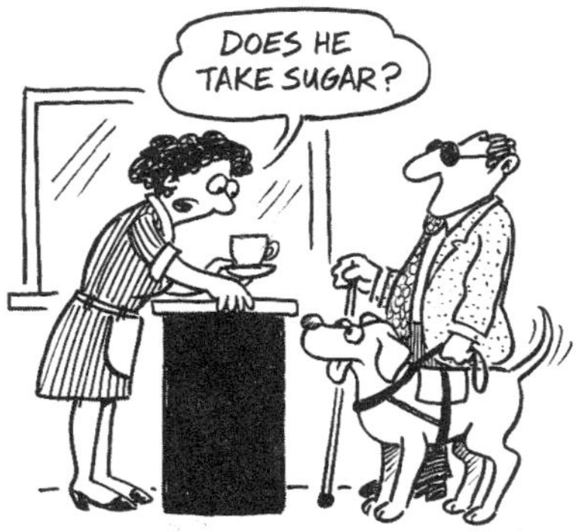

Figure 4.25 This is an example of direct discrimination

Case study: a problem with direct discrimination

One social services department had to address the problem of overt racism from one of their clients. The client in question was 85 years old. The care plan indicated that domiciliary support (home help) was needed on a daily basis. A support worker was allocated the task.

The support worker was Afro-Caribbean whilst the client was white. The client insisted that the support worker was not acceptable because of her race. The social services department was in a cleft stick. Client choice should give the right to accept or reject the worker. However, to accept the client choice would be to condone the racist attitude of the client. The client would not accept the worker on any terms.

What options were open to the social services department?
How would you have dealt with it?
Role play some of the possibilities with others in your group; in particular think about the individual's feelings.
Did you reach a satisfactory conclusion?

Case study: James

James had used a wheelchair for most of his life. He had struggled to lead a normal life and looked forward to employment.

He was advised to go to university and get a good degree because people would recognise his qualifications and not worry about his disability.

He went to Cambridge University and obtained the highest level of degree in mathematics.

He could not obtain a job. He was advised to get a vocational qualification because people would recognise his qualifications and not worry about his disability.

He trained and qualified as an accountant but still had problems finding a job. Eventually he was employed by a small company. Within a short time he was a senior manager and, because of his skills, the company began to expand. Eventually they moved to a bigger factory. The factory required some modifications to make the office accessible to James in his wheelchair. The company applied for a grant, explaining how valuable James was and his great importance in running the company.

When the access had been provided a representative from the grant-providing organisation visited. He walked into James' office and in a very loud voice asked, 'How are we today, then?'

How had James suffered from discrimination during his life?
How had the visitor demonstrated discrimination against James?

Indirect (covert) discrimination

This form of discrimination is one of the cruellest. It involves the use of things such as tone of voice and body language to convey the discriminatory message. It is often difficult to identify and is very difficult to prove. This means that the recipient of the discrimination has little clear evidence, yet feels, and is, disempowered. Sometimes the discrimination involves the person being discriminated against apparently being supported but actually being set up to fail. Because it is so hidden it is also the most damaging to an individual's self esteem.

Indirect discrimination can be demonstrated by:
- tone of voice
- body language
- avoidance of contact – trying not to have to speak to or work with an individual
- making assumptions about the help, advice and support a person needs.

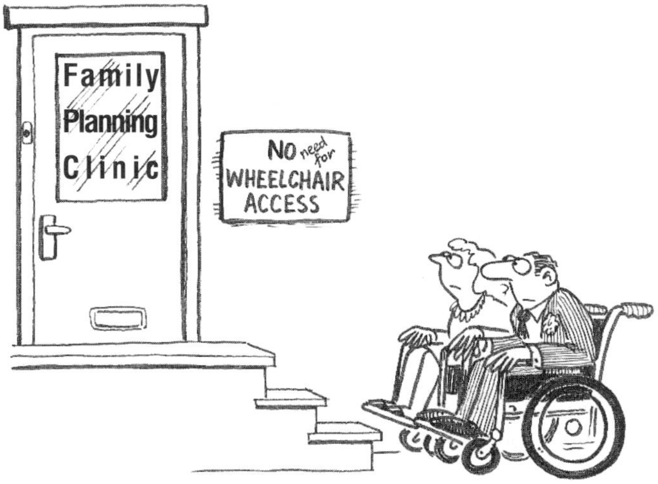

Figure 4.26 Making assumptions can be discriminatory

Effects of discrimination

A person suffering from discrimination suffers in two ways. The first is because of the attack on his or her individuality. The second relates to their position in society, particularly in employment.

Effects on individuality

You are special. Your need to be special is important to you and also to your relationship with others. That special nature is built around your own life history and, to be useful, is about liking yourself (self-esteem). It also contributes to how you feel about other people.

When a person is discriminated against, one of the first responses may be **anger**. This anger may be directed at the person doing the discrimination but often it cannot be expressed. A woman being discriminated against by her male boss may not be able to express her anger for fear of losing her job.

A later response may be to feel that the discriminatory behaviour was a true reflection of the situation. In other words, the person may lose self-confidence. With this comes a loss of **self-esteem** (liking oneself). All of these can have the effect of making the discrimination appear reasonable. A person who is called stupid often enough may eventually lose so much confidence they are unable to carry out simple tasks. In doing this, the person lives down to the description of being stupid.

Prejudice and discrimination in employment may lead to jobs and promotion being barred. If the discrimination is on the grounds of race, sex or religion (in Northern Ireland) the discrimination is illegal. Many women would say that in order to compete with men for employment they have to be able to do things 50% better than the men applying.

Whatever the type of discrimination, the effects are often the same:
- anger
- lack of self-esteem
- lack of motivation.

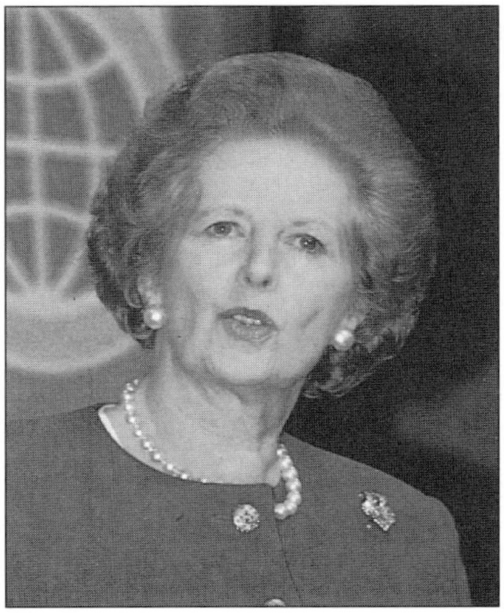

Figure 4.27 Margaret Thatcher – did she have to be 50% better than her male colleagues?

Communication and relationships

▶ Anti-discriminatory legislation, Appendix III, page 229

Legislation relating to equality of opportunity:
- The Race Relations Act 1976
- Public Order Act 1986 and Public Order (NI) Order 1987
- The Sex Discrimination Act 1975 and 1986
- Sex Discrimination (NI) Order 1976
- The Equal Pay Act 1970 (amended 1988)
- Equal Pay Act (NI) 1970 (amended 1988)
- The Chronically Sick and Disabled Persons Act 1970
- Disabled Persons/services, Consultation and Representation Act 1986
- The Fair Employment Act. (N.I.) 1989

Details of the acts are included in Appendix III.

Working with people in health and social care

What does caring mean? If you care for new-born babies, then you must do everything for them. As the children grow, you demonstrate care by enabling them to do more and more for themselves. It is very easy to see, and possibly for you to remember, how you established yourself and became more and more independent of your parents.

Once a person has demonstrated a level of independence, then to be in need of care can have a range of effects. It is important to recognise these effects and work to develop a **caring relationship**. The following case study gives an example of how a caring relationship can develop and change.

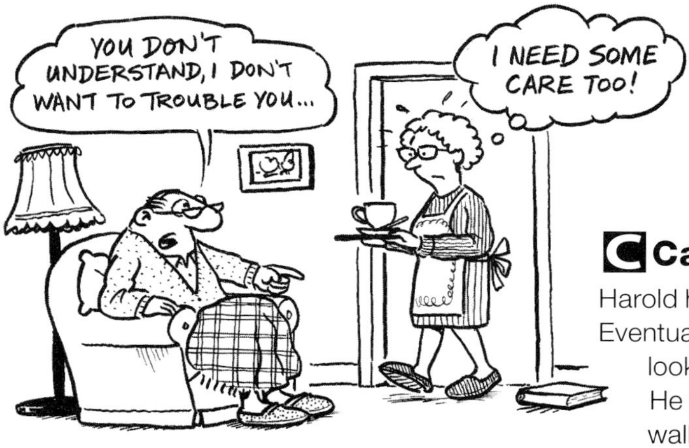

Figure 4.28 Caring relationships can develop and change with circumstance

Case study: Harold's hip

Harold had been developing problems in his hip for many years. Eventually he was called into hospital to have an artificial hip. He was looking forward to increased movement and reduction of the pain. He was not looking forward to the operation and learning to walk again.

The operation went very well and Harold was soon back on the ward. At this time the nurses were being very attentive to his needs. If he needed anything the staff would get it as he was unable to do much for himself other than feed and drink. Harold was reasonably happy with this. He had been in hospital before and accepted the help in things like using a bed pan with its loss of privacy.

Eventually he was moved to another hospital where he was to learn to walk again. The physiotherapist worked with him and started him walking using a frame and then sticks. She insisted that he dress himself and provided guidance but did not do things for him. This was a change from the time before the operation when Harold's wife had had to put Harold's shoes and socks on him. Generally the other care staff continued to provide for Harold's needs and he could easily call them during the day and night for help whenever he thought he needed it.

Two weeks after the operation Harold returned home. Here there were no full-time nurses or physiotherapists. Harold's wife had to take on a major caring role. Harold called for her, as he had called for the nurses. At night his wife got little sleep because he woke her fifteen times or more to get drinks, adjust the bedding, help him to sit up, roll over, fetch and clean the urine bottle he used. During the day he said he could not dress himself and wanted to return to the situation before his operation. He called regularly for food and drink. He also needed help going to the toilet, or using the urine bottle. He was very anxious if his wife left to go to the shops or neighbours as he was worried he would fall or want something he could not reach.

Harold's wife was becoming exhausted. She was becoming in need of care herself and so contacted the social services department. They came round and fixed some rails in the bungalow for Harold to hold as he moved around. They also considered the possibility of providing some domiciliary support for a couple of weeks while Harold was improving his walking skills. Harold was unhappy about strangers coming into his house and refused the help saying that his wife could do what was necessary.

There are many things you may think about Harold but you should consider the nature of the caring relationships.

How did Harold show dependence on carers?
Who encouraged Harold to do things for himself?
Why do you think Harold was unable/unwilling to do things for himself and be self managing?
How equal was his relationship with the carers?
How did Harold exercise power over his carers?

The behind-the scenes activity that supported Harold

Harold's story is only half told in the case study. Underpinning the situation is a series of letters, records, report and memoranda. Figure 4.30 illustrates some of the formal communications that enabled Harold and his wife to receive the services that they did.

In the communications you see an example of how individual care planning starts. What is not included is any detail of how the services would be paid for, and how Harold's means would be assessed to determine how much he would have to pay for the support recommended by Social Services.

In the case study you were asked to consider many features of a caring relationship. We will consider some of those in more detail.

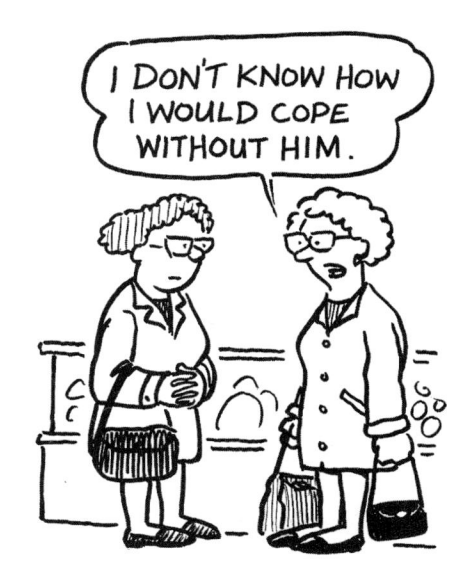

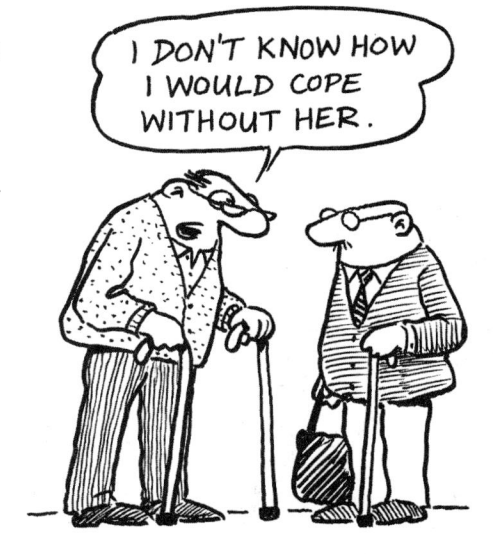

Figure 4.29 Dependence can be in both directions

Anti-discrimination legislation, Appendix III, page 229

Communication and relationships

St David's Hospital Trust
Halcyon Street, Mexborough ME2 5AB

Mr Harold Lipman　　　　　　　　　　　　　　　　　6 March 1995
58 Worral Avenue
Mexborough
ME8 1PN

Dear Mr Lipman

Further to your recent visit to the clinic of Mr Stratton, I am writing to inform you that a date has now been arranged for your operation.

Please go to **Ward 16** on **Wednesday 15 March** at **10 am** and report to the ward clerk.

Enclosed is a copy of the Patient's Information Booklet which we recommend you read before your admission. It gives advice about what you will need to bring into hospital with you, as well as important information like visiting times and the Trust's no-smoking policy.

It is suggested that you telephone the ward between 8 am and 9.30 am on the day of admission to confirm the availability of a bed.

Yours sincerely

Cheryl Warburton (ms)
Secretary to Mr Stratton
(Orthopaedic Surgeon)

Mexborough City Council
Director of Social Services

HOME ASSESSMENT REPORT

Subject:	Mr H and Mrs V Lipman 50 Worral Avenue Mexborough, WEG 1PN
By:	Martin Grainger, Elderly Persons Services
For:	Jane Swales, Senior Social Worker, Mexborough East Team Leader
Referred by:	Memorandum from Jane Swales, 19 May 1995
Personal profiles:	Attached
Procedure:	A one-hour visit was made, 23 April 1995: all rooms in the house were visited in the company of Mrs Lipman. Mr and Mrs. Lipman were interviewed jointly and separately.
Observations:	(a) The house is a three-bedroom, 1960s semi on two floors with two reception rooms on the ground floor. One of the rooms is in use as a temporary bedroom for Mr. Lipman. There is also a toilet off the entrance hall. There are no steps to front or rear. The house is in good repair, comfortably furnished, clean and generally tidy. (b) Mr Lipman declared himself 'a martyr to' his wife as well as in her absence that he was not getting the care and attention he needed and deserved. During the assessment visit he called on his wife to carry out 12 separate tasks, all trivial all requiring her to get up and move across the room. Once, he asked her to help him from his armchair to a chair at the dining table, and one to help him to and from the toilet. He did not thank her on any occasion. He has and uses a stick. He has the loan of a zimmer, but says he cannot be doing with it. (c) Mrs Lipman gave him all the help he asked for and anticipated some likely requests. She looked exhausted and once or twice, close to tears. She said, interviewed alone. She was not sure how long she could continue to provide care for her husband: she felt certain it would not be for much longer.
Conclusions:	1. That Mr Lipman needs to be encouraged to be more independent in his own interests as well as his wife's. At present a genuine degree of mobility difficulty exits and he needs some support in moving about the house 2. Mrs Lipman's health seems likely to suffer from physical exhaustion and emotional stress without intervention of social work support.
Recommendations	1. That rails be fitted to the ground-floor toilet, upstairs bathroom toilet and landing and staircase (opposite wall to existing handrail) 2. That a home care support worker attend for one hour each day to give Mrs Lipman physical and emotional respite. 3. That the situation be monitored initially by a following visit one month from this date by a social welfare officer from Elderly Persons Services
Signed	Martin Grainger
Date	24th May 1995

Communication and relationships

Mexborough City Council
Director of Social Services

Client's Personal Profile

Name:	Harold Lipman
Address:	58 Worral Avenue
	Mexborough
Postcode:	ME8 1PN
Tel no:	Mex 490670
DOB:	21 / 04 / 20

Married ☑ **Single** ☐ **Divorced** ☐ **Separated** ☐ **Widowed** ☐ **Other** ☐

Next of kin*:	Mrs Cynthia Walker	(*Apart from spouse)
Relationship:	Daughter	
Address:	9 Bulpitt Street	
	Mexborough	
Postcode:	ME17 5RT	
Tel no:	Mex 628098	

Social worker:	Martin Grainger	(provisional)
Tel no:	Mex 493681	
GP:	Dr A C Brooke	
Tel no:	Mex 744777	
Religion:	C of E	

Mexborough City Council
Director of Social Services

Client's Personal Profile

Name:	Violet Lipman
Address:	58 Worral Avenue
	Mexborough
Postcode:	ME8 1PN
Tel no:	Mex 490670
DOB:	18 / 05 / 21

Married ☑ **Single** ☐ **Divorced** ☐ **Separate** ☐ **Widowed** ☐ **Other** ☐

Next of kin*:	Mrs Cynthia Walker	(*Apart from spouse)
Relationship:	Daughter	
Address:	9 Bulpitt Street	
	Mexborough	
Postcode:	ME17 5RT	
Tel no:	Mex 628098	

Social worker:	Martin Grainger	(provisional)
Tel no:	Mex 493681	
GP:	Dr A C Brooke	
Tel no:	Mex 744777	
Religion:	C of E	

Mexborough City Council
Department of Social Services

Memorandum

From:	Jane Swales, Senior Social Worker,
	Mexborough East, Team Leader
To:	Martin Grainger, Elderly Persons Services
Subject:	Home Assessment
Date:	19th May 1995

Please arrange to visit Mr and Mrs Lipman of 58 Worral Avenue, Mexborough, and make an assessment of the position. Mrs Violet Lipman has written to the Director, claiming that since her husband's hip replacement operation in March she is unable to cope alone with him. There is an indication that the situation is one which may require some social work support for both parties. I would hope to recieve your report within the week.

JS

Mexborough
ME 1PN
17 May 1995

Mr G. P. Wallace
Director of Social Services
Mexborough

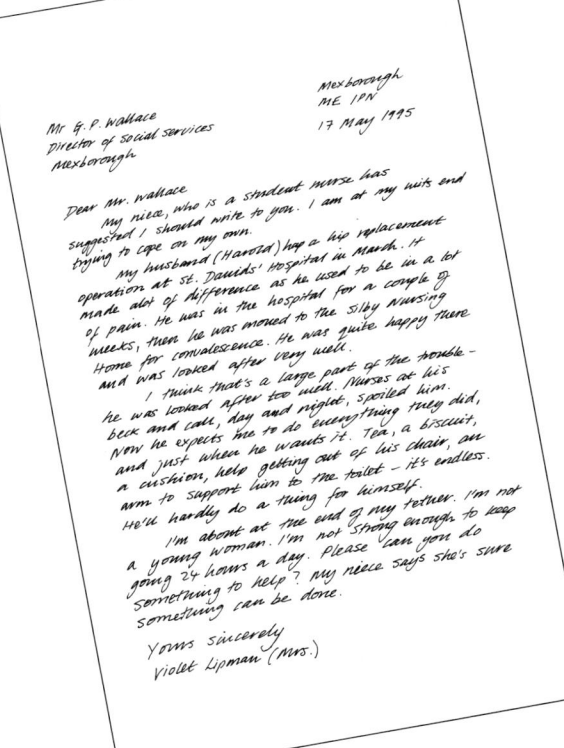

Dear Mr Wallace,

My niece, who is a student nurse has suggested I should write to you. I am at my wits end trying to cope on my own.

My husband (Harold) had a hip replacement operation at St. Davids' Hospital in March. It made a lot of difference as he used to be in a lot of pain. He was in the hospital for a couple of weeks, then he was moved to the Silby Nursing Home for convalescence. He was quite happy there and was looked after very well.

I think that's a large part of the trouble – he was looked after too well. Nurses at his beck and call, day and night, spoiled him. Now he expects me to do everything they did, and just when he wants it. Tea, a biscuit, a cushion, help getting out of his chair, an arm to support him to the toilet – it's endless. He'll hardly do a thing for himself. I'm not I'm about at the end of my tether. I'm not a young woman. I'm not strong enough to keep going 24 hours a day. Please can you do something to help? My niece says she's sure something can be done.

Yours sincerely
Violet Lipman (Mrs.)

Figure 4.30 This shows how Harold's care planning progressed

Communication and relationships

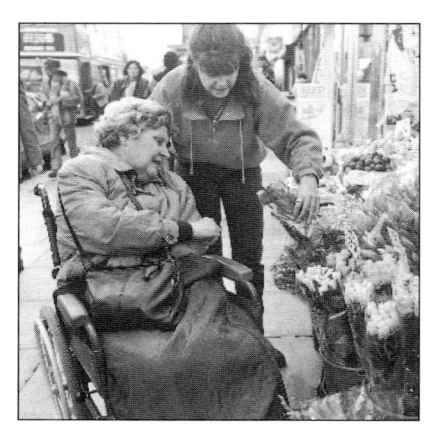

4.31 Giving people choice and respecting it is important

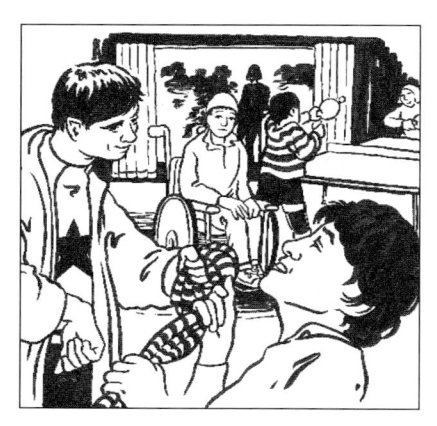

Figure 4.32 People can be relaxed and happy in a caring situation. Others may be depressed

Dependence

Clients often come to depend upon their carers. They rely on the carer to do things, and become unwilling or lose the ability to do things for themselves. There is also a level of emotional dependence. This can express itself in the client doing things to attract the carer's attention and seeking praise (or in some cases provoking anger). The latter situation occurs with some people, especially disturbed adolescents, where they need attention and they do not mind if it is positive or negative.

The carer can also gain from the relationship emotionally. There can be a dependence of the carer on the client for positive emotional support. In these situations the care provision can damage the client because of the dependence. In extreme cases such a situation can actually lead to the carer's dismissal.

Power relationships

The ideal caring relationship is one in which the client does as much as possible for him or herself. The client is fully involved in decision making. The care given is determined with the needs and wants of the client being seen as of greatest importance.

It is very easy to take over from the client and make decisions for them. At very simple levels the client should be allowed choice of clothes, food and activities wherever possible. Supporting the client to use this power to control his or her life is supporting self empowerment of the client.

At the same time, the client can exercise power over the carer: the client can use the need for care as an emotional weapon. Often this can be by causing feelings of guilt in the carer, especially if the carer is a member of the family or a close friend.

How people respond to care

Imagine you were taken away from your family by someone who you did not know very well. Imagine also that you did not really understand why you were being taken away. How would you feel? The emotions of anger, fear and frustration may describe many of your feelings. People who need health and social care may feel many of these emotions. There can also be a feeling of embarrassment and failure associated with the need to seek help.

If you think about the way you experience the emotions suggested, you will have some ideas about the ways that clients can respond to the stress and distress they feel in care situations. There may also be **positive** emotions relating to relief and the knowledge of the caring support being given. In summary, people respond in both positive and negative ways:

- **positive feelings:**
  - feeling relaxed about the situation, having been well prepared for entering care
  - feeling relieved about the reduced stress and about the improved ability to cope

- **negative feelings:**
  - fear, for example at being admitted to a hospice
  - anger at the carers or at the reasons that care was needed
  - being aggressive and abusive; not just as an expression of anger but

also as a plea to be noticed as an individual
- becoming withdrawn - often this presents itself as having settled in the care situation but it is a symptom of depression.

Types of support

Different **types of support** can bring different responses from clients. The support offered affects the interaction between client and carer. To be offered advice, as an equal, gives the client the opportunity to take or ignore the advice.

Care may also involve social interaction with others. This means that the client will have to adapt to fit into the social situation. In many cases this is seen by the client as a positive benefit. The carer is seen as somebody who enables the client to participate in the social interaction. In these cases the caring role is one of supporting social interaction and providing materials (such as food and equipment).

Often the major needs of the client are for help in providing the resources needed. In the case study of Harold, rails were provided to enable him to move around. Similarly the case study of James showed the use of funds to support access to an office. The support can be simply providing the funds to purchase and fit equipment or providing the facilities themselves. In either case the care delivered was limited to the physical resource being provided. The client may feel unhappy about the 'charity' aspect of the care but is empowered by the provision of the resource.

Resources can be provided on a regular basis. Support can be provided to support the client in undertaking the activities of daily living. In this case the relationship between carer and client assumes a greater importance. The carer is in some ways standing in for the client to carry out some activities. In providing the support there is a risk that the carer will assume power and disempower the client.

The final aspect of support to be considered is the support that was offered to Harold but in reality was to support his wife. She was offered the emotional support and recognition of the strain of being a carer. By being offered domiciliary support she was being offered respite from the caring role. This factor is often the last to be considered in care provision. The client is offered care in a different situation, thus providing care for the carer.

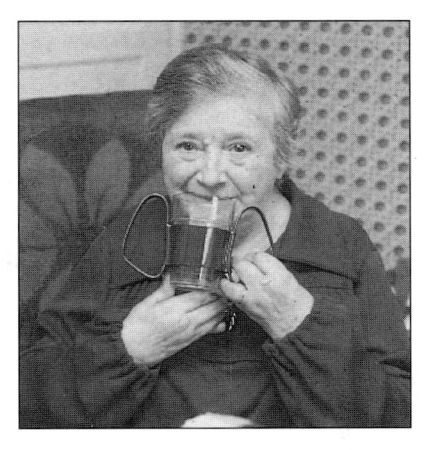

Figure 4.33 Adapted equipment can help people maintain their independence

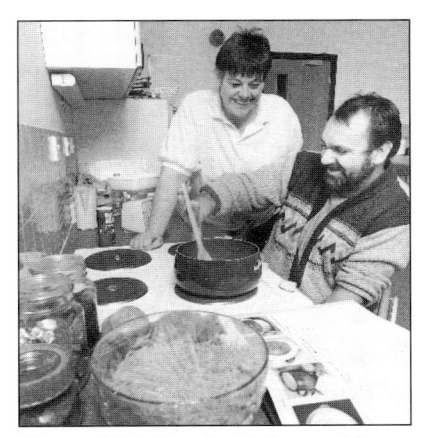

Figure 4.34 Regular visits provide necessary help and support

The importance of effective interaction

Who are you? What do you think makes you different from other people? How do you describe yourself? Religion, race, likes, dislikes and life experience all contribute to the unique nature of yourself – your individuality.

Not only do you have your own individuality but so does everybody else. Some people, however, have difficulties with feeling special, or with their own self-esteem. They may have been abused and damaged at some point in their life. A person exercising power in a damaging way can destroy a person's self-esteem and lead to a loss of individuality. For any caring situation to be effective there is a need to recognise each person's individuality.

The Value Base and individual rights, Appendix II, page 220

Communication and relationships

As a carer it is important for you to understand why you have chosen the caring professions. You must recognise not only that everyone is an individual but that because people are seeking care they may well be vulnerable. You will be in a position of power over them and as such they will be disempowered. It is a vital part of your role that you do not abuse your power by taking away their rights. At the same time you must work to enable them to exercise their rights and seek to help them to establish their voice and power (**empowerment**).

Communicating respect

Although you can choose your friends you cannot necessarily choose who you are going to work with. You may have many things in common with friends but you may find that you share little with work colleagues and clients. However, it is important that you can communicate with and support the wide range of people you will meet in your life. You need to be able to respect them as individuals even though you may not wish to choose them as friends. You should acknowledge their personal beliefs and identity. By communicating your respect for them you are also contributing to their self-esteem and empowerment.

If you respect someone, what they say and do is important to you. Simple things such as remembering and using a person's name helps this process. Spending time listening and remembering what has been said helps to build up a rapport and respect for each other.

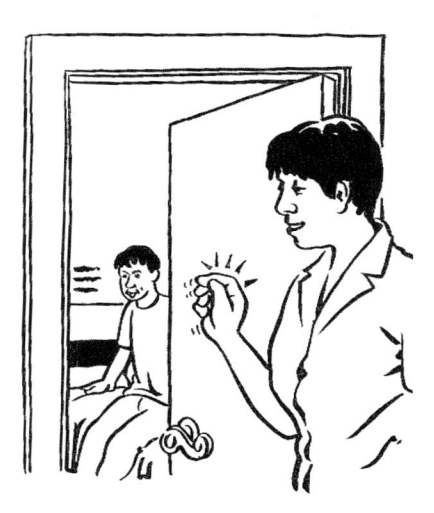

Figure 4.35 The simple act of knocking before entering a room communicates respect

A Golden Park Home

Imagine that you are the Deputy Care Manager at Golden Park Home, a residential home for older people. You receive the following memo:

1 From your observations, and from discussions within your group, list examples of the ways in which clients of social care can be spoken to, or talked about, that fail to respect their individuality, dignity or privacy.
2 As a group, explore ideas for making carers aware of how they should communicate with and about clients.
3 As the Deputy Care Manager, send a memo to your manager detailing how you have carried out the requests.
4 Within your own group, devise your own code of practice. The one for Golden Park Home will give you some starting points.
5 Try to arrange an interview with the care manager or other appropriate person in a care establishment you know of, to discuss the importance of their code of practice. Write an account of the interview.

memo

To: Care manager
Deputy care manager
Subject: Dignity of residents

It has been drawn to my attention that on a number of occasions over the last two or three weeks, the way some of our residents have been spoken to, or referred to, has not been consistent with the high standards we set ourselves. I am afraid the complaints I have recieved have been supported by my own observations. Please draw the attention of all care assistants to our Code of Practice, and let me know by the end of the week the steps you have taken to ensure that all our team will be giving our residents that respect for their dignity we acknowledge as so important.

Speaking to clients

One area that can cause a breakdown in communication is in how you speak to, and about, clients. To be over-familiar, by using a first name without permission, can cause offence. Similarly to call all women clients 'darling' takes away some of their individuality.

Many of your duties as a carer may involve potentially embarrassing situations. Often technical or shorthand terms are used which degrade the action. To say to a colleague, 'I'm going to toilet Mr Jones' can be upsetting. You could be overheard and also it implies that you are going to do something to Mr Jones. A better phrase would be 'to assist Mr Jones to use the toilet'. This has the effect of helping Mr Jones maintain his dignity and also shows that you are encouraging him to do as much as possible for himself.

You can communicate respect by:
- treating a person as an individual
- recognising and valuing their views
- not being judgmental
- understanding that we all have very different life experiences
- recognising that people's views are based on their own unique life experience.

Being non-judgmental
Being non-judgmental can be difficult. It is easy to be non-judgmental with people who have similar views to your own. This will not always be the case in your work. It would be wrong of a carer who was vegetarian to make it clear to clients that she thought eating meat was distasteful.

A positive relationship must be based on:
- trust
- respect
- communication.

In this context a very warm relationship can develop between people who have very different views but who are very strong and happy with their own individuality. The relationship can develop, acknowledging the differences but also each person's individuality.

Self-esteem
People who have high self-esteem are likely to be happy, successful and healthy. It is important to have an inner core of feeling of self-worth and to have this acknowledged by others. People with low self-esteem lack self confidence, feel insecure and can have poor health.

When working in care situations it is important to recognise the power you have. People who need care, in most cases, do so because they are unable to care fully for themselves. They do not necessarily need you to do everything for them. They may, because of this need to be cared for, or because of their personal histories, have a lowered self-esteem. They could start to develop negative feelings of alienation and distrust. It is very easy to take over and do things for them that they are able to do. This has the effect of lowering self-esteem and starting to develop dependency.

To promote self-esteem it is useful to be able to:
- say positive things about the person
- take time to listen to and value what is being said
- recognise that whilst they may be slow at doing something, it is important for them to do things for themselves.

The praise should be genuine and not patronising: to use a standard formula of words without meaning it is insulting.

An example of promoting self esteem

A young child in a nursery brings you a picture with a scribbled circle on it and says it is a picture of you. It is the first mark-making this child has done. It would be reasonable to praise this. If the child continues to produce similar pictures over the next few weeks then to repeat the praise may be of little benefit. Continued, repetitive praise would be insulting as it would have less and less meaning. You know the child should be developing and so praise can be changed to encourage development. You could say, 'That is very colourful, but do I really look like that? What about drawing some arms and legs?'. The child has received a boost, with praise, but is also being helped to move on. A new picture with arms and legs drawn in will be a new achievement and build up the child's self-esteem.

Independence and self-esteem

Independence and self-esteem are linked. Being able to do something for yourself gives you a boost. With young children where there are regular steps towards independence it can be easy to boost self-esteem. With older people who are moving towards dependence it can be more difficult. It is important to try to help maintain self-esteem by assisting the older person to maintain as much independence as possible. Where a person is having difficulties in doing something it is very easy to be in a hurry and take over. You should always ask if your help is needed. It may be that you can think of a way that will help the person maintain independence.

An example of maintaining independence

An arthritic person may have difficulty putting on slippers and so either has to ask for help or walk around with them not fully on. From a safety point of view, it is important that they are worn properly. To provide a long-handled shoe horn might help maintain the person's independence and promote self esteem.

The Care Value Base and individual rights, Appendix II, page 220

Ethical issues in care

Within caring professions there is a value base that underpins all actions. Within this value base is a right of clients to expect information given by them to remain confidential. The client has the right to know who should share the information being given. To break confidentiality destroys the client's trust and removes the right to choose who knows the information.

Confidentiality

Confidentiality can create many ethical dilemmas. When working in a caring situation it is useful to use the following guidelines which should be explained to the client at the outset.

Confidentiality can be maintained apart from two types of situation:
- if you demonstrate that you are a risk to yourself
- if you demonstrate that you are a risk to society.

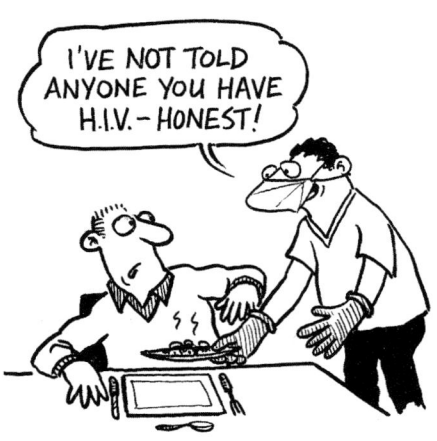

Figure 4.36 Actions can lead to breaches of confidentiality even if you say nothing

There are situations in which the carer becomes concerned and feels the need to break a confidence. In most of these it is important to seek the client's permission before speaking to someone else. An example of this could be a client who has money worries. The carer may not be competent to advise on financial matters and may seek permission to approach somebody for help. In doing so the carer is seeking to retain the trust of the client and helping to establish links with the necessary support.

There are other situations in which the request for confidentiality needs to be over-ridden. A client who says that he has stored up sleeping tablets and is intending to commit suicide has put the carer in a very difficult situation. It is a situation where the right to confidentiality can be broken and a responsible person informed.

Other situations where confidentiality may need to be broken include where the information given by the client means that other people are in danger. A client revealing that he or she is HIV positive does not necessarily fall into this category. If normal hygiene is being followed, then there are no risks. If the client is proposing to have unprotected sex

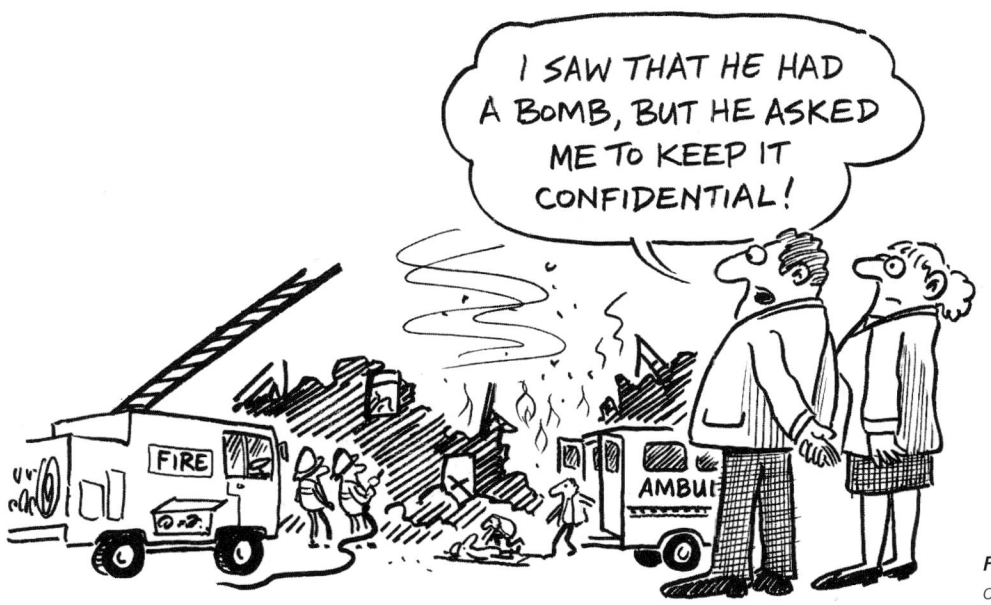

Figure 4.37 Situations occur where confidentiality needs to be broken

with a person who is unaware of the situation, then confidentiality may be breached by seeking advice.

Ethical dilemmas are largely based around the balance between the client's rights and those of others. There are no easy answers and there are few situations where it is essential to breach confidentiality. What is important is to recognise that if you do choose to breach confidentiality you should do so in a responsible way. Talk to a person who has the power to act (a manager or supervisor): do not gossip to others.

Putting it all together

The following section provides some guidance in working in caring situations. It draws on the rest of the unit and provides some sample role plays. Working through this you will be using your practical competence in communication and be developing interpersonal relationships.

As a care worker, it is important for you to be aware of strategies for working in close contact with your clients. The value base defines the underpinning values you should bring to your work. The skills of verbal and non-verbal communication provide the means for you to interact with colleagues and clients. What worries people most when starting to work in caring or when meeting a new client is, 'How does it all fit together?'.

Communication and relationships

A check-list

You need to establish a rapport
Even if you are going to see a person only once it is important to communicate your interest, understanding and empathy.
- Never make assumptions, always ask before doing anything. For example, ask what the person likes to be called.
- Don't intimidate. Ways of intimidating include:
  - making a person stand whilst you are sitting
  - standing over them whilst they are sitting
  - sitting behind a desk with the client opposite
  - interrupting – talking over the client.

The first approach
Whoever you are working with is an individual with feelings and rights. In order to work with them you need to establish a relationship involving trust.

Establishing contact
Crucially, all the messages you communicate must be open.
Verbally Introduce yourself. Check what the person would like you to call them. Initially use one or two closed questions.
Non-verbally Use eye contact or other means (knocking on doors) to gain permission to approach. Adopt an open posture – do not have arms folded, fists clenched. Smile – naturally and with your whole face. Use your senses - eyes, ears, smell. To try to understand how the person is feeling – is he or she: nervous, upset, happy, confused.
If the person is coming to meet you, stand to greet them – do not ignore them – make safe body contact, for example shake hands if appropriate.

Maintaining the flow
Verbally Use sensitive probes to check the messages you received by observing the client's non-verbal behaviour. Start asking open questions. Do not assume – always check.
Non-verbally Try not to dominate – establish a rapport: get down to the level of the person – sit, if necessary, with permission – if you have to stand over the client stay in view to reduce the threat – if you are sitting, try to sit at an angle to the client – if you are sitting at a table try to ensure that the table is not between you – make brief physical contact and use 'safe to touch' areas – shoulders, forearms – use your skills of listening, and prompts, to encourage conversation.

Seeking more information
Verbally Use open questions. Allow for silence when the person needs time to think. Do not jump in with the answers.
Non-verbally Constantly check the non-verbal feedback you are getting. In particular check for signs of openness or build-up of stress (becoming more closed).

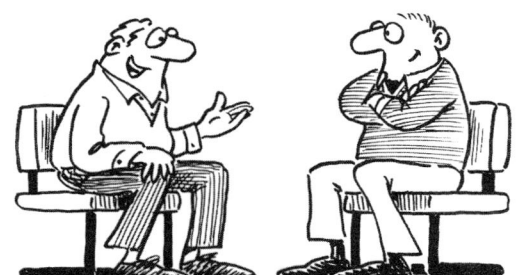

COMFORTABLE

is better than

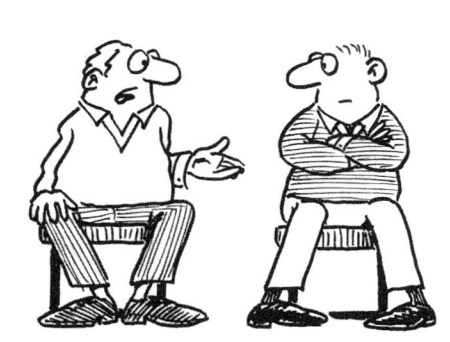

UNCOMFORTABLE

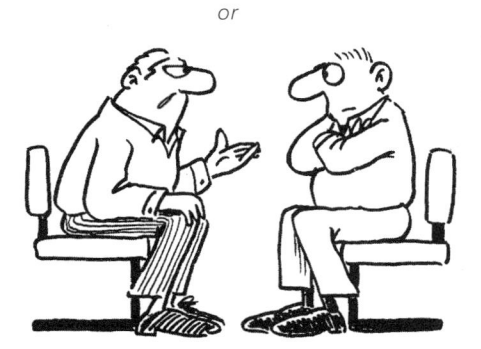

or

A CONFRONTATION

Communication and relationships

A — Practice role play

Role play 1

Student 1
You are working in a day centre with older people. A new member has just arrived. Welcome the person and help settle them in.

Student 2
You have been living with your son and daughter-in-law. They have insisted that you come to the day centre so that they can have some time off. You didn't want to come and are angry with your son. You are also worried that this may be the first move towards getting you into residential care. You do not feel like co-operating.

Role play 2

Student 1
You are working in a nursery as an assistant. You notice Martin(a) is upset and appears to have had a 'toilet accident'. S/he has been playing with a best friend who has just gone to the toilet.

Student 2
You are Martin(a), a 4 year old in the nursery. You were so engrossed in drawing that you forgot to go to the toilet, and wet yourself. You do not want other children to know because they will tease you.
If asked directly – deny that you have wet yourself. You really meant to talk to the assistant in the quiet corner – away from the other children, and do not want to go near the toilet until your best friend has left.

Role play 3

Student 1
You are working in a residential home and notice Mrs Smith is withdrawn and not talking to her friends.

Student 2
You are upset because it is the anniversary of your first husband's death. He was killed whilst preparing for D Day. There has been a lot in the news about the VE Day anniversary. You want to be able to talk about your feelings and show someone photographs of him in uniform.

▶ Role play – debriefing, page xxi

Having carried out the practice role plays, the next step is to 'go live' and do it for real. Hopefully you will have this opportunity by working in care environments. When you do, try to remember the things you have learned in this unit. Most important of all, always think before you act and be clear about your role and if you are unsure, ask. You could ask your co-workers but in most cases you can learn a lot by talking with those for whom you are caring.

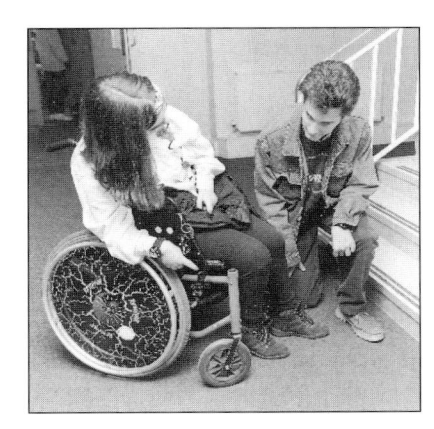

Figure 4.38 Always be prepared to ask

Assignment

A COMMUNICATION RECORD

Setting the scene
This assignment is deliberately very open ended. Your potential work as a carer means that you must develop the skills of communicating with individuals. The opportunities for you to communicate on the course and in your work or workplace are endless. You could set up role plays to demonstrate a particular skill (which is what many of the activities in the unit ask you to do). However, the evidence required should come from your records of communication, which in many ways may reflect the progressive development of the skill.

Task 1
In order to achieve this element it is important to maintain a record of communication. This could include audio and videotapes of the activities undertaken as part of the chapter. You should also have written notes made by a responsible person (for example, a work or workplace supervisor or your tutor) who has observed you communicate with others.

Task 2
Beyond the activities in the unit you should identify an opportunity to record your communication with someone who is not one of the students on the course. This could be an adult or a child.

Task 3
Analyse some of your records collected together from Task 1, and evaluate your communication skills. In doing this you should identify and tag in some way the point at which you are demonstrating that you meet the performance criteria. You will need to select a few examples (a minimum of two) of your activities demonstrating communication to provide the evidence necessary. In your evaluation you should identify clearly the importance of communication in the examples you give.

The product of this assignment will be a written evaluation of your communication skills backed up by the evidence in the form of audio tape, video or written feedback from somebody other than yourself.

Opportunities to collect evidence
On completing these tasks you will have the opportunity to meet the following requirements for Intermediate GNVQ Health and Social Care.
Unit 4
Element 4.1 PCs 1,2,3,4,5

Core skills
The core skill of communication is the one that will be most readily available.

Communication and relationships

Grading
Planning will be important in identifying opportunities for gathering the evidence. You will also return to your action plans following evaluation of your performance.

Evaluation is essential as part of the process of selecting the evidence that meets the needs of the element.

Quality of outcomes will be available in assessing your written evaluation of your skills. In particular, you will need to identify clearly and explain how you are meeting the performance criteria.

Assignment

DISCRIMINATION

Setting the scene
Read the following case studies. In each case identify and describe:
- the behaviour that indicated discrimination
- how different groups were stereotyped
- the possible long-term and short-term effects of the discrimination
- the equality of opportunity rights which may have been flouted (defied). (Ensure you consider up-to-date legislation.)

You may present a summary of the answers as a table but you should write a more detailed explanation of the possible long-term and short-term effects of the discrimination on the person being discriminated against. Also try to say how the discrimination might affect the person doing the discrimination.

Case study 1
Robert was a tall child with one parent who was Afro-Caribbean and the other who was white. He started school in a small city where he was almost the only black, mixed-race child.

In school he worked hard and completed his work quickly. He then got bored and messed about. His teacher complained that he was always messing about and was too lazy to find things to do. At a parents' evening his teacher failed to talk about his academic ability but constantly referred to his athletic ability. She used phrases like, 'Well of course you would expect him to be athletic' and 'What do you expect of people like him.'

Case study 2
Laura was an unusual woman in many ways. She was extremely well qualified as both a scientist and a teacher. She had two children, both of whom were at school. She gave up a well-paid job in the civil service to teach in a reception class.

At the job interview she was asked about her family and what her husband thought about her becoming a teacher. She was also asked about how she would cope when her school's holidays did not exactly fit in with those of her children.

Case study 3

Marsha had just been admitted to hospital. When her details were taken her religion was recorded as Jewish. This was true but she had not been strictly orthodox for many years and she did not observe the dietary requirements. One day on the ward she had marked up her menu card with boiled ham, potatoes and broad beans for dinner. The health care assistant who collected her card started to walk down the ward and then realised that Marsha had asked for ham. She turned round and called to Marsha, 'I think you must have made a mistake. You're Jewish and you've asked for ham. Shall I change it to chicken?'

Until that time Marsha had not discussed religion on the ward. Afterwards the person in the next bed kept telling stories and jokes about Jews.

Case study 4

John was eleven years old and had just started secondary school. He was a diabetic who regularly needed insulin. He injected himself with insulin during the day, while he was in school. Whilst he did not hide the fact that he was injecting himself, he did not make it very public.

One day he was seen injecting himself, by a parent. The parent immediately assumed that John was injecting illegal drugs. The parent warned his child not to play with John as he was a drug addict who most probably had AIDS. The parent had jumped to this conclusion about AIDS because he had attended a parents' evening to inform parents about their children's health education classes. The parents had been told these classes would cover such topics as sex, drugs and sexually transmitted diseases.

Soon the rumour spread round the school that there was a pupil with AIDS. The rumour also identified John as the person. The rumour was at its peak when John fell and cut his knee badly. Many children made faces and ran away shouting that the blood was deadly and everybody should keep away as they might 'get AIDS'.

Opportunities to collect evidence

On completing these tasks you will have the opportunity to meet the following requirements for Intermediate GNVQ Health and Social Care.
Unit 4
Element 4.2 PCs 1,2,3,4,5

Core skills

Communication will be reflected in written work. Information technology can come from selecting appropriate software and producing both the written work and the table using a computer. It may also be possible to search data bases for information about legislation.

Grading

Planning will be important in identifying the types of discrimination and meeting your evidence requirements. You will also return to your action plans following evaluation of how you have met the performance criteria.

Information seeking and information handling will be important identifying the legislation and how it applies to the case studies.

Evaluation is essential as part of the process of selecting the evidence that meets the needs of the element. Quality of outcomes will be available from the table and written work that you produce. In particular, you will need to use appropriate language to show an understanding of the effects of discrimination.

Assignment

WORKING WITH CLIENTS

Setting the scene

You are working in a caring situation and have been asked to provide information for a new member of staff. This information is to be in the form of a list of important things for them to remember at work. You have also been asked to prepare an information sheet for new members of staff that builds on this list.

Note. You may be able to use work placement experience to help you to carry out this assignment. Make use of any skills that you have learned in the workplace to help you to prepare the list. If you can, talk to staff in a caring workplace to get a better understanding of the caring work role.

Task 1
Draft the list. Use the headings in Task 3 to guide you.

Task 2
Talk to people who are working in caring situations about the different headings on your own list. Ask them what they consider to be important information for a new worker. They may give you further ideas for your list.

Task 3
Use word processing or desk-top publishing to prepare an information sheet for new members of staff. You should include examples of things to do and things not to do. The information should address these five areas:
- the caring relationship
- different ways that people respond to care
- different types of support
- the basics for good communication
- the need for confidentiality and when it might be breached.

Opportunities to collect evidence
On completing these tasks you will have the opportunity to meet the following requirements for Intermediate GNVQ Health and Social Care.
Unit 4
Element 4.3 PCs 1,2,3,4,5,6

Core skills
This assignment develops communication core skills. Tasks 1 and 3 address written core skills communication, whereas task 2 addresses oral core skills communication and note-taking.

Grading
The themes of planning (in organising the sequence of your work and arranging to speak with people in the workplace), information seeking and information handling (in gathering and presenting appropriate material on the information sheet) may be demonstrated in this assignment. Quality of outcomes (in the use of appropriate language in a form that meets the needs of the junior staff member on the information sheet) may also be shown.

Questions

Note: *There will be no Unit Test for Unit 4, but these questions can be used to help you check your understanding.*

Each question shows more than one possible answer, **a, b, c** and **d**; only **one** is correct.

1. Seeing a person or a group of people as inferior on the grounds of their race or ethnicity is called:
   a sexism
   b racism
   c ageism
   d class.

2. Not admitting a child to a nursery on grounds of his/her race is:
   a direct discrimination
   b indirect discrimination
   c inequality
   d stereotyping.

3. Indirect discrimination is discrimination which is:
   a highly visible
   b written down
   c hidden
   d fair.

4. Refusing to give somebody a job because they are 'too old' is known as:
   a sexism
   b ageism
   c nepotism
   d socialism.

5. Body language and tone of voice play the largest part in how we communicate. Which one of the following activities is an example of body language?
   a talking
   b singing
   c facial expression
   d writing.

6. A group of people of a similar age and with similar interests is called:
   a a peer group
   b a pressure group
   c a public group
   d a private group.

7. A person's social position relative to others in the group is:
   a their status
   b their stance
   c their beliefs
   d their individuality.

8. In relation to body language, which one of the following statements is **true**
   a our physiology plays no part in the communication process
   b there are cultural differences in interpretation of body language
   c body language behaviours are the same for all cultures
   d we only ever use language to communicate.

9. Which one of the following questions is an example of a closed question?
   a Do you like reading?
   b What books have you read?
   c When do you like to read?
   d Where do you like to read?

10. Open-ended questions are those which:
    a allow the respondent to give broad unstructured answers
    b require no response
    c require the respondent to choose from a small number of possible responses
    d have no correct answer.

11. Appraisal and feedback from others are methods of:
    a appreciation
    b evaluation
    c questioning
    d non-verbal communication.

12. Treating people differently, some favourably and others unfavourably on the basis of particular criteria is known as:
    a discrimination
    b deprivation
    c detention
    d dyslexia.

13. Verbal abuse and physical abuse are examples of:
    a indirect forms of discrimination
    b indiscriminate behaviour
    c direct forms of discrimination
    d body language.

14. To label somebody or categorise someone, and not consider individual characteristics, is called:
    a socialising
    b stereotyping
    c subculture
    d equality.

15 Some books portray boys and girls, women and men in roles which are rigid and very often outdated. Depicting males and females in such roles is referred to as:
a positive stereotyping
b scapegoating
c socialism
d sexual stereotyping.

16 Sexism refers to:
a discrimination against the female sex
b discrimination against the male sex
c discrimination against both sexes
d discrimination against older people.

17 The problems that members of a particular cultural group experience in society because of their race or ethnicity is referred to as:
a sexual disadvantage
b gender disadvantage
c racial disadvantage
d age disadvantage.

18 The effects of discrimination are widespread; studies have shown that discrimination affects a person's life chances in:
a education
b housing
c employment
d all of the above areas.

19 Which one of the following statements is **true**?
'A carer:
a must maintain absolute confidentiality of information at all times
b must always tell their supervisor the information
c may need to disclose information if it endangers the life of the client or others
d must always inform the client's closest relative.

20 Which one of the following instances is best described as an example of social support? Arranging:
a a bank overdraft for a client
b a doctor's appointment at the surgery
c for a stairlift to be fitted in the clients home
d for the client to go to the theatre with friends.

Glossary

Balanced diet: a diet consisting of sufficient nutrients to maintain and promote good health.

Centile charts: graphs that show the average pattern of growth (height, weight, head circumference, etc.). Each chart has statistical details of the normal ranges for the growth pattern displayed.

Closed questions: questions which allow only a limited fixed range of responses.

Cohabiting parents: parents who live together as husband and wife, but are not married.

Complementary health service: people who practice forms of health care that are often related to ideas that have little scientific support. This does not mean that they do not work, it just means that they are not part of mainstream medical provision.

Developmental age: the developmental age is the age indicated by the social, emotional and intellectual behaviour together with physical development.

Emotional support: the support and respect for feelings, needs and beliefs.

Empathy: understanding and experiencing how a person is feeling – putting yourself in their place.

Fund-holding GPs: have money allocated by Regional Health Authorities to provide for a variety of health requirements. The GP must identify the priorities for the health care of his/her patients. Fund-holding GPs are becoming more common. A non fund-holding GP relies on the services for patients that are purchased by the other authorities.

Hazard: something that is dangerous (see risk).

Leading questions: questions phrased in such a way as to give the person who will reply information about the expected answer. This can be achieved both in the words used and the tone and pitch of the voice.

Life chances: opportunities within your life. These are affected by social stratification (class). The higher up the social class scale the greater the life chances.

Macronutrients: the nutrients we take in largest quantities.

Means-tested benefits: a person's income and savings are taken into account and a charge determined based, in theory, on the ability to pay.

Menarche: the first menstruation. The first time that the lining of the uterus is shed with some blood loss.

Menopause: the time during which the ovaries stop producing eggs. During the menopause egg production becomes irregular and the production of hormones by the ovaries comes to an end.

Micronutrients: substances we need in small amounts.

Open questions: questions without a yes/no or simple answer; they ask the speaker to think about the answer and expand upon it. They give more opportunity to explore the detail of what is being talked about, and enable the speaker to think further about the subject. In many cases open questions help the speaker to gain a new perspective on the situation.

Passive smoking: being exposed to the tobacco-smoke of a smoker. This has a similar range of effects to actually smoking the tobacco. The effect is controlled by the amount of exposure.

Prejudice: not an easy concept to define. The dictionary offers: a judgement or opinion formed beforehand or without due examination; bias; injury or hurt; disadvantage.

Pressure point: where an artery can be compressed against a bone to cut off the blood supply to the limb.

Probe: a short question used to help a person expand on a previous answer. Probes can help bring out issues that a client needs to talk about, but is afraid to do so. A probe is used to reveal what a person is concealing.

Prompt: a short question or statement used to focus on an area. Prompts can help lead a conversation. They can also refocus a rambling conversation. A prompt is an invitation to elaborate on what has been said.

Providers: the organisations and people who deliver the care that is bought by the purchasers. In some cases a purchaser may also be a provider. A fund-holding GP may provide care through a contract with the Family Health Services Authority (a purchaser). The GP may also purchase care (e.g. an operation) from a hospital trust (a provider of care). In social care similar systems exist but often the local authority may be a purchaser of care as well as a provider (e.g. the authority may purchase nursery day care for a child as well as provide the care in a Social Services-run day nursery).

Psychotropic drugs: drugs that change our mood or the way our senses work, e.g. they may cause hallucinations.

Purchasers: the organisations or parts of organisations that fund the care. They buy (purchase) the caring services from an organisation that undertakes caring. To do this they need to have systems (plans) to predict the needs for care in the areas for which they are responsible.

Reference Nutrient Intakes (RNI): typical amounts of the various nutrients to form a balanced diet. The figures are related to the age and gender (sex) of an individual and represent figures that would supply 97% of the group with sufficient of a given nutrient.

Reflective listening: a technique in which important things that are being said to you are repeated in order to encourage the speaker to say more. It involves a combination of skills.

Rehabilitation: returning a person to as near normal a state of health as possible.

Risk: an assessment of the likelihood of a hazardous incident taking place (see hazard).

Social group: the groups of people which can be defined by things such as family ties, living together, place of employment, school or college membership and leisure interests.

Social interaction: any activity involving several people. The interaction may be very formal (e.g. a business meeting) or very informal (e.g. a party).

Socialisation: the process by which social contacts with other people develop and shape our personalities, values, norms and roles. Because the process takes place throughout our lives we come to behave, feel and think in similar ways to those around us.

Social mobility: movement up or down the social ladder, between social classes.

Social role: your position in society defined by what you are and what you do. Roles include parent, sibling, child, employed, unemployed or unpaid worker, neighbour, voter and taxpayer.

The statutory sector: organisations that have been set up by law. It includes the Health (under the NHS), Social, Probation and Education Services.

Summarising: restating in your own words what you have heard. In doing so you should identify what you think is important in what has been said. It helps to confirm to the speaker that you have understood what was said.

Bibliography/ useful addresses

1 Useful organisations and their addresses

Action for ME
PO Box 1302
Wells
Somerset BA5 2WE

Action on Smoking and Health (ASH)
109 Gloucester Place
London W1H 3PH

Age Concern
Astral House
1268 London Road
London SW16 4ER

Alcohol Concern
Waterbridge House
32–36 Loman Street
London SE1 0EE

Alzheimer's Disease Society
158–160 Balham High Road
London SW12 9BN

Arthritis and Rheumatism Council
Copeman House
St Mary's Court
St Mary's Gate
Chesterfield S41 7TD

Asthma Research Council
St Thomas's Hospital
Lambeth Palace Road
London SE1

Barnardos
Tanners Lane
Barkingside
Ilford IG6 1QG

British Diabetic Association
10 Queen Anne Street
London W1M 0BD

British Heart Foundation
14 Fitzhardinge Street
London W1H 4DH

Carers National Association
20/25 Glasshouse Yard
London EC1A 4JS

Centre for Policy on Ageing
25–31 Ironmonger Row
London EC1V 3QP

Child Poverty Action Group
4th Floor, 1–5 Bath St
London EC1V 9PY

Commission for Racial Equality
Elliot House
10–12 Allington Street
London SW1E 5EH

Coronary Prevention Group
Plantation House
31–35 Fenchurch Street
London EC3M 3NN

Council for Education and Training in Social Work
Derbyshire House
St Chad's Street
London WC1H 8AD

Cruse (Bereavement Care)
126 Sheen Road
Richmond TW9 1UR

Cystic Fibrosis Trust
Alexandra House
5 Blyth Road
Bromley BR1 3RS

Department of Health
The Adelphi
1–11 John Adam Street
London WC2N 6HT

Disability Alliance
1st Floor East
Universal House
88–94 Wentworth Street
London E1 7SA

Disabled Living Foundation
380–384 Harrow Road
London W9 2HU

Down's Syndrome Association
155 Mitcham Road
Tooting
London SW17 9PG

English National Board for Nursing and Midwifery
170 Tottenham Court Road
London W1P 0HA

Equal Opportunities Commission
Overseas House
Quay Street
Manchester M3 3HN

Family Planning Association
27–35 Mortimer Street
London
W1N 7RJ

Family Welfare Association
501–505 Kingsland Road
Dalston
London E8 4AU

Health and Safety Executive
PO Box 1999
Sudbury CO10 6FS

Health Education Authority
Hamilton House
Mabledon Place
London WC1H 9JP

Health Visitors' Association
50 Southwark Street
London SE1 1UN

Help the Aged
St James's Walk
London EC1R 0BE

HMSO Books Publicity
St Crispins
Duke Street
Norwich NR 3 1PD

Institute for Complementary Medicine
PO Box 194
London SE16 1QZ

Institute of Chiropodists
27 Wright Street
Southport PR9 0TL

Institute of Race Relations
2–6 Leek Street
King's Cross Road
London WC1

Invalid Children's Aid Nationwide
Allen Graham House
198 City Road
London EC1V 2PH

Leukaemia Research Fund
43 Great Ormond Street
London WC1N 3JJ

Low Pay Unit
9 Upper Berkeley Street
London W1H 8BY

MENCAP
(Royal Society for Mentally Handicapped Children and Adults)
National Centre
123 Golden Lane
London EC1Y 0RT

MIND
(National Association for Mental Health)
Granta House
15–19 Broadway
Stratford
London E15 4BQ

National Association of Citizens Advice Bureaux
Myddelton House
115–123 Pentonville Road
London N1 9LZ

National Asthma Campaign
Providence House
Providence Place
London N1 0NT

National Childminding Association
8 Masons Hill
Bromley
Kent BR2 9EY

NCH Action for Children
85 Highbury Park
London N5 1UD

National Council for One Parent Families
255 Kentish Town Road
London NW5 2LX

National Council of Voluntary Organisations
Regent's Wharf
8 All Saints Street
London N1 9RL

National Dairy Council
5–7 John Prince's St
London W1M 0AP

National Deaf Children's Society
45 Hereford Road
London W2 5AH

National Osteoporosis Society
PO Box 10
Radstock
Bath
Avon BA3 3YB

National Schizophrenia Fellowship
28 Castle Street
Kingston-upon-Thames
Surrey KT1 1SS

NSPCC
(National Society for the Prevention of Cruelty to Children)
National Centre
42 Curtain Road
London EC2A 3NH

Parentline
Endway House
The Endway
Benfleet
Essex
SS7 2AN

Parkinson's Disease Society of the UK
22 Upper Woburn Place
London WC1H 0RA

PHAB (Physically Handicapped and Able Bodied)
PHAB England Ltd
12–14 London Road
Croydon
Surrey CR0 2TA

Relate
(National Marriage Guidance)
Herbert Gray College
Little Church Street
Rugby
Warwickshire CV21 3AP

Release (drugs and legal helpline)
169 Commercial Street
London E1 6BW

RNIB
(Royal National Institute for the Blind)
224 Great Portland Street
London W1N 6AA

RNID
(Royal National Institute for the Deaf)
105 Gower Street
London WC1E 6AH

RoSPA
(Royal Society for the Prevention of Accidents)
Cannon House
Priory Queensway
Birmingham B4 6BS

Royal Society for the Promotion of Health
RSH House
38A St George's Drive
London SW1V 4BH

Samaritans
10 The Grove
Slough
Berkshire SL1 1QP

Scope
(for people with cerebral palsy)
12 Park Crescent
London W1N 4EQ

Shelter
(National Campaign for Homeless People)
88 Old Street
London EC1V 9HU

Sickle Cell Society
54 Station Road
London NW10 4UA

Society of Chiropodists and Podiatrists
53 Welbeck Street
London W1M 7HE

Speak out and Listen
PO Box 7
Winchcombe
Cheltenham GL54 5HY

Terrence Higgins Trust
(AIDS and HIV)
52–54 Gray's Inn Road
London WC1X 8JU

The Butter Council
Tubs Hill House
London Road
Sevenoaks
Kent TN13 1BL

The Chartered Society of Physiotherapy
Room 422 Fulton House
Jessop Avenue
Cheltenham GL50 3SH

The Community Affairs Department
The Wellcome Foundation Ltd
PO Box 129
160 Euston Road
London NW1 2BP

Voluntary Council for Handicapped Children
8 Wakley Street
Islington
London EC1V 7QE

Voluntary Organisations Liaison Council for Under-Fives (VOLCUF)
77 Holloway Road
London N7 8JZ

Women's Aid Federation
PO Box 391
Bristol BS99 7WS

2 Bibliography

Anderson, J.
Health Skills for Life Key Stage 4
Nelson
1994

Association of the British Pharmaceutical Industry
Medicines, Health and You poster series
1991 and 1993

Association of the British Pharmaceutical Industry
Medicines and Drugs – The Facts
1994

Beashel, B. and Taylor, J.
Sport Examined
Nelson
1992 and 1995

Beecham, Y. et al.
Childhood – a study in Socialisation
Nelson
1980

Black Report
Inequalities in Health
Penguin
1980

Brimicombe, M., Ellis, R., Gadd, K., Reiss, M.
Intermediate GNVQ Science
Nelson
1995

British Medical Association
Complete Family Health Encyclopaedia
Dorling Kindersley
1992

Clegg, F.
Simple Statistics: A Course Book for the Social Sciences
Cambridge University Press
1982

Collins, M. and Wood-Robinson, V.
Human and Social Biology
Nelson Blackie
1993

Comfort, A.
The Biology of Senescence, 3rd edn
Churchill Livingstone
1979

Commission for Racial Equality
From Cradle to School: a Practical Guide to Race Equality and Childcare
Commission for Racial Equality
1990

Davies, B. M.
Community Health and Social Services
Edward Arnold
1991

Equal Opportunities Commission
An Equal Start…Guidelines on Equal Treatment for the Under-eights
Equal Opportunities Commission
1992

Family Welfare Association
Guide to the Social Services
Family Welfare Association
1995

Foster, J.
Basic Health, Hygiene & Safety
Nelson
1992

Foulger, R. and Routledge, E.
The Food Poisoning Handbook
Chartwell Bratt
1981

Fox, E. L.
Sports Physiology, 2nd edn
Wm. C. Brown
1988

Griffin, M. and Redmore, A.
Human Systems
Nelson Blackie
1993

Hayes, N.
A First Course in Psychology, 3rd edn
Nelson
1993

HMSO
Dietary Reference Values for Food Energy & Nutrients for the UK
HMSO
1994

HMSO
Manual of Nutrition, 10th edn
HMSO
1995

HMSO
Social Trends
HMSO
1995

Hunt, A. (ed.)
Satis 14–16 Books 1–12
Association for Science Education
1986–91

Hunt, A. (ed.)
SATIS 16–19 files 1–4
Association for Science Education
1990–92

Hutchinson, G. and Oliver, S.
Child Development
Nelson Blackie
1989

Jupe, J. et al.
Child development and the Family
Macmillan Education
1985

Katz, J.
Fitness Works!
Leisure Press Publications
1988

MacKean, D. and Jones, B.
Human and Social Biology, 3rd edn
John Murray
1993

Madden, D.
Food and Nutrition
Gill and Macmillan
1980

Mansfield, P.
The Good Health Handbook
Grafton Books
1988

McAvoy, B. R. and Donaldson, L.J. (eds)
Health Care for Asians
Oxford Medical Publications
1990

McCommon, S. et al.
Your choice (series of books)
Nelson
1992

Morris, D.
Manwatching
Triad Granada
1978

National Association of Health Authorities and Trusts
NHS Handbook
JMH Publishing
1994

O'Donnell, M.
A New Introduction to Sociology
Nelson
1992

O'Donnell, M. and Garrod, J.
Sociology in Practice
Nelson
1990

Oppenheim, C.
Poverty: the Facts
Child Poverty Action Group
1990

Roberts, M.
Biology For Life
Nelson
1986

Rowntree, D.
Statistics without Tears
Penguin
1983

Science Museum
Health Matters
Science Museum
1994

Secretary of State for Health
The Health of the Nation: A strategy for Health in England
HMSO
1992

Smith, A. and Jackson, B. (eds)
The Nation's Health: A Strategy for the 1990s. (A report from an Independent Multidisciplinary Committee)
King Edward's Hospital Fund for London
1988

St John Ambulance, St Andrew's Ambulance Association and British Red Cross
First Aid Manual, 6th edn
Dorling Kindersley
1993

Swain, J. Finkelstein, V. French, S. and Oliver, M.
Disabling Barriers: Enabling Environments
Sage
1993

Taylor, D.
Human Physical Health
Cambridge University Press
1989

Tossell, D. and Webb, R.
Inside the Caring Services,
Edward Arnold 2nd edn
1994

Tossell, D. and Webb, R.
Social Issues for Carers
Edward Arnold
1991

Tunniclife, H.
Basic Food Hygiene Certificate – Coursebook
The Institute of Environmental Health Officers (IEHO)
1993

Various
The Thomson Directory Community Pages
Thomson Directories Ltd
Annual

Wallwork, J. and Stepney, R.
Heart Disease: What it is and How it's Treated
Basil Blackwell
1987

Appendix I – Table of nutrients

Table. Composition per 100 g of edible portion.

No.	Food	Inedible waste%	Water (g)	Energy (kJ)	Energy (kcal)	Protein (g)	Fat (g)	Saturated fatty acids (g)	Carbohydrate (g)	Total sugars (g)	Fibre NSP (g)	Calcium (mg)	Iron (mg)	Sodium (mg)	Vitamin A (μg)	Thiamin (mg)	Vitamin C (mg)	No.
	Cereals																	
1	Flour, plain, white	0	14.0	1450	341	9.4	1.3	0.2	77.7	1.5	3.1	140	2.0	3	0	0.31	0	1
2	Flour, wholemeal	0	14.0	1318	310	12.7	2.2	0.3	63.9	2.1	9.0	38	3.9	3	0	0.47	0	2
3	Oats, porridge, raw	0	8.2	1587	375	11.2	9.2	1.6	66.0	1.1	7.1	52	3.8	9	0	0.90	0	3
4	Rice, brown, boiled	0	66.0	597	141	2.6	1.1	0.3	32.1	0.5	0.8	4	0.5	1	0	0.14	0	4
5	Rice, white, boiled	0	68.0	587	138	2.6	1.3	0.3	30.9	0.0	0.1	18	0.2	1	0	0.01	0	5
6	Spaghetti, white, boiled	0	73.8	442	104	3.6	0.7	0.1	22.2	0.5	1.2	7	0.5	0	0	0.01	0	6
	Breads																	
7	Brown bread, average	0	39.5	927	218	8.5	2.0	0.4	44.3	3.0	3.5	100	2.2	540	0	0.27	0	7
8	White bread, average	0	37.3	1002	235	8.4	1.9	0.4	49.3	2.6	1.5	110	1.6	520	0	0.21	0	8
9	White bread 'with added fibre' (soft grain)	0	40.0	978	230	7.6	1.5	0.4	49.6	3.3	3.1	150	2.3	450	0	0.20	0	9
10	Wholemeal bread, average	0	38.3	914	215	9.2	2.5	0.5	41.6	1.8	5.8	54	2.7	550	0	0.34	0	10
	Breakfast cereals																	
11	Bran flakes	0	3.0	1353	318	10.2	1.9	0.4	69.3	18.7	13.0	50	20.0	1000	0	1.0	25	11
12	Corn flakes	0	3.0	1535	360	7.9	0.7	0.1	85.9	8.2	0.9	15	6.7	1110	0	1.0	0	12
13	Muesli, Swiss style	0	7.2	1540	363	9.8	5.9	0.8	72.2	26.2	6.4	110	5.8	380	0	0.5	0	13
14	Weetabix	0	5.6	1498	352	11.0	2.7	0.4	75.7	5.2	9.7	35	7.4	270	0	0.9	0	14
	Biscuits																	
15	Chocolate biscuits, full coated	0	2.2	2197	524	5.7	27.6	16.7	67.4	43.4	2.1	110	1.7	160	0	0.03	0	15
16	Cream crackers	0	4.3	1857	440	9.5	16.3	N	68.3	0.0	2.2	110	1.7	610	0	0.23	0	16
17	Crispbread, rye	0	6.4	1367	321	9.4	2.1	0.3	70.6	3.2	11.7	45	3.5	220	0	0.28	0	17
18	Digestive biscuits, plain	0	2.5	1978	471	6.3	20.9	8.6	68.6	13.6	2.2	92	3.2	600	0	0.14	0	18
19	Semi-sweet biscuits	0	2.5	1925	457	6.7	16.6	8.0	74.8	22.3	1.7	120	2.1	410	0	0.13	0	19
	Buns and cakes																	
20	Currant buns	0	27.7	1250	296	7.6	7.5	N	52.7	15.1	N	110	1.9	230	0	0.37	0	20
21	Fruit cake, rich	0	17.6	1438	341	3.8	11.0	3.4	59.6	48.4	1.7	82	1.9	200	125	0.08	0	21
22	Jam tarts, retail	0	14.4	1551	368	3.3	13.0	4.8	63.4	36.0	N	72	1.7	130	N	0.06	0	22
23	Madeira cake	0	20.2	1652	393	5.4	16.9	8.8	58.4	36.5	0.9	42	1.1	380	N	0.06	0	23
24	Swiss rolls, chocolate, individual	0	17.5	1421	337	4.3	11.3	N	58.1	41.8	N	77	1.1	350	N	0.12	0	24
	Puddings																	
25	Bread pudding	0	29.3	1252	297	5.9	9.6	5.9	49.7	33.1	1.2	120	1.6	310	107	0.10	0	25
26	Cheesecake, frozen	0	44.0	1017	242	5.7	10.6	5.6	33.0	22.2	0.9	68	0.5	160	N	0.04	0	26
27	Custard made up with whole milk	0	75.5	495	117	3.7	4.5	2.8	16.6	11.4	0.0	130	0.1	81	63	0.04	1	27
28	Fruit crumble	0	54.8	835	198	2.0	6.9	2.1	34.0	21.3	1.7	49	0.6	68	88	0.05	3	28
29	Fruit pie, pastry top and bottom	0	47.9	1089	260	3.0	13.3	4.8	34.0	12.0	1.8	59	0.8	200	74	0.08	3	29
30	Rice pudding, canned	0	77.6	374	89	3.4	2.5	1.6	14.0	8.2	0.2	93	0.2	50	N	0.03	0	30
31	Trifle	0	67.2	674	160	3.6	6.3	3.1	22.3	16.8	0.5	79	0.5	53	75	0.06	4	31
	Milk and milk products																	
32	Cream, fresh, single	0	73.7	817	198	2.6	19.1	11.9	4.1	4.1	0.0	91	0.1	49	336	0.04	1	32
33	Cream, fresh, double	0	47.5	1849	449	1.7	48.0	30.0	2.7	2.7	0.0	50	0.2	37	654	0.02	1	33
34	Dried skimmed milk	0	3.0	1482	348	36.1	0.6	0.4	52.9	52.9	0.0	1280	0.27	550	351	0.38	13	34
35	Evaporated milk, whole	0	69.1	629	151	8.4	9.4	5.9	8.5	8.5	0.0	290	0.26	180	122	0.07	1	35
36	Ice cream, non-dairy, vanilla	0	65.3	746	178	3.2	8.7	4.4	23.1	19.2	0.0	120	0.1	76	2	0.04	1	36
37	Semi-skimmed milk, average	0	89.8	195	46	3.3	1.6	1.0	5.0	5.0	0.0	120	0.05	55	23	0.04	1	37
38	Skimmed milk, average	0	91.1	140	33	3.3	0.1	0.1	5.0	5.0	0.0	120	0.06	54	1	0.04	1	38
39	Whole milk, average	0	87.8	275	66	3.2	3.9	2.4	4.8	4.8	0.0	115	0.06	55	55	0.03	1	39
40	Yogurt, whole milk, plain	0	81.9	333	79	5.7	3.0	1.7	7.8	7.8	N	200	0.01	80	31	0.06	1	40
41	Yogurt, whole milk, fruit ('thick and creamy')	0	73.1	441	105	5.1	2.8	1.5	15.7	15.7	N	160	0	82	42	0.06	1	41
42	Yogurt, low fat, fruit	0	77.0	382	90	4.1	0.7	0.4	17.9	17.9	N	150	0.1	64	11	0.05	1	42

Table of nutrients

No.	Food	Inedible waste%	Water (g)	Energy (kJ)	Energy (kcal)	Protein (g)	Fat (g)	Saturated fatty acids (g)	Carbo-hydrate (g)	Total sugars (g)	Fibre NSP(g)	Calcium (mg)	Iron (mg)	Sodium (mg)	Vitamin A (µg)	Thiamin (mg)	Vitamin C (mg)	No.
	Cheese																	
43	Brie	0	48.6	1323	319	19.3	26.9	16.8	0.0	0.0	0.0	540	0.8	700	320	0.04	0	43
44	Cheddar, average	0	36.0	1708	412	25.5	34.4	21.7	0.1	0.1	0.0	720	0.3	670	363	0.03	0	44
45	Cheese spread, plain	0	53.3	1143	276	13.5	22.8	14.3	4.4	4.4	0.0	420	0.2	1060	293	0.05	0	45
46	Cottage cheese, plain	0	79.1	413	98	13.8	3.9	2.4	2.1	2.1	0.0	73	0.1	380	46	0.03	0	46
47	Feta	0	56.5	1037	250	15.6	20.2	13.7	1.5	1.5	0.0	360	0.2	1440	225	0.04	0	47
48	Fromage frais, fruit	0	71.9	551	131	6.8	5.8	3.6	13.8	13.8	0.0	86	0.1	35	N	0.02	0	48
	Eggs																	
49	Eggs, chicken, boiled	0	75.1	612	147	12.5	10.8	3.1	0.0	0.0	0.0	57	1.9	140	190	0.07	0	49
50	Eggs, chicken, fried in vegetable oil	0	70.1	745	179	13.6	13.9	4.0	0.0	0.0	0.0	65	2.2	160	215	0.07	0	50
	Fats and oils																	
51	Butter	0	15.6	3031	737	0.5	81.7	54.0	0.0	0.0	0.0	15	0.2	750	887	0.00	0	51
52	Low-fat spread	0	49.9	1605	390	5.8	40.5	11.2	0.5	0.5	0.0	39	0.0	650	501	0.00	0	52
53	Margarine, polyunsaturated	0	16.0	3039	739	0.2	81.6	16.2	1.0	1.0	0.0	4	0.3	800	946	0.00	0	53
54	Sunflower seed oil	0	0.0	3696	899	0.0	99.9	11.9	0.0	0.0	0.0	0	0.0	0	0	0.00	0	54
	Meat and meat products																	
55	Bacon, rasher, lean and fat, raw back	6	40.5	1766	428	14.2	41.2	16.2	0.0	0.0	0.0	7	1.0	1470	0	0.35	0	55
56	Bacon, rasher, lean and fat, grilled, back	0	36.0	1681	405	25.3	33.38	13.2	0.0	0.0	0.0	12	1.5	2020	0	0.43	0	56
57	Beef, lean only, raw, average	0	74.0	517	123	20.3	4.6	1.9	0.0	0.0	0.0	7	2.1	61	0	0.07	0	57
58	Beef, mince, stewed	0	59.1	955	229	23.1	15.2	6.5	0.0	0.0	0.0	18	3.1	320	0	0.05	0	58
59	Beef, stewing steak, lean and fat, raw	4	68.7	736	176	20.2	10.6	4.5	0.0	0.0	0.0	8	2.1	72	0	0.06	0	59
60	Beef, stewing steak, lean and fat, stewed	0	57.1	932	223	30.9	11.0	4.7	0.0	0.0	0.0	15	3.0	360	0	0.02	0	60
61	Beefburgers, frozen, fried	0	53.0	1099	264	20.4	17.3	8.0	7.0	1.4	N	33	3.1	880	0	0.2	0	61
62	Black pudding, fried	0	44.0	1270	305	12.9	21.9	8.5	5.0	0.0	N	35	20.0	1210	41	0.09	0	62
63	Bolognese sauce	36	74.7	602	145	8.0	11.1	3.1	3.7	3.3	1.0	23	1.4	430	213	0.07	4	63
64	Chicken, raw, meat and skin	0	64.4	954	230	17.6	17.7	5.9	0	0.0	0.0	10	0.7	70	0	0.08	0	64
65	Chicken, roast, meat only	0	68.4	621	148	24.8	5.4	1.6	0.0	0.0	0.0	9	0.8	81	0	0.08	0	65
66	Chicken, roast, meat and skin	0	61.9	902	216	22.6	14.0	4.2	0.0	0.0	0.0	9	0.8	72	0	N	0	66
67	Corned beef, canned	0	58.5	905	217	26.9	12.1	6.3	0.0	0.0	0.0	14	2.9	950	0	0.00	0	67
68	Ham, canned	0	72.5	502	120	18.4	5.1	1.9	0.0	0.0	0.0	9	2.9	1250	0	0.52	0	68
69	Kidney, pig, raw	0	78.8	377	90	16.3	2.7	0.9	0.0	0.0	0.0	8	5.0	190	160	0.32	14	69
70	Kidney, pig, stewed	0	66.3	641	153	24.4	6.1	2.0	0.0	0.0	0.0	13	6.4	370	46	0.19	11	70
71	Lamb, lean only, raw, average	0	70.1	679	162	20.8	8.8	4.2	0.0	0.0	0.0	7	1.6	88	0	0.14	0	71
72	Lamb roast, meat only	0	55.3	1106	266	26.1	17.9	8.9	0.0	0.0	0.0	8	2.5	65	0	0.12	0	72
73	Liver, lamb, raw	0	67.3	748	179	20.1	10.3	2.9	1.6	0.0	0.1	0.0	9.4	76	38644	0.27	10	73
74	Liver, lamb, fried	0	58.4	970	232	22.9	14.0	4.0	3.9	0.0	0.0	12	10.0	190	57300	0.26	12	74
75	Paté, liver	0	50.6	1308	316	13.1	28.9	8.4	1.0	0.3	0.0	15	7.1	790	7352	0.13	N	75
76	Pork, lean only, raw, average	0	71.5	615	147	20.7	7.1	2.5	0.0	0.0	0.0	8	0.9	76	0	0.89	0	76
77	Pork chops, loin, lean, only grilled	0	56.1	945	226	32.3	10.7	3.8	0.0	0.0	0.0	9	1.2	84	0	0.88	0	77
78	Salami	0	28.0	2031	491	19.3	45.2	N	1.9	0.0	0.1	10	1.0	1850	0	0.21	0	78
79	Sausages, beef, grilled	0	47.9	1104	265	13.0	17.3	6.7	15.2	2.4	0.7	73	1.7	1100	0	0.00	0	79
80	Sausages, pork, grilled	0	45.1	1320	318	13.3	24.6	9.5	11.5	1.8	0.7	53	1.5	1000	0	0.02	0	80
81	Sausages, low fat, grilled	0	50.1	959	229	16.2	13.8	5.0	10.8	0.9	1.5	130	1.3	1190	0	0.00	0	81
82	Steak and kidney pie, individual	0	42.6	1349	323	9.1	21.2	8.4	25.6	2.3	0.9	53	2.5	510	N	0.12	0	82
83	Turkey, roast, meat and skin	0	65.0	717	171	28.0	6.5	2.1	0.0	0.0	0.0	9	0.9	52	N	N	0	83
	Fish and fish products																	
84	Cod in batter, fried in blended oil	0	60.9	834	199	19.6	10.3	0.9	7.5	0.1	0.3	80	0.5	100	N	0.20	0	84
85	Fish fingers, grilled	0	56.2	899	214	15.1	9.0	2.8	19.3	0.0	0.7	52	0.8	380	0	0.10	0	85
86	Haddock, steamed, flesh only	24	75.1	417	98	22.8	0.8	0.2	0.0	0.0	0.0	55	0.7	120	0	0.08	0	86
87	Herring, grilled	0	65.5	828	199	20.4	13.0	3.7	0.0	0.0	0.0	33	1.0	170	34	0.09	0	87
88	Mackerel, fried	0	65.6	784	188	21.5	11.3	2.3	0.0	0.0	0.0	28	1.2	150	43	0.09	0	88
89	Pilchards, canned in tomato sauce	0	70.0	531	126	18.8	5.4	1.1	0.7	0.6	0.0	300	2.7	370	32	0.02	0	89
90	Prawns, boiled	0	70.0	451	107	22.6	1.8	0.4	0.0	0.0	0.0	150	1.1	1590	0	0.02	0	90
91	Sardines, canned in oil, drained	17	58.4	906	217	23.7	13.6	2.8	0.0	0.0	0.0	550	2.9	650	11	0.04	0	91
92	Tuna, canned in brine, drained	19	74.6	422	99	23.5	0.6	0.2	0.0	0.0	0.0	8	1.0	320	N	0.02	0	92

Table of nutrients

No.	Food	Inedible waste%	Water (g)	Energy (kJ)	Energy (kcal)	Protein (g)	Fat (g)	Saturated fatty acids (g)	Carbo-hydrate (g)	Total sugars (g)	Fibre NSP (g)	Calcium (mg)	Iron (mg)	Sodium (mg)	Vitamin A (µg)	Thiamin (mg)	Vitamin C (mg)	No.
	Potatoes and potato products																	
93	Chips, homemade, fried in blended oil	0	56.5	796	189	3.9	6.7	0.6	30.1	0.6	2.2	11	0.8	12	0	0.24	9	93
94	Oven chips, frozen, baked	0	58.5	687	162	3.2	4.2	1.8	29.8	0.7	2.0	12	0.8	53	0	0.11	12	94
95	Potato crisps	0	1.9	2275	546	5.6	37.6	9.2	49.3	0.7	4.9	37	1.8	1070	0	0.11	27	95
96	Potatoes, new, average, raw, flesh only	11	81.7	298	70	1.7	0.3	0.1	16.1	1.3	1.0	6	0.3	11	0	0.15	16	96
97	Potatoes, old, average, raw, flesh only	20	79.0	318	75	2.1	0.2	0.0	17.2	0.6	1.3	5	0.4	7	0	0.21	11	97
98	Potatoes, old, baked, flesh and skin	0	62.6	581	136	3.9	0.2	0.0	31.7	1.2	2.7	11	0.7	12	0	0.37	14	98
99	Potatoes, old, boiled in unsalted water	0	80.3	306	72	1.8	0.1	0.0	17.0	0.7	1.2	5	0.4	7	0	0.18	6	99
100	Potatoes, old, roast in blended oil	0	64.7	630	149	2.9	4.5	0.4	25.9	0.6	1.8	8	0.7	9	0	0.23	8	100
	Vegetables																	
101	Aubergine, raw	4	92.9	64	15	0.9	0.4	0.1	2.2	2.0	2.0	10	0.3	2	12	0.02	4	101
102	Beans, baked, canned in tomato sauce	0	71.5	355	84	5.2	0.6	0.1	15.3	5.9	3.7	53	1.4	530	12	0.09	0	102
103	Beans, red kidney, canned, drained	36	67.5	424	100	6.9	0.6	0.1	17.8	3.6	6.2	71	2.0	390	1	0.21	0	103
104	Beans, runner, boiled in unsalted water	0	92.8	76	18	1.2	0.5	0.1	2.3	2.0	1.9	22	1.0	1	20	0.05	10	104
105	Beetroot, boiled in salted water	20	82.4	195	46	2.3	0.1	0.0	9.5	8.8	1.9	29	0.8	110	5	0.01	5	105
106	Brussels sprouts, boiled in unsalted water	20	86.9	153	35	2.9	1.3	0.3	3.5	3.0	3.1	20	0.5	2	53	0.07	60	106
107	Cabbage, raw, average	23	90.1	109	26	1.7	0.4	0.1	4.1	4.0	2.4	52	0.7	5	64	0.15	49	107
108	Cabbage, boiled in unsalted water, average	0	93.1	67	16	1.0	0.4	0.1	2.2	2.0	1.8	33	0.3	8	35	0.08	20	108
109	Carrots, old, boiled in unsalted water	0	90.5	100	24	0.6	0.4	0.1	4.9	4.6	2.5	24	0.4	50	1260	0.09	2	109
110	Cauliflower, boiled in unsalted water	0	90.6	117	28	2.9	0.9	0.2	2.1	1.8	1.6	17	0.4	4	10	0.07	27	110
111	Celery, raw	9	95.1	32	7	0.5	0.2	0.1	0.9	0.9	1.1	41	0.4	60	8	0.06	8	111
112	Courgette, raw	12	93.7	74	18	1.8	0.4	0.1	1.8	1.7	0.9	25	0.8	1	100	0.12	21	112
113	Cucumber	3	96.4	40	10	0.7	0.1	0.0	1.5	1.4	0.6	18	0.3	3	10	0.03	2	113
114	Lentils (red, dried) boiled in unsalted water	0	72.1	424	100	7.6	0.4	0.0	17.5	0.8	1.9	16	2.4	12	3	0.11	0	114
115	Lettuce, average	26	95.1	59	14	0.8	0.5	0.1	1.7	1.7	0.9	28	0.7	3	59	0.12	5	115
116	Mycoprotein, Quorn	0	75.0	360	86	11.8	3.5	0.6	2.0	1.1	4.8	N	N	240	0	36.6	0	116
117	Mushrooms, raw	3	92.6	55	13	1.8	0.5	0.1	0.4	0.2	1.1	6	0.6	5	0	0.09	1	117
118	Onions, raw	9	89.0	150	36	1.2	0.2	0.0	7.9	5.6	1.4	25	0.3	3	2	0.13	5	118
119	Parsnips, boiled in unsalted water	0	78.8	278	66	1.6	1.2	0.2	12.9	5.9	4.7	50	0.6	4	5	0.07	10	119
120	Peas, frozen, boiled in unsalted water	0	78.3	291	69	6.0	0.9	0.2	9.7	2.7	5.1	35	1.6	2	67	0.26	12	120
121	Peppers (green, raw)	16	93.3	65	15	0.8	0.3	0.1	2.6	2.4	1.6	8	0.4	4	44	0.01	120	121
122	Plantain, boiled in unsalted water	0	68.5	477	112	0.8	0.2	0.1	28.5	5.5	1.2	5	0.5	4	58	0.03	9	122
123	Processed peas, canned, re-heated, drained	35	69.6	423	99	6.9	0.7	0.1	17.5	1.5	4.8	33	1.8	380	10	0.10	0	123
124	Spinach, frozen, boiled in unsalted water	0	91.6	90	21	3.1	0.8	0.1	0.5	0.3	2.1	150	1.7	16	640	0.06	6	124
125	Sweetcorn kernels, canned, re-heated, drained	0	74.7	358	84	1.1	0.3	0.1	20.5	11.6	2.3	23	0.7	32	660	0.07	17	125
126	Sweetcorn kernels, canned, re-heated, drained	18	72.3	519	122	2.9	1.2	0.2	26.6	9.6	1.4	4	0.5	270	19	0.04	1	126
127	Tofu, soya bean, steamed	0	85.0	304	73	8.1	4.2	0.5	0.7	0.3	N	510	1.2	4	0	0.06	0	127
128	Tomatoes, raw	0	93.1	73	17	0.7	0.3	0.0	3.1	3.1	1.0	7	0.5	9	105	0.09	17	128
129	Turnip, boiled in unsalted water	0	93.1	51	12	0.6	0.2	0.0	2.0	1.9	1.9	45	0.2	28	3	0.05	10	129
130	Watercress	38	92.5	94	22	3.0	1.0	0.3	0.4	0.4	1.5	170	2.2	49	420	0.16	62	130
131	Yam, boiled in unsalted water	0	64.4	568	133	1.7	0.3	0.1	33.0	0.7	1.4	12	0.4	17	0	0.14	4	131
	Fruit																	
132	Apples, eating, average, raw, flesh and skin	11	84.5	199	47	0.4	0.1	0.0	11.8	11.8	1.8	4	0.1	3	3	0.03	6	132
133	Apricots, ready-to-eat	0	29.7	674	158	4.0	0.6	N	36.5	36.5	6.3	73	3.4	14	91	0.00	1	133
134	Apricots, canned in syrup	0	80.0	268	63	0.4	0.1	0.0	16.1	16.1	0.9	19	0.2	10	25	0.01	5	134
135	Avocado, average, flesh only	29	72.5	784	190	1.9	1.95	4.1	1.9	0.5	3.4	11	0.4	6	3	0.10	6	135
136	Bananas, flesh only	34	75.1	403	95	1.2	0.3	0.1	23.2	20.9	1.1	6	0.3	1	3	0.04	11	136
137	Blackcurrants, stewed, without sugar	0	80.7	103	24	0.8	0.0	0.0	5.6	5.6	3.1	51	1.1	2	14	0.02	130	137
138	Cherries, raw, weighed without stones	17	82.8	203	48	0.9	0.1	0.0	11.5	11.5	0.9	13	0.2	1	4	0.03	11	138
139	Dates, dried, weighed without stones	16	14.6	1151	270	3.3	0.2	0.1	68.0	68.0	4.0	45	1.3	10	7	0.07	0	139
140	Figs, dried, ready to eat	0	23.6	889	209	3.3	1.5	N	48.6	48.6	6.9	230	3.9	57	10	0.07	1	140
141	Gooseberries, cooking, stewed without sugar	0	78.9	310	73	0.4	0.2	N	18.5	2.5	2.0	23	0.3	2	7	0.01	11	141
142	Grapefruit, raw, flesh only	32	89.0	126	30	0.8	0.1	0.0	6.8	6.8	1.3	23	0.1	3	3	0.05	36	142
143	Grapes, seedless	5	81.8	257	60	0.4	0.1	0.0	15.4	15.4	0.7	13	0.3	2	3	0.05	3	143
144	Kiwi fruit, flesh and seeds	14	84.0	207	49	1.1	0.5	N	10.6	10.3	1.9	25	0.4	4	6	0.01	59	144
145	Mangoes, ripe, raw, flesh only	32	82.4	245	57	0.7	0.2	0.1	14.1	13.8	2.6	12	0.7	2	300	0.04	37	145

218

Table of nutrients

No.	Food	Inedible waste %	Water (g)	Energy (kJ)	Energy (kcal)	Protein (g)	Fat (g)	Saturated fatty acids (g)	Carbohydrate (g)	Total sugars (g)	Fibre NSP (g)	Calcium (mg)	Iron (mg)	Sodium (mg)	Vitamin A (µg)	Thiamin (mg)	Vitamin C (mg)	No.
146	Melon, honeydew, flesh only	37	92.2	119	28	0.6	0.1	0.0	6.6	6.6	0.6	9	0.1	32	8	0.03	9	146
147	Oranges, flesh only	30	86.1	158	37	1.1	0.1	0.0	8.5	8.5	1.7	47	0.1	5	5	0.11	54	147
148	Peaches, raw, flesh and skin	10	88.9	142	33	1.0	0.1											148
149	Peaches, canned in syrup	0	81.1	233	55	0.5	0.0	0.0	14.0	16.4	0.9	3	0.2	4	13	0.01	5	149
150	Pears, average, raw, flesh and skin	9	83.8	169	40	0.3	0.1	0.0	10.0	10.0	2.2	11	0.2	3	3	0.02	5	150
151	Pineapple, canned in juice	9	86.8	200	47	0.3	0.0	0.0	12.2	12.2	0.5	8	0.5	1	2	0.09	11	151
152	Plums, average, raw, flesh and skin	6	83.9	155	365	0.6	0.1	0.0	8.8	8.8	1.6	13	0.4	2	49	0.05	4	152
153	Prunes, ready-to-eat	0	31.1	601	141	2.5	0.4	N	34.0	34.0	5.7	34	2.6	11	23	0.09	0	153
154	Raspberries, raw	0	87.0	109	25	1.4	0.3	0.1	4.6	4.6	2.5	25	0.7	3	1	0.03	5	154
155	Rhubarb, stewed with sugar	0	84.6	203	48	0.9	0.1	0.0	11.5	11.5	1.2	33	0.1	1	5	0.03	5	155
156	Strawberries, raw	5	89.5	113	27	0.8	0.1	0.0	6.0	6.0	1.1	16	0.4	6	1	0.03	77	156
157	Sultanas	0	15.2	1171	275	2.7	0.4	N	69.4	69.4	2.0	64	2.2	19	2	0.09	0	157
	Nuts																	
158	Almonds, flesh only	63	4.2	2534	612	21.1	55.8	4.7	6.9	4.2	7.4	240	3.0	14	0	0.21	0	158
159	Coconut, desiccated	0	2.3	2492	604	5.6	62.0	53.4	6.4	6.4	13.7	23	3.6	28	0	0.03	0	159
160	Peanut butter, smooth	0	1.1	2581	623	22.6	53.7	11.7	13.1	6.7	5.4	37	2.1	350	0	0.17	0	160
161	Peanuts, roasted and salted	0	1.9	2491	602	24.5	53.0	9.5	7.1	3.8	6.0	37	1.3	400	0	0.18	0	161
	Sugars and preserves																	
162	Chocolate, milk	0	2.2	2214	529	8.4	30.3	17.8	59.4	56.5	0.0	220	1.6	120	7	0.1	0	162
163	Honey	0	23.0	1229	288	0.4	0.0	0.0	76.4	76.4	0.0	5	0.4	11	N	0.0	0	163
164	Jam, fruit with edible seed	0	29.8	1114	261	0.6	0.0	0.0	69.0	69.0	N	24	1.5	16	N	0.0	10	164
165	Marmalade	0	28.0	1114	261	0.1	0.0	0.0	69.5	69.5	0.6	35	0.6	18	8	0.0	10	165
166	Peppermints	0	0.2	1670	392	0.5	0.7	N	102.2	102.2	0.0	7	0.2	9	0	0.0	0	166
167	Sugar, white	0	0.0	1680	394	0.0	0.0	0.0	105.0	105.0	0.0	2	0.0	9	0	0.0	0	167
168	Syrup, golden	0	20.0	1269	298	0.3	0.0	0.0	79.0	79.0	0.0	26	1.5	270	0	0.0	0	168
	Beverages																	
169	Cocoa powder	0	3.4	1301	312	10.5	21.7	12.8	11.5	0.0	12.1	130	10.5	950	7	0.16	0	169
170	Coffee, infusion, 5 minutes	0	N	8	2	0.2	0.0	0.0	0.3	0.3	0.0	2	0.0	0	N	0.00	0	170
171	Coffee, instant powder	0	3.4	424	100	14.6	0.0	0.0	11.0	6.5	0.0	160	4.4	41	N	0.00	0	171
172	Drinking chocolate powder	0	2.1	1554	366	5.5	6.0	3.5	77.4	73.8	N	33	2.4	250	N	0.06	0	172
173	Tea, Indian, infusion	0	N	2	0	0.1	0.0	0.0	0.0	0.0	0.0	0.0	0	0.0	N	0.00	0	173
	Soft drinks and juices																	
174	Coca-cola	0	89.8	168	39	0.0	0.0	0.0	10.5	10.5	0.0	4	0.0	8	0	0.00	0	174
175	Lemonade, bottled	0	94.6	90	21	0.0	0.0	0.0	5.6	5.6	0.0	5	0.0	7	0	0.00	0	175
176	Orange drink, undiluted	0	71.2	456	107	0.0	0.0	0.0	28.5	28.5	0.0	8	0.1	21	N	0.00	0	176
177	Orange juice, unsweetened	0	89.2	153	36	0.5	0.1	0.0	8.8	8.8	0.1	10	0.2	10	3	0.08	39	177
178	Pineapple juice, unsweetened	0	87.8	177	41	0.3	0.12	0.0	10.5	10.5	0.0	8	0.2	8	1	0.06	11	178
179	Baking powder	0	6.3	163	693	5.2	0.8	0.0	37.8	0.0	0.0	1130	0.0	11800	0	0.00	0	179
180	Curry powder	0	8.5	979	233	9.5	0.7	N	26.1	N	23.0	640	58.3	450	17	0.25	0	180
181	Marmite	0	25.4	730	172	39.7	75.6	N	1.8	0.0	0.0	95	3.7	4500	0	3.10	N	181
182	Mayonnaise, retail	0	18.8	2843	691	1.1	8.2	11.1	1.7	1.3	0.0	8	0.3	450	103	0.02	0	182
183	Mustard, smooth	0	63.7	579	139	7.1	0.6	0.5	9.7	7.8	N	70	2.9	2950	N	N	0	183
184	Pickle, sweet	0	58.9	572	134	0.6	31.0	0.0	34.4	32.6	1.2	19	2.0	1700	42	0.03	0	184
185	Salad cream	0	47.2	1440	348	1.5	3.3	3.9	165.7	16.7	N	18	0.5	1040	12	N	0	185
186	Soup, cream of tomato, canned, ready to serve	0	84.2	230	55	0.8	0.0	N	5.9	2.6	N	17	0.4	460	35	0.03	0	186
187	Soy sauce	0	67.6	266	64	8.7	0.0	0.0	8.3	N	0.0	19	2.0	1700	42	0.03	0	187
188	Tomato ketchup	0	64.8	420	98	2.1	0.0	0.0	24.0	22.9	0.9	2.5	1.2	1120	38	1.00	2	188
	Composition per 100 ml Alcoholic drinks																	
189	Beer, bitter, keg	0	93.5	129	31	0.3	0.0	0.0	2.3	2.3	0.0	8	0.01	8	0	0	0	189
190	Cider, dry	0	93.2	152	36	0.0	0.0	0.0	2.6	2.6	0.0	8	0.5	7	0	0	0	190
191	Lager, bottled	0	94.9	120	29	0.2	0.0	0.0	1.5	1.5	0.0	4	0.0	4	0	0	0	191
192	Spirits, 40% volume	0	63.3	919	222	0.0	0.0	0.0	0.0	0.0	0.0	0	0.0	0	0	0	0	192
193	Wine, white, medium	0	86.3	311	75	0.1	0.0	0.0	3.4	3.4	0.0	14	1.2	21	0	0	0	193
194	Wine, red	0	88.0	284	68	0.2	0.0	0.0	0.3	0.3	0.0	7	0.9	10	0	0	0	194

N = not determined

Appendix II

The Value Base and individual rights

The Value Base is central to the way in which people employed in health and social care pursue their work and it should be demonstrated daily in the ways in which they perform.

The value base components are:
- promotion of anti-discriminatory practice
- maintaining confidentiality of information
- promoting and supporting individual rights to dignity, independence, choice and health and safety
- acknowledging individuals' personal beliefs and identity
- supporting individuals through effective communication.

Promotion of anti-discriminatory practice

This value is about not stereotyping and treating people differently because of their colour, race, religion, sex, gender, age or ability. There are two broad categories of discrimination; direct and indirect. Direct discrimination refers to treating people less favourably than others because of their race, gender, etc. Indirect discrimination is where conditions are set that exclude certain groups, for example assuming that all people have a Christian name. Most people have a first name, but not all people are Christian!

In reality, we all discriminate in some ways. Where this discrimination is open and reasonable, such as in personal choice of friends, there should be no problems. However, when we are providing care for people who are vulnerable, disadvantaged or distressed it is important that we all need to identify unreasonable discrimination: the type of discrimination based on stereotypes that is dangerous and hidden (covert).

Discrimination can be expressed verbally in the words used and the tone of voice, and non-verbally through body language.

Summary
- No assumptions should be made about an individual (do not use stereotypes to guide your behaviour).
- Language used should be at a level consistent with the client's understanding.
- The carer's behaviour should be non-exploitative.
- The carer should identify his/her own prejudices and challenge them.

Legislation
Legislation relating to discrimination in England and Wales includes:
- The Race Relations Act 1976
- The Public Order Act 1986 and the Public Order (NI) Order 1987
- The Sex Discrimination Acts 1975 and 1986
- The Chronically Sick and Disabled Persons (Services, Consultation and Representation) Act 1986
- The Education Acts 1980 and 1981
- The Disabled Persons Act 1970
- The Equal Pay Act 1970

There is no legislation relating to religious discrimination in England and Wales. In Northern Ireland the Fair Employment Act 1989 covers this area.

Maintaining confidentiality of information

If a care worker is to be trusted by the client then that person will expect information not to be passed on to others. This area creates some professional conflicts because the information given by the client may mean that the client or someone else is at risk. In most cases it is essential that the client knows what you intend to do with any information before it is passed to you. Each individual agency will have its own specific policies.

If you are involved in taking personal details, then the reason for needing the details and who will see them needs to be explained. If a client says that s/he does not want information passed to a close relative then those wishes should be respected.

Most agencies have a code of practice which says that confidentiality could not be maintained in this situation but would explain how it would be handled, for example the client would be told that the information would be taken elsewhere.

Summary
- Confidentiality is important.
- An individual's choice regarding confidentiality should be respected as far as possible.
- Who will have access to information should be established at the first meeting.

Legislation
Legislation relating to confidentiality:
>The Data Protection Act 1984 (This relates only to data that is stored electronically, for example on computers.)
>The Access to Personal Files Act 1987
>The Access to Health Record Act 1990

Professional codes of practice and charters also describe standards of confidentiality. This is particularly important where maintaining confidentiality puts the client in danger. Where you are told by a client that s/he intends to commit suicide there might be a requirement to break confidentiality. The Samaritans have a code of practice that says confidentiality should not be broken in such situations.

Promoting and supporting individual rights to dignity, independence, choice and health and safety

Whenever a person is receiving care there can be a tendency for the carer to take over and make decisions for the client. There is also a tendency to assume that the needs of the care organisation take precedence over the needs of the client. Carers often ignore the client, and ask the relatives questions that could be answered by the client. Walking into a bedroom without knocking is unacceptable, but has been commonplace in some care establishments. The health and safety of clients is a key area where there is a shared responsibility between the client and the carer. Where a client is highly dependent on the carer for support, then the carer also takes on more responsibility for health and safety. However, where a client is able to take responsibilities s/he should be encouraged to do so.

Summary
- The recognition of rights and choice is important.
- It is important to encourage individuals to express their needs and wishes.
- Individuals should be encouraged to be as self-managing as possible.

Legislation
Legislation that relates to these areas:
>The Health and Safety at Work Act 1974.
>The Children Act 1989
>The Education (Handicapped Children) Act 1981
>National Health Service and Community Care Act 1990
>The Chronically Sick and Disabled Persons (Services, Consultation and Representation) Act 1986

There is no specific legislation that defines these rights. However, parts are covered in the Children Act 1989. Professional codes of practice and charters also describe standards to be maintained.
Individuals should be encouraged to exercise informed choice.

Acknowledging individuals' personal beliefs and identity

One area where people can clearly differ is in personal (including religious) beliefs. It is very easy to make the mistake of assuming people hold the same beliefs as you. This can be expressed in simple ways such as allowing no choice on diet: this would fail to take account of religious needs (Jews, Muslims and Hindus), cultural needs (different food preferences), personal preference or conscience (vegetarians), and dietary needs which have a medical base. There can also be conflicts where a client's beliefs are at odds with your own. This may express itself in many aspects of daily living such as personal hygiene, diet, clothing and worship.

Summary
- An individual's personal preferences and beliefs are important.
- It is important to encourage individuals to express their personal beliefs and preferences, provided this does not adversely affect the rights of others.
- Recognising and supporting a client's rights to his/her beliefs is important.

Legislation
Legislation that relates to these rights:
>The Race Relations Act 1976
>Sex Discrimination Acts 1975 and 1986
>The Children Act 1989

There is no legislation relating to religious discrimination in England and Wales. In Northern Ireland, Fair Employment legislation covers this area. Professional codes of practice and charters also describe standards to be maintained.

Supporting individuals through effective communication

Effective communication is the key to promoting equality for all individuals. Communication should be used to help you learn about others and to help them learn about you. For it to be effective it must recognise their needs and ability to understand. As a care worker you will need to recognise barriers to effective communication and seek ways to overcome them. Translators for oral language or sign can be an asset here.

Summary
- Communication should be modified for individuals.
- Your communication should be consistent with the client's understanding and preferred language.
- You should confirm information you have been given with the client.
- You should develop strategies to support your listening skills.
- Communication should recognise the importance of body language (non-verbal communication).

Legislation
The Children Act 1989
Professional codes of practice and charters often describe standards to be maintained.

The effects of removal of an individual's rights

This can be summarised in two phrases:
- loss of self esteem
- disempowerment.

All of these have the effect of increasing client dependence on the carer. They also cause physiological changes leading to increased risk of illness and increased healing times. Psychologically, it leads to depression.

Your roles

Your roles are important. You should:
- challenge discrimination wherever and whenever it occurs
- strive to maintain client dignity
- promote client independence
- maximise client choice and assist them to speak up for themselves
- maintain client confidentiality and promote trust
- work to ensure and maintain a safe environment.

Appendix III

Key legislation

The framework of the law

British law is a very large and complex system involving four countries and at least two very different legal systems. However, most of the law which you will need to know about will have come from an *Act of Parliament*, such as the National Health Service and Community Care Act 1990.

An Act of Parliament will usually have been introduced by the government of the day and then debated, voted upon and possibly changed by both Houses of Parliament. During this stage it is called a Bill. It is only known as an Act once it has passed through Parliament and been given royal assent.

However, before the government takes proposed legislation to Parliament it will usually have gone through a period of consultation, starting with what is known as a *Green Paper,* a document published by the government in order to test opinion. Alternatively, the government may ask a committee or an individual to produce a report. An example of this is the Griffiths Report which proposed the community care structure introduced as part of the NHS and Community Care Act.

The next stage will probably be what is known as a *White Paper,* which is a statement of what the proposed legislation will be about. The White Paper can often be an important means of understanding the philosophy which may lie behind an Act of Parliament.

Not all Acts of Parliament are proposed by the government. Some are introduced by individual Members of Parliament who may be working on behalf of groups of interested organisations in order to change the law. These are called *Private Members Bills*. An important example is the Chronically Sick and Disabled Persons Act 1970, which had the support of many organisations representing the interests of people with disabilities. This path will often also be used for socially controversial legislation on which the government wishes to take a neutral stance, such as the abolition of capital punishment or the Sexual Offences Act 1967, which legalised homosexual acts between men over twenty-one.

Acts of Parliament may contain powers which allow the government to introduce them a piece at a time. So, just because an Act has been passed, you should not assume that everything in it is current law. This is particularly likely to happen where there are resource implications to introducing the whole Act at one time. An example of an Act which has been implemented in part only is the Disabled Person's Act 1986.

An Act of Parliament may include a clause which gives the senior Minister involved (usually called the Secretary of State) the power to introduce at a later date *Regulations* which give more detailed law on specific areas covered by the Act. This is done by means of a *Statutory Instrument* which is placed before Parliament but is usually not debated. The Children Act 1989 has many examples of Regulations, such as the Foster Care Regulations which lay down the way in which foster carers are to be approved, reviewed and supervised.

With major pieces of legislation, such as the Children Act, *Guidance* may be introduced at a later stage. Whilst this does not have the force of law, it explains, clarifies and amplifies the law and defines what may be considered to be good practice and must therefore be considered very seriously by practitioners.

Because the structure of the law and service provision in Scotland is different from England and Wales, Scottish legislation must often be treated differently. Sometimes this is done within the main Act by explaining how it will be applied in Scotland, and defining specifically Scots terminology. On other occasions there will be a separate Act for Scotland.

In the case of Northern Ireland, legislation must be introduced by *Order in Council*. This is because it had a separate legislature (the Northern Ireland Assembly) until 1972, when its powers were taken over by the Secretary of State for Northern Ireland. Although this power lies with the Secretary of State there is a consultative process and, as a result, there is usually a time lag between the appearance of the main Act and its Northern Irish equivalent. The Order itself, once put before Parliament, cannot be amended, but simply accepted or rejected.

Local Authority Social Services Act 1970

This Act, which followed the Seebohm Report on the provision of personal social services, established unified Social Services Departments in England and Wales, covering the provision of personal social services for all children and adults. The same thing had been done for Scotland two years earlier in the **Social Work (Scotland) Act 1968,** which established Social Work Departments. They include the probation service which, in England and Wales, is under the direct control of the Home Office. In Northern Ireland the relevant legislation is the **Health and Personal Social Services (NI) Order 1972** which established four Health and Social Services Boards to administer both health and personal social services provision.

The Local Authority Social Services Act also confers the powers under which the Secretary of State can issue Guidance (*see above*).

Children Act 1989

The Children Act is a large and very complex piece of legislation which brought together the law relating to children in a single Act. It covers the law relating to public child care (the means by which children are looked after by local authorities), the powers and duties of local authorities to protect children from abuse, and the law relating to custody in private matters such as contested divorce proceedings. The basic belief which underlies the Act is that:

'...children are generally best looked after within the family with both parents playing a full part and without resort to legal proceedings.'

A central concept of the Act is that of *parental responsibility* which defines the rights and duties which a parent has in regard to a child and which can only be lost in the event of the child being adopted by someone else. The Act also says that when a court makes decisions about the future of a child the child's interests must be *paramount*.

The Act places on local authorities a general duty to safeguard and promote the welfare of children who are in need within their area, and to promote the upbringing of those children by their families. Therefore, a resort to legal proceedings must always be seen as an act of last resort. It follows from this that, where caring agencies are involved with parents, it must be in *partnership* and that parents must be encouraged to *participate* in all decision making.

Amongst their many responsibilities, local authorities must: keep a register of *children in need* (defined as 'children whose health and welfare may suffer significantly without support'); provide services for children in need; to publish information of the services they have available for children in need; and provide a complaints system for their service users. (All children with disabilities are automatically assumed to be in need.)

Finally, the Act requires local authorities to consider a child's race, religion, culture and linguistic background when making decisions about the services that will be offered to meet its needs.

There have been a number of Regulations made following the Act, in particular on fostering, adoption, child minding and children's homes. The Act applies to England, Wales and Scotland (although in the latter within a separate court structure) and will be applied to Northern Ireland in 1995 through the **Children (NI) Order 1993.**

Criticisms of the Act are that, although it makes a major statement of intent about meeting the needs of children in need, it still leaves it to local authorities to define who those children are. It has also introduced a court framework for child care proceedings which can be very long and cumbersome, leaving children in a state of uncertainty for an unnecessarily long time.

Criminal Justice Act 1991

The aim of this Act was to keep more people out of prison through a new sentencing framework, although, because of public criticism, there were major changes in 1993 which retreated from this objective. It also placed a duty on those administering criminal justice to avoid discrimination on the grounds of race or sex and established a youth court to deal with criminal proceedings against children and young people.

Education (Handicapped Children) Act 1981

Following the recommendation of the Warnock Report, a government enquiry into the educational needs of 'disabled children', this Act sought to integrate *children with special educational needs* into mainstream education wherever possible. Special educational need is seen as including a wide range of learning difficulties, as well as physical disabilities, ill health and emotional problems. Local authorities are expected to ensure that no child is discriminated against on the basis of their special needs.

Any child is entitled to an assessment and statement of their educational needs which must be completed within six months of the request being made, and local authorities must endeavour to ensure that those needs are met. The **Education Reform Act 1988** allows children with statements of special educational needs to be excluded from the national curriculum, although reasons must be given for doing so.

The 1993 Education Act reinforces the 1981 Education Act on Special Education in advocating integration. It proposes a 'code of practice' to guide Local Authorities and schools in Special Education Needs cases.

The relevant Act for Scotland is the **Education (Scotland) Act 1981** but the Act has not been applied to Northern Ireland.

The intention behind the Act was that, so far as possible, those needs would be met by putting the necessary resources into mainstream schooling. In practice this has not happened to the extent intended, partly because of the shortage of resources, partly because of the resistance of the parents of many children with special educational needs, who have preferred the idea of separate provision as providing a safer and more protective environment.

Mental Health Act 1983

The main aim of this Act was to provide a framework which would protect the rights of the mentally ill. The Act requires that the professionals who are involved in compulsory admissions to psychiatric hospitals must have received special training. They are known as Approved Doctors and Approved Social Workers. The Act provides protection for patients regarding treatment and compulsory admission and treatment. It also lays down an appeals structure, with an independent element, for people who have been compulsorily detained.

The application of the Act was extended to Scotland by the **Mental Health (Scotland) Act 1984** and to Northern Ireland by the **Mental Health (NI) Order 1986.**

A serious omission of this Act is that it fails to acknowledge that cultural differences in the use of language and in behaviour may lead to misdiagnosis. It is argued that, as a result, some cultural groups are over-represented amongst compulsorily detained patients.

Another problem is that, although it predates the NHS & Community Care Act, it encouraged discharge of patients into the community, but without the care management structure which exists in the later legislation.

The National Health Service and Community Care

The National Health Service, with a comprehensive pattern of free medical care, was established by the **National Health Service Act 1946.**

The structure of the National Health Service has been amended several times since, most recently by the **National Health Service and Community Care Act 1990** which covers England, Wales and Scotland (and was extended to Northern Ireland by the **Health and Personal Social Services (NI) Order 1991**) and which affected both the Health Service and local authority Social Services Departments. Central to its philosophy is the split between 'service purchasing' and 'service provision' and the interdependency of social care agencies – whether statutory, voluntary or private – and their need to work collaboratively.

In the NHS it brought about major structural changes, introducing the internal market, allowing the establishment of Health Trusts and allowing GP practices to become fund-holders.

The other main thrust of the act was to encourage the provision of care in the community rather than in institutions. The responsibility for this was placed with local authorities who must prepare and publish community care plans and employ 'care managers' who will assess an individual's need for care, and design and implement a care package to meet those needs. Local authorities must also establish 'arm's length' Inspection and Registration Units and complaints procedures (which have also incorporated the same responsibilities for children's homes and childminders).

Central to the philosophy underpinning the Act is an emphasis on the equal opportunities of service users and their right to choice and dignity. It also recognises the important role played by carers.

In the Act the Sections on community care occupy a relatively small amount of space as the services which local authorities provide had already been established through earlier legislation. They include the **National Assistance Act 1948,** which requires local authorities to promote the welfare of 'persons who are ... substantially and permanently handicapped,' and the **Health Services and Public Health Act 1968**, which does the same for 'old people'. The 1948 Act enables local authorities to set up residential homes, whilst the 1968 Act enables the provision of Home Helps, Meals on Wheels, adaptations to the home and social work support.

The **Chronically Sick and Disabled Persons Act 1970** strengthened these earlier Acts so far as people with disabilities are concerned, requiring local authorities to identify those in need within their areas and to publish information on the services they provide. The intention of the Act was to enable those people identified in the National Assistance Act to live reasonably independent lives. The relevant legislation for Northern Ireland is the **Chronically Sick and Disabled Persons (NI) Act 1978.**

The **Disabled Person's (Services, Consultation and Representation) Act 1986**, which has only been implemented in part, embraced the principles of individual rights and self-determination for people with disabilities and, for the first time, recognised the needs of carers. The Act established four main rights for people with disabilities: the right to *assessment*; to be provided with *resources* to permit as independent a life as possible; where they are unable or limited in their ability to speak for themselves, people with disabilities are entitled to *representation* by another person, either a friend or an independent advocate; and, recognising that individual needs change over time, *monitoring and review*. The Act was extended to Northern Ireland in the **Disabled Persons (NI) Act 1989**.

The requirement to register all homes in a local authority area, built upon in the NHS and Community Care Act, was established in the **Registered Homes Act 1984.**

The community care aspects of the NHS and Community Care Act have run into controversy, not because of the intentions of the Act, but because it has created expectations which cannot be met within the resources available. This has been further exacerbated because, whilst the Act creates a right to an assessment, it does not extend that right automatically to a service.

Health and safety at work

The **Health and Safety at Work Act 1974**, as amended by the **Management of Health and Safety at Work Regulations 1992**, imposes a set of duties on both employers and employees. An employer must: provide a safe and healthy workplace for everyone on their premises, whether worker, client or visitor; produce a written policy statement, including who is responsible for implementing it; provide employees with training in health and safety; and, in larger organisations, ensure that there is a staff Health and Safety Representative.

However, the Act also recognises that we all have some responsibility, both for ourselves and others. Therefore, employees: have a responsibility for the safety of themselves, colleagues, clients, and anyone else on the premises; must co-operate with their employers to ensure that the Regulations are kept; and must not interfere with or damage equipment provided in the interests of safety (for example, fire extinguishers).

Also important to health and safety at work is the **Control of Substances Hazardous to Health Regulations 1988** which require employers to assess risks caused by dangerous substances and provide guidelines for storing and using them. In practice this means that employers, and by extension their employees, must be aware not just of the dangers presented by individual substances but also of how they might react when combined with each other.

Both of these Regulations, which are required under European Community law, apply to the whole of the United Kingdom. They are of particular importance in health-care work where there are likely to be many people whose frail health, physical disabilities or mental state means that safety codes must be exacting and rigorously enforced. However, there may be conflicts between the Regulations and individual rights, for example, fire doors that frail elderly people are unable to open.

Anti-discriminatory legislation

The **Race Relations Act 1976** makes it illegal to discriminate in housing, education, employment, membership of public or private clubs, entertainment, or the provision of goods or services, on the grounds of race, colour, nationality or ethnic origin. The Act defines discrimination as being direct, indirect or victimisation. Under this Act the Commission for Racial Equality (CRE) was established. The CRE publishes information, carries out research and can investigate the practices and procedures of organisations and pursue action to redress discriminatory practices.

The Act also places upon local authorities a duty to ensure that their functions are carried out with due regard to the need to eliminate unlawful discrimination and to promote good relations between people of different racial groups. Services must be provided in a non-discriminatory way. You may have seen job advertisements saying that because a particular group are poorly represented 'applications will be invited from ...'. This is because employers are allowed to take positive action in order to encourage the participation of a particular group if they have been under-represented or to ensure the welfare of a particular group.

You may also come across reference to 'Section 11 money'. This is special government money, made available to local authorities under Section 11 of the **Local Government Act 1966**, to work with people from the New Commonwealth.

Neither of the previous two Acts applies to Northern Ireland, where the issues of discrimination have a very specific local character relating to intercommunal conflict, and with roots far back in history. Because of this, the **Fair Employment Act (NI) 1989** made it unlawful to discriminate in employment against someone on the grounds of their religious beliefs or political opinions.

Under the **Public Order Act 1986** and **Public Order (NI) Order 1987** it is illegal to stir up hatred against, or arouse fear of, groups because of their colour, race, nationality, national origin or (in Northern Ireland) religious beliefs.

Whilst the law provides safeguards and legal redress against discrimination, there is much evidence that discrimination continues, albeit in more covert forms than in the past.

The **Sex Discrimination Act 1975** makes it illegal to discriminate or give favourable treatment on the grounds of sex or marital status and covers both men and women in its scope. As with the Race Relations Act it allows for positive action in order to address imbalance. It also permits gender to be used as a specific qualification for a job in certain circumstances, for example a woman working in a women's refuge, where it is a *Genuine Occupational Qualification*. It can also permit the provision of women-only occupational courses in work areas where they may be seriously under-represented.

The Act also established the Equal Opportunities Commission which provides advice and undertakes research on the promotion of equality of opportunity between the sexes. It applies in England, Wales and Scotland and in Northern Ireland is covered by the **Sex Discrimination (NI) Order 1976.**

The **Sex Discrimination Act 1986** which applies to England, Wales and Scotland makes it illegal for an employer to distinguish between men and women on retirement age.

The **Equal Pay Act 1970 (amended 1988)** requires that women must be paid equally with men when they are doing broadly similar work (covered in Northern Ireland by the **Equal Pay Act (NI) 1970 (amended 1988)**). Whilst both the Sex Discrimination and Equal Pay Acts may be considered landmark legislation for women's rights, the statistical evidence suggests that discrimination continues in employment (where women are much more likely to accept part-time work), pay and education.

Confidentiality and access to records

Public concern about the growth of computerisation and the dangers to individual freedom led directly to the **Data Protection Act 1984.** This places restrictions on what can be kept on computer about individuals. Its main provisions are that information must be: obtained legally; only used for the purposes given when collected; only disclosed to those who have a right to see it; relevant and no more than is necessary for its purpose; accurate and up-to-date; and kept no longer than is necessary. Individuals should be entitled to see what is kept on them and there must be appropriate security measures to prevent unauthorised access.

Although the Act does not apply to written records, it could be said that its measures provide an appropriate model for good practice for all files. The Act does not apply to Northern Ireland.

Unlike many other Western countries the United Kingdom does not have freedom of information legislation which assumes an automatic right of access to all information unless there are strong reasons not to give it. However, there have been some moves so far as personal information is concerned. The **Access to Personal Files Act 1987** gives individuals a right of access to information kept on them by local authorities or those acting on the authorities' behalf (such as agencies supplying community care). However, certain kinds of information may still be kept confidential and the Act does not apply retrospectively, that is, it only applies to information kept since the date of its passage. **The Access to Personal Files (Social Services) Regulations 1989** offers more detailed regulations for the application to Social Services files. The **Access to Personal Files (Social Work) (Scotland) Regulations 1989** applies the Regulations to Scotland. Under these regulations, where information refers to a third party (such as the applicant's parent) then that person's permission to disclose must be sought. This can create conflicts of interest.

The **Access to Health Records Act 1990** makes similar provision for Health Service files, there having been much criticism of the fact that, where social work files contained medical records, such as psychiatric reports, they had to be kept confidential. Both of the above two Acts have now been applied to Northern Ireland by means of a single Order.

One of the most positive results of these acts is that greater care is now taken to record accurate, rather than speculative, information.

Answers

Unit 1
1. **d** high in fibre
2. **b** cereals and sugar
3. **c** airway, breathing, circulation
4. **a** arteries
5. **c** wholemeal bread
6. **c** smoking
7. **a** unprotected sex
8. **b** an audio-visual presentation
9. **a** proteins, carbohydrates, fats, vitamins, minerals, water, fibre.
10. **b** inactivity
11. **c** fats
12. **b** personal hygiene
13. **d** your target group
14. **c** obtaining feedback
15. **a** a toddler
16. **d** assess the situation, make the area safe, give emergency aid, get help
17. **c** a haemorrhage
18. **a** the circulatory system
19. **b** less salt, less sugar, more fibre and less fat
20. **c** lighter fluid
21. **d** addiction

Unit 2
1. **b** mid-life
2. **d** hormones
3. **a** self-concept
4. **d** a compliment
5. **a** community
6. **c** socio-economic factors
7. **c** cognition
8. **d** puberty
9. **a** physical changes
10. **c** emotional developments
11. **a** adolescence
12. **c** gender roles
13. **a** the life cycle
14. **c** culture
15. **d** a role
16. **c** age
17. **a** an increase in the number of one parent families
18. **d** find it difficult to establish a loving relationship
19. **a** wider family
20. **b** bonding
21. **c** self-concept

Unit 3
1. **d** statutory organisations
2. **b** filling any gap in statutory provision
3. **a** respite care
4. **d** Social Services
5. **d** nursing homes
6. **c** the health visitor
7. **a** the independent sector
8. **a** self-governing
9. **c** the family
10. **c** National Health Service
11. **b** District Health Authorities
12. **a** personal social services
13. **a** practice nurse
14. **d** children, parents, friends, neighbours
15. **b** home help
16. **d** empowerment of the client
17. **a** an acute illness
18. **b** hospital services
19. **b** those members of the population who pay the full cost of the services
20. **d** the Local Social Services

Unit 4
1. **b** racism
2. **a** direct discrimination
3. **c** hidden
4. **b** ageism
5. **c** facial expression
6. **a** a peer group
7. **a** their status
8. **b** there are cultural differences in interpretation of body language
9. **a** Do you like reading?
10. **a** allow the respondent to give broad unstructured answers
11. **b** evaluation
12. **a** discrimination
13. **c** direct forms of discrimination
14. **b** stereotyping
15. **d** sexual stereotyping
16. **c** discrimination against both sexes
17. **c** racial disadvantage
18. **d** all of the above areas
19. **c** may need to disclose information if it endangers the life of the client or others
20. **d** for the client to go to the theatre with friends

A more common version of the poem

Twinkle, twinkle little star
How I wonder what you are
Up above the world so high
Like a diamond in the sky

Index

abuse
    in childhood 94–5
    drugs 138
    sexual 138
    solvents 25
Access to Health Records Act (1990) 221, 230
Access to Personal Files (Social Services) Regulations (1989) 230
Access to Personal Files (Social Work) (Scotland) Regulations (1989) 230
Access to Personal Files Act (1987) 221, 230
accidents 9
    see also casualties; emergencies
accommodation
    residential 124, 133, 142, 146
    temporary 106
    see also housing
Acts of Parliament 224
acupuncturists 133
adolescence 68, 76, 85–6
adoption 94
adrenalin 21
adulthood 68
    growth 75, 76
    learning difficulties 141
    relationships 97
    stages 68, 75, 86–7
    see also old age
advocacy 145
AIDS 9, 26
airway, unblocking 44, 47
alcohol 18, 23
amino acids 10
amphetamines 24
anaemia 19
anorexia nervosa 19

anti-discriminatory measures 220–1, 229–30
artery 44, 51
arthritis, tools 142
ATP 21

babies: see infancy
bacteria 28–9
Barnardo's 139
befriending 7
birth 68
bleach 39
bleeding 51–5
    controlling 52–4
    severe 52, 53
blood pressure 18
blood supply 21, 51
body position, mirroring 186
bonding 77, 79
boredom 6
brachial pressure point 54
breathing 21, 44, 45
BTEC National Diploma 154
bulimia 19

calcium 13, 75, 76
calories 13
cancer prevention 17
cannabis 24
capillary 51
carbohydrates 10–11, 21
cardiac compression 46, 47, 51
cardiovascular system 21
care
    children and families 124, 137–40
    cultural factors 143–4
    delivery of 147–54
    ethical issues 201–2
    payment 145–6
    responses 197
care assistants 153

care in community 129
care needs 125–7, 136–7
care planning 125, 129, 148, 196
carers xiii, 153, 155–6, 188
    duties 199–200
    informal 134–5
    roles 223
    support for 154–5
    training 155
caring relationships 194, 195, 197
carotid artery 44
case studies
    child development 83
    dependence 194–6
    discrimination 192, 207–8
    family relationships 93–5
    informal carers 134–5
    language acquisition 80–1
casualties 42
    assessment 43
    cardiac compression 46, 47, 51
    examining 48–51
    five checks 43, 44, 45, 46
    LIONEL 44
    mouth-to-mouth resuscitation 45–7
    pulse/no pulse 46–7
    recovery position 47–8
    shock 54–5
    wounds and treatment 51–5
cell membranes 11
centile charts 70–1, 83
cerebral palsy 184
ceremony 91–2
Certificate of Qualification in Social Work 153
Certificate in Social Service 153

Certificates in Caring Services 154
change
    effects 97
    relationships 96–7
    support needed 91–2
charades 82
charitable organisations 124, 131
charters 144, 221
chest compression 46, 47, 51
child-care 124, 137–40
    Health Service professionals 138, 140
    Social Services professionals 138–40
childhood 68
    ages five-plus 84–5
    development 40, 81–3
    families 137–40
    growth 69–71, 74, 76
    special needs 141
Children Act (1989) 139, 222, 223, 224, 225–6
Children Learn What They Live (Dorothy Law Nolte) 92
children in need 226
Children's Departments, Local Authorities 124
Chinese whispers 172, 173
chiropractors 133, 134
choice 197
cholesterol 11, 20
Chronically Sick and Disabled Persons (NI) Act (1978) 228
Chronically Sick and Disabled Persons Act (1970) 194
Chronically Sick and Disabled Persons Act (1986) 220, 222, 224, 228
circulatory system 21, 44, 51

Index

Citizen's Advocacy 145
class: *see* social class
clients
    communication breakdown 199
    individual rights 222–3
co-ordination, hand-eye 72
cocaine 22, 24
codes of practice 221
cohabitation 93
COMA Report No. 46 18
Commission for Racial Equality 229
communication 168–70
    breakdown 200
    non-verbal 173, 182–5, 204
    respect shown 199–200
    supportive 170, 223
    verbal 204
    see also conversation
community care 123, 129
community psychiatric nurses 152
community-based mental handicap nurses (RNMH) 152
complementary medicine 133–4
complex sequential scans 149
conception 68
confidentiality 1, 202–3, 221, 230
contraceptives 26
Control of Substances Hazardous to Health Regulations (1988) 228
conversation
    body mirroring 186
    controlling 185
    feedback 174
    probes/prompts 181–2
    skills 171–2
    verbal/non-verbal language 176, 185–6
    see also questioning
Councils for Voluntary Service 131
counselling 92, 139, 174–5
crack cocaine 24
Criminal Justice Act (1991) 226
cross infection, prevention 52
culture
    care for elders 143–4

learned 99
in society 97–8
values 98

D-lysergic acid diethylamide 24
Data Protection Act (1984) 221, 230
death 91
dental care 28, 103, 138
dentists 121
dependence 194–6, 201–2
deprivation, cycle of 104
deviance 99–100
diet
    balanced 10–11, 14–15
    calories 13
    costs 105
    eating patterns 15, 17
    fibre 17, 18
    food groups 16
    health risks 18–20
    monitoring 32–3
    nutrient content 10, 14, 19
    Reference Nutrient Intakes 12–13
    see also food composition tables
digestive system 17
Diploma in Social Work 153
disabilities, physical/sensory 140
Disabled Persons (NI) Act (1989) 228
Disabled Persons Act (1986) 220, 224, 228
discrimination 191–4, 207–8, 220–1, 229–30
disempowerment 193, 223
District Health Authorities 121–2
divorce 225
doctors 148
    see also general practitioners
drugs
    abuse 138
    alcohol 23
    controlled/illegal 24
    dangers 25
    psychotropic 22
    tobacco 22

eating patterns 15, 17, 19

ecstasy 24
education 84, 85, 103–4
Education (Handicapped Children) Act (1981) 222, 226
Education (Scotland) Act (1981) 226
Education Acts (1980, 1981) 220
Education Reform Act (1988) 226
elderly people: *see* old age
emergencies 3
    five checks 43, 44, 45, 46
    flow chart 44
    making area safe 42
    see also casualties
emergency services 44, 55–7
emotions
    in adolescence 85
    development 77–9
    expressing 182–3
    needs 136–7
    positive 197
    support for 168
empathy 171
empowerment 197, 199
energy
    from food 11
    use 20
England, NHS structure 120, 121
Equal Opportunities Commission 229–30
Equal Pay Act (1970, amended 1988) 194, 220, 230
Equal Pay Act (NI) (1970, amended 1988) 230
equality of opportunity, legislation 194, 220, 230
ethical issues 201–2
exercise 20–1
expression, facial 182–3
eye contact 185, 186

Fair Employment Act (1986) 220, 222
family 93–5, 137–40
Family Health Service Authorities 121–2
fats 10, 11, 18, 21
fatty acids 11

feelings, positive/negative 197
femoral pressure point 54
fibre 11, 16, 17, 18
First Course in Psychology (Hayes) 104
fitness 20–1, 32
flies 28, 29
foetal development 68, 69
food composition tables 216–19
food groups 16
food-poisoning 28–9
food storage 30, 31
Foster Care Regulations 224
foster carers 133, 138, 161
fridges 30
funerals 91

garden, hazards 40, 41
gaseous exchange 21, 45
general practitioners 121, 148, 151–2
    fund-holding 127, 227
glycerol 11
glycogen 11, 21
GNVQ portfolio xvii
grazing 15
Green Paper 224
group membership 96, 98, 102
group roles 97–106
growth 69–71
    adulthood 75, 76
    childhood 69–71, 74, 76
    puberty 74

hair hygiene 27, 31
Hayes, N. 104
hazards 39, 40
Hazchem symbols 56
headlice 27
health
    hygiene 26
    personal 3, 27, 31
    and safety 39–41
    social well-being 2
Health Care Assistants 148–9, 151
health centres 151–2
Health Commissions 128–9
Health of the Nation Project 8–9
Health and Personal Social Services (NI) Order

233

Index

(1991) 227
health promotion 2, 9, 35–8
health risks 8, 18–20, 102
Health and Safety at Work Act (1974) 222, 228–9
health services 118–19
    class differences 103–6
    community-based 151–2
    deliverers 147
    formation 120
    subdivisions 123–4
Health Services and Public Health Act (1968) 227–8
health and social care
    access 143
    organisations 119
    provision of services 116–17
    working with people 194–5
Health and Social Care workers 147
Health Trusts 227
health visitors 149, 152
hearing/listening 172
heart disease prevention 9, 17, 18
heart rate 20
height charts 76
height/weight chart 19
hepatitis 24
heroin 24
HIV 9, 24, 26
home
    hygiene 31
    importance for well-being 106
    risks 39, 40, 41
homeopaths 133
homosexuality 224
hormone replacement therapy 75
hormones 11, 74–5
hospitals 136, 148–51
housing
    social class 102
    well-being 106
hygiene
    care establishments 31
    food preparation 28, 30
    and health 26
    levels 28–31
    personal 3, 27–8, 31

public eating places 30
treatment for bleeding 51

identity 222
    see also self-concept
imagining 177
immunisation 137
independence 201
individual rights 220–3, 222–3
individuality 65–6, 189–90, 193
inequality, and social class 103–4
infancy 68, 70, 76
infant mortality rates 102, 103
intellectual development 77–9
interaction, effective 199–200
intestine 17
Ireland, Northern 121, 220, 225, 226, 227

key-workers 154

language
    development 80–1
    mother tongue and second language 81, 144, 145
    for questioning 181
    and relationships 96
laws and conventions 98–9
learning difficulties 141
legal system in Britain 224–5
life chances 102
life events, major 91
life preservation 43
life stages 67–8
lifestyles 4–5, 7
LIONEL, help summons 44
listening
    active 174
    barriers 174
    reflective 175–6
    skills 172–6
    styles 173–4
liver 11, 25
living standards 104–6
local authorities, social services 124
Local Authority Social Services Act (1970) 225
Local Government Act (1966) 229
love 79

LSD 24
lungs, exercise 20

macronutrients 10
magnetic resonance imaging 149, 150
malnutrition 19
Management of Health and Safety at Work Regulations (1992) 228
manipulative skills 73
marginalisation 105
marriage 92
mass media 101
masseurs 133
means testing 143, 146
menarche 74
menopause 75, 76
mental health 9, 142, 152
Mental Health (NI) Order (1986) 227
Mental Health (Scotland) Act (1984) 227
Mental Health Act (1983) 124, 227
mental hospitals, closed 129
mental stimulation 6
metabolic rate 20
micro-organisms 27
micronutrients 10, 19
midwives 149, 152
minerals 10, 11
mirroring, body position 186
motor development 72
mouth-to-mouth resuscitation 45–7
muscles 20, 75
myelin 11

National Advisory Committee on Nutrition Education 18
National Assistance Act (1948) 227
National Council for Voluntary Organisations 131
National Curriculum 84
National Health Service (NHS) 119, 120
National Health Service Act (1946) 227
National Health Service and Community Care Act (1990) 120, 122, 125, 129, 222, 227–8
National Health Trusts 122
National Nursery Examinations Board 154
National Society for the Prevention of Cruelty to Children 139
nature/nurture debate 92
Nolte, D. L. 92
non-judgmental behaviour 201
non-verbal communication 173, 182–5, 204
Northern Ireland: see Ireland, Northern
not-for-profit services 134
nursery nurses 158–9
nurses 148–9
nursing homes 142

obesity 18, 19–20
occupational therapists 150
oestrogen 74, 75
old age 68
    diet 13
    elasticity loss 76
    role 87–8
    services 141–2
opticians 122
osteopaths 133, 134
osteoporosis 75
oxygen 20

paracetamol 25
parenthood 86, 87
peer groups 86, 101
personal beliefs 222
personal development 69
personal health
    assessment 32–3
    improvements 33–5
    promotion 31, 33–5
personal safety 40
personal space 186–8
pharmacists 122
physical abuse 138
physical activity 5
physical care needs 136
physical development 69–76
physiotherapists 150
poverty risks 105

Index

power relationships 197
pregnancy 26, 68, 69, 149
prejudice 190–1
presentations, health advice 35–8
pressure points, bleeding 54
preventative medicine 123
primary care 123–4
Primary Health Care Team 147
private health care 133
Private Members Bills 224
private sector 132–3, 146
probes 181–2
progesterone 74, 75
Project 2000 149, 151
Project Headstart 104
prompts 181–2
protein 10
puberty, growth 74
Public Order (NI) Order (1987) 229
Public Order Act (1986) 194, 229
pulses 18
purchasers/providers 127–8, 129–30

questioning 176, 177–82
questions
    complexity 180
    leading 178
    open/closed xvii–xviii, 177–8
    organised sequences 179–80
    probes/prompts 181–2

Race Relations Act (1976) 194, 220, 222, 229
radiographers 149
radiotheraphy 149
rapport 203
records, access 221, 230
recovery position 47–8
reference groups 100
Reference Nutrient Intakes 12–13
referral 138, 143
reflecting 174–5
reflective listening 175–6
refrigerators 30
Regional Health Authorities 120, 121
Registered Homes Act (1984) 228
Registrar General, social class scale 102
Regulations 224
rehabilitation 123
rejection 79
relationship charts 95
relationships 170–1
    behaviour 95
    bonding 77, 79
    caring professions 194, 195, 197
    changes 96–7
    courtship 79
    family 93–5
    groups 86, 97–106
    language 96
    marriage 92
    outside family 96
    parenthood 86, 87
    power 197
    social 15, 17
    and well-being 92
religion 101, 222
residential accommodation 124, 133, 142, 146
respect, communicating 199–200
respiratory system 21, 45
respite care 142
resuscitation 45–7
risks 39
    to children 40
    health 8
    sexual 26
role play 1, 184–5, 204
roles
    group 97–106
    old age 87–8
    social 88, 99
roughage 10, 11
    see also fibre
rules 98–9

safety
    in emergencies 42, 44
    health 39–41
    at work 222, 228–9
Salmonella bacteria 28, 29
salt 18
Samaritans 221
school 84, 85, 103–4
Scotland 121, 225, 226, 230
screening checks 137
sebum 27
secondary care 123
Seebohm Report 225
self-concept 88–90
self confidence 171
self-esteem 193, 201–2, 223
sensory development 73
Sex Discrimination (NI) Order (1976) 230
Sex Discrimination Act (1975) 194, 220, 222, 229
Sex Discrimination Act (1986) 220, 222, 230
sex hormones 74
sex organs 74
sexual abuse 138
sexual behaviour 26
Sexual Offences Act (1967) 224
sexually transmitted diseases 9, 26
shock 54–5
sleep 5–6
smoking 9, 22
social class 101–2, 103–6
social development 77–9
social interaction 7, 99, 137, 198–9
social mobility 102
social services
    deliverers 118–19, 147
    formation 124–5
    homes for elderly 142
    personnel 152–4
    purchasers/providers 129–30
    range 130
    see also health and social care
Social Services Committees 124
Social Trends 103
social well-being 2, 66
Social Work (Scotland) Act (1968) 225
social workers 152, 153, 154, 155, 157
socialisation 99, 100–1, 191
society, and culture 97–8
solvent abuse 25

somatotropin 74
Special Health Authorities 122
special needs 141
specialist services 148–51
speech therapy 140, 150
starches 10, 11
State Enrolled Nurse 148
State Registered Nurse 148
status 98
Statutory Instrument 224
statutory sector 119–30, 145–6
stereotyping 100, 155, 189, 190
strokes 9
sugars 10, 11
suicide 202, 221
summarising 174–5
support, types 154, 198–9

talking 172
teeth 28, 103, 138
temporary accommodation 106
tertiary care 123
testosterone 74
tobacco 9, 22
toilet, hygiene 28, 30
toys 82

ultrasound scans 149
underclass 105

Value Base xiii, 220–3
values, cultural 98
vein 51
vitamins 10, 11, 13, 18
voluntary sector 131–2, 139, 146

Wales, NHS 121
water, bodily needs 10
weight loss 20
weight/height chart 19
well-being 2, 66, 92, 106
White Paper 224
wounds, treatment 51–5

X-rays 149, 150